Form Follows Fever

Christopher Cowell's account of British Hong Kong offers the most detailed account yet of the crucial first decade of the colony's existence. Focusing on the urban realm, it skilfully employs analysis of the built environment as a lens through which to understand the colonial mentality in relation to social organisation and commercial expansion against the backdrop of disease, in a place where the prospects of either seemed hopelessly bleak. Cowell's engagement with the medley of actors, from across the globe, that contributed to the colony's ultimate success is both intriguing and revealing.

It is an excellent case study in how British colonial practices strove to overcome initial and potentially terminal difficulties, and is thus a brilliant miniature of colonial urban development in action.

—**Alex Bremner**, Edinburgh School of Architecture and Landscape Architecture, University of Edinburgh

This is an important and timely book. Cowell provides carefully researched, vivid analysis of an extensive array of textual and visual material, much of which has not been previously studied or published. The result is a wonderfully rich and detailed architectural history of Hong Kong's first decade as a British colony that sheds new light on the consequential effects of disease and climate on what was built, by whom, and why.

—**Cole Roskam**, Department of Architecture, The University of Hong Kong
International Editor, *Journal of Architecture*

Drawing on a rich trove of sources, *Form Follows Fever* shows how Hong Kong's path from a so-called 'barren island' to a thriving port city was often a perilous one. Malaria plagued the young colony so badly that it became known as 'Hong Kong fever'. With a historian's flair for narrative and an architect's eye for detail, Christopher Cowell shows how a cast of Chinese and foreign personalities from all walks of life both built and imagined early colonial Hong Kong from the ground up.

Packed with images, and written in a fluid and engaging style, *Form Follows Fever* is a wonderfully original and insightful study that weaves together an unlikely melange of urban history, military engineering, and medical history.

—**John M. Carroll**, Department of History, The University of Hong Kong
Author of *The Hong Kong–China Nexus: A Brief History*

This is a beautifully written book that explores the formation of Hong Kong in its first decade of development. Through careful analysis of extensive historical sources, Cowell offers fresh perspectives on how malaria played a decisive role in shaping the forms of the colonial built environment and the future course of the city. It is a must-read for anyone interested in Hong Kong history and urbanism, who will learn key insights from a perceptive scholar and gifted writer.

—**Cecilia L. Chu**, School of Architecture, The Chinese University of Hong Kong

FORM FOLLOWS FEVER

MALARIA AND THE CONSTRUCTION OF HONG KONG, 1841–1849

Christopher Cowell

The Chinese University of Hong Kong Press

Form Follows Fever: Malaria and the Construction of Hong Kong, 1841–1849
By Christopher Cowell

ISBN: 978-988-237-290-0

First edition 2024
Second printing 2025

The Chinese University of Hong Kong Press
The Chinese University of Hong Kong
Sha Tin, N.T., Hong Kong
Fax: +852 2603 7355
Email: cup@cuhk.edu.hk
Website: cup.cuhk.edu.hk

Printed in Hong Kong

PAUL MELLON CENTRE
for Studies in British Art

This publication was supported by a Publications Grant from the Paul Mellon Centre for Studies in British Art.

To my loving parents,
Max and Elizabeth Cowell,
and my lovable brothers,
Simon and Damian.

Here is a book none of you will read.

Contents

List of Illustrations

Preface

The completion of this book marks a double tragedy. The second, our recent pandemic has reanimated my writing on the first, a deadly epidemic and its effects on the colonisation of Hong Kong Island in the mid-nineteenth century. It was an outbreak that indelibly altered the fledgling city. I began reviewing my work on this subject just as we started experiencing the early stages of Covid-19, the first global pandemic since the Spanish Flu. Our local sense of society and space had become fractured and cellular in extended lockdowns that stretched from the eastern to western hemispheres, revealing the constructed fragility of our communities. As a distant echo, Hong Kong's urban beginnings along the northern shore of its island were also fragmented and secluded. Immediately forged in uncertainty, its community staggered through a series of crises, first political and economic, and shortly after, epidemic. It was a tragedy of lost lives and squandered opportunities. Yet this forming, rupture, and reforming across the 1840s infused the city's muscle memory with a formal resilience, one through which we can trace stubborn examples of its physical language, including relentless land reclamation, building climate control, and vertiginous construction. The population's evolving conception of disease and its relations to the terrain, innate and made, was foundational to this transformation.

This study is the first in-depth historical account of the beginnings of Hong Kong society and its urbanism. It is a rare thing for a historian to be able to examine any city's formation and determine its constituent elements. But Hong Kong's circumstances were also highly peculiar, the basis for its existence intentionally uncertain. When I wrote the core of the manuscript more than a decade ago, while studying at the Department of

History at The University of Hong Kong (HKU), my initial intention had been to uncover and explain the motives and politics of colonists that drove the early construction of the settlement on the island. Surprisingly, what best tied the materials together as history was the outbreak of an epidemic, waves of malarial attacks stretching from the summer of 1841 onwards, though cresting in 1843. It turned out that the most poignant way one might attempt to explain the architecture and urban pattern of the young city was as manifestations that recorded in their making both the fears and opportunities of settlers brought about by a precariousness of life wrought by the disease. During the first half of this decade, the 1840s, the island gained a terrible reputation as a diseased and deadly location. Visual evidence of the time conveys as much about the paranoia and perils of life on the island as the textual, and both have been used interconnectedly throughout the book. The disease also accentuated the brutal colonial politics of race and class and the contours of privilege traced in well-timed land grabs that disempowered vulnerable sections of the community in favour of others. Imagery is never innocent. This study emphasises how Hong Kong's 'construction' was, by necessity, both physical and imagined, as it altered over time. So, my project mutated into a landscape history wherein settlers re-evaluated the topography, geology, society, and building of the early city settlement along the northern shoreline of Hong Kong Island in a desperate attempt to understand the nature and causes of a sickness that was killing them. This leveller was called 'malaria', as in 'bad air', believed to be a gaseous emanation from the land. Since malaria was considered a low-lying gas, it soon compelled the young city to be conceived of in 'section' as a divided community living at differing heights and atmospheres. Disease, therefore, added this vital third dimension to colonial urban space and division. When it comes down to it, histories of urban epidemics are, in fact, histories of political opportunity, separation, and social change. The question is, into whose hands does this power fall?

The research and writing of this book have involved the help and generous advice of many friends, colleagues, and institutions, and I sincerely apologise to those I have missed. I must begin my thanks with Dr. Peter Cunich. He was head of the Department of History at HKU when I joined it more than fifteen years ago. I was already a design tutor at the Department of Architecture, and moving into history as a discipline was daunting for me, but Peter took me under his wing. He became more than a supervisor; he became a mentor and a friend. I thank him for his patience, methodological care and training, his passion for history, and, equally, his compassion towards his students. Peter's approach has indelibly shaped my early training as a historian. Professor John Carroll, one of our great Hong Kong historians, had just joined the department. John shared with me, on countless occasions, detailed advice and the sum of his experiences, ranging from archival approaches to writers and the broader field of research. I have enjoyed our many warm discussions. He generously reviewed this manuscript in its earliest form, chapter by chapter. Early in my work, Dr. Elizabeth Sinn at HKU's Centre of Asian Studies (now part of Hong Kong Institute for the Humanities and Social Sciences) kindly shared her research into early Chinese culture, especially concerning the dim pre-colonial history of stonemasonry on the island. This insight led to my understanding of a relatively sophisticated culture of construction labour and building contracting within the region that the British used rather than created. As I wrote the manuscript, I had the privilege of many enjoyable conversations with Jonathan Wattis, Hong Kong's preeminent map dealer. His boundless passion and imagination for Hong Kong history and his expertise in regional paintings, drawings, and maps have challenged, provoked, and inspired my interpretations. Dr. Graham Mooney, at the Institute of the History of Medicine at Johns Hopkins University, has kindly shared his expertise on the literature of malaria and medicine concerning urbanism. It has, I hope, made this work stronger, as it has enriched my sense of the lines of research within this specialist field.

Despite my subsequent doctoral research at Columbia University having shifted emphatically towards India, Hong Kong history occasionally stormed back in. The most significant incursion began with a surprise communication I received from Derek McDonnell, founding director of Hordern House, Sydney, and one of the world's leading antiquarian book dealers. Ironically, he contacted me just as I was heading back to New York from a conference in Sydney, so we failed to meet. A recent trove of long-lost watercolours by the architect Edward Ashworth surfaced in Australia. Purchased by Hordern House, Derek asked for attribution and help in identifying each painting, its date, its context for the artist, and its relationship to Ashworth's movements. The peripatetic English architect has proved to be an outsized figure in colonial urban history, not just for early Victoria in Hong Kong but for Auckland and Sydney. He provides a rare linkage to the nascent construction industry on Hong Kong Island and is a crucial illustrator of the city's growth. And so, the second phase in my research work on this period of Hong Kong began and of a more intense architectural and scenographic nature. I completed the catalogue in late 2014, and to my delight, the Hong Kong Museum of Art purchased the Hong Kong portion of the collection. The book benefits immeasurably from their inclusion, and apart from the catalogue, these works have not been published before nor situated in their proper context against other visual evidence. I must thank Derek for reviving my explorations into early Hong Kong and opening up further dimensions from which this book has benefited.

I thank my friends and fellow travellers on the historian's path. Dave Macri, then completing his PhD in the department, inspired me with his meticulous attention to detail and his forensic approach towards research, all churning within his ever-growing database. I have been fortunate to share experiences and insights with Cecilia Chu, Chang Jiat-Hwee, and Cole Roskam, architectural historians then at Berkeley and Harvard, respectively, who all coincidentally converged in London just when I needed them the most and was finding my feet in the various archives. They have, perhaps unwittingly, planted the seeds of many disciplinary branches in my secondary literature knowledge. I must also mention two good friends, Humphrey Yuen and Lawrence Tse, whose passion for the dwindling built heritage of Hong Kong corresponds with my own and with whom I have spent many hours thinking about the history of Hong Kong from various vantage points. At HKU's Department of Architecture, I must thank Zhu Tao and Eunice Seng, who gave me much helpful advice on extending my research. Tao became a sounding board, helping me to frame my broader thoughts and providing critical and theoretical insights. If Tao and Elaine Zhu had not approached me in 2020 to contribute an article on disease and urbanism in Hong Kong for their SpaceAction China blog, this book would likely not have come about. In parallel, as part of this unfortunate zeitgeist, I was invited by Ian Tan, co-editor, to contribute an abridged form of my earlier writing on malaria and early Hong Kong for the *Hong Kong Institute of Architects* (HKIA) *Journal* later that year, further signalling reader interest in a book.

I must also thank several archives and staff for their generous help. Though in a fragmented state, the Hong Kong SAR Government's Public Records Office stands out among these, with thoughtfulness and care from the staff that I was more than eager to receive while adrift in historical drawing materials. Most fortunate has been the discovery of T. B. Collinson's family letters and valuable references contained in the card files of the Carl T. Smith Collection. Also within Hong Kong, The University of Hong Kong's Special Collections had become a months-long nocturnal home for me. The Morrison Collection's mid-nineteenth-century newspapers and the library's extensive microfilm and microfiche collections have proved extremely valuable. The British Library in London was essential for various rare nineteenth-century publications, particularly travel journals and periodicals, including the *Professional Papers* of the Royal Engineers. The Royal Institute of British Architects (RIBA) Library and its staff assisted me in exploring specialist architectural journals of the period, such as *The Builder*, Edward Ashworth's dictionary entry on Chinese architecture, and other valuable contemporary commentary within the discipline. Staff at the Caird Library and Archive at the National Maritime Museum, Greenwich, London, helped with my investigations into various naval materials, particularly surgeon Edward Cree's extraordinary illustrated diaries. I got lost in The National Archives at Kew, particularly among its CO 129 materials (the Colonial Office's enduring code for Hong Kong) and the War Office's visual documentation. This repository has proved vast and vital for almost all governmental correspondence between Hong Kong and Britain, contained in reports, memos, ordinances, legislation, and various maps, plans, and drawings, much of their counterparts destroyed in the invasion of Hong Kong during WWII. Outside of London, I must thank the Institution of Royal Engineers for permission to spend some days at the archive and library adjacent to their museum and barracks at Chatham, Kent, a space they specially opened for my use. The library has offered a wealth of further published and unpublished materials on their endeavours. I must also thank Matheson & Co., London, for granting access to the substantial Jardine Matheson Archives at The Department of Manuscripts and University Archives, Cambridge University Library, revealing the ambitions and fears of colonisation by the most significant single investor on the island.

For the compiling of this book, I must thank the following institutions and individuals for their kind permission to use various visual sources: The National Archives, Kew, London; the Hong Kong Museum of Art, Hong Kong; the Caird Library and Archive, National Maritime Museum, Greenwich, London; the Peabody Essex Museum, Salem, Massachusetts; the Public Records Office of Hong Kong, Hong Kong; the British Library, London; the Alexander Turnbull Library, National Library of New Zealand, Wellington, New Zealand; the Yale Center for British Art, Yale University, New Haven, Connecticut; the Baker Library Special Collections and Archives, Harvard University, Cambridge, Massachusetts; the Wellcome Collection, London; Mr. Anthony Hardy, Sze Yuan Tang Collection, Hong Kong; Mr. Richard Castle, Castle Fine Arts Inc., Sacramento, California; the UK Hydrographic Office Archive, Taunton, Somerset;

the Victoria & Albert Museum, London; and the Barry Lawrence Ruderman Map Collection, Stanford University, Stanford, California.

I understand this book to be pioneering in the oeuvre of The Chinese University of Hong Kong Press (CUHKP), introducing colonial architecture and urban history in Asia as new strands in the publisher's long-standing work on Chinese art and architecture. I was keen to approach them, recognising CUHKP's unique mission to publish their works in English and Chinese and desiring the book to reach beyond the English-speaking world. And so, I must thank the Press for their unstinting dedication and care in realising this project, first here, for the English edition of the book. I thank Director Qi Gan and Acquisitions Editor Minlei Ye, both of whom, to my delight, immediately saw the work's worth and remained committed and enthusiastic throughout the lengthy peer review. At the other end of production, I am very grateful to Zoe Ross, my indexer based in Edinburgh, for her careful eye and for working extremely hard to finish the work within a tight timeframe. But, in particular, I must thank my editor, Brian Yu, for his sensitive and patient efforts as he accompanied me through the various stages of production. I must apologise to him and his colleagues for the numerous delays on my side as I juggled teaching commitments and moved country. But the result speaks for itself: a product surpassing expectations. This book has been generously supported by a publications grant from the Paul Mellon Centre for Studies in British Art and a second grant from the Trinity College Dublin Association and Trust. I am both glad and relieved that this hitherto neglected yet strange and fascinating early history of colonial Hong Kong can now be read, pondered, debated, and imagined across the English- and Chinese-speaking worlds in all its rapid and raw drama, and hopefully make better sense of modern Hong Kong.

Chris Cowell

London, December 2023

A Note on Names

For consistency, most Chinese location names, names of persons, and other proper nouns will appear either in Pinyin or, if localised and of current Hong Kong familiarity, in the English spelling customarily used. However, discrepancies will arise, for instance, when a proper noun gains familiarity within contemporary (mid-nineteenth-century) English literature, such as the 'Treaty of Nanking' or the island of 'Chusan' ('Zhoushan' in Pinyin). Where there are multiple contemporary variants, such as the unratified 'Treaty of Chuenpeh' or 'Chuenpee', which is also spelt 'Chuenpei' or 'Chuenpi' in modern phoneticised English from Cantonese, I have used Pinyin as the final arbiter: 'Chuanbi'. Personal Chinese names, such as those of well-known Chinese officials, are spelt using Pinyin (for example, 'Qiying' instead of the contemporary British 'Keying'), whereas those of, say, local Chinese in early Hong Kong, for want of alternative Chinese documents, adopt the spellings given to them in the original English sources, such as Loo Aqui and Tam Achoy.

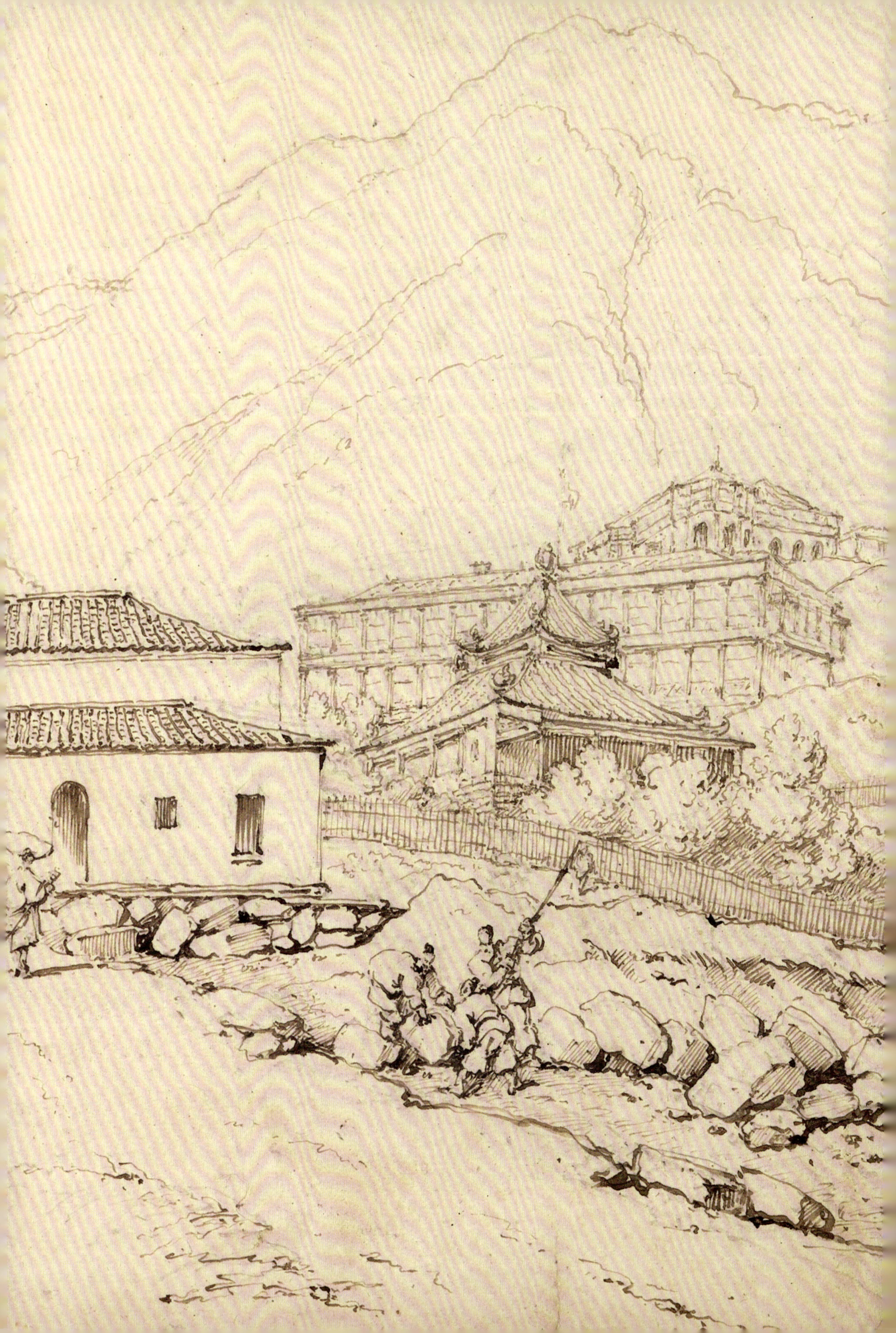

CHAPTER 1

Introduction

> When to the foregoing calendar of horrors, we add the malignant fever, which swept off foreigners by the score, due, as was supposed, to the noxious gases exhaled from the surfaces of decomposed granite laid bare during the erection of the city, we must admit that the island fairly earned its reputation as the grave of Europeans.
>
> Both it and the native inhabitants have undergone marvellous changes within the last twenty-five years. A splendid town has been built out of its barren rocks; and the hill-sides are covered with trees, which not only enhance the picturesqueness of the place, but are of great value in purifying the air, and improving the health of the population.
>
> —John Thomson, 'Hong Kong', *Illustrations of China and Its People*, 1873.

When the Scottish photographer John Thomson wrote his entry for Hong Kong before embarking on his pioneering journey into China, the port city had become a haven for foreign residents and flocks of curious tourists. For many westerners, including Thomson, encounters with China began now with Hong Kong. It served both as a basecamp and gateway. It framed the vast mainland in sharp juxtapose as a first point of reference. The grand arcades and terraced streets balanced, in their solid assurance, the transience of the island community. The recent afforestation of the once-stark hillsides filled the air with a moist fragrance as if a city within a garden oasis. Trade was humming. Crime was containable. It was now a colony with a counterpart, Kowloon, beaming at it across the harbour (**fig. 1.1**). But old-timers did not have to cast their memories that far back to recall how this transformation had been far from certain; how, in fact, Hong Kong had nearly failed.

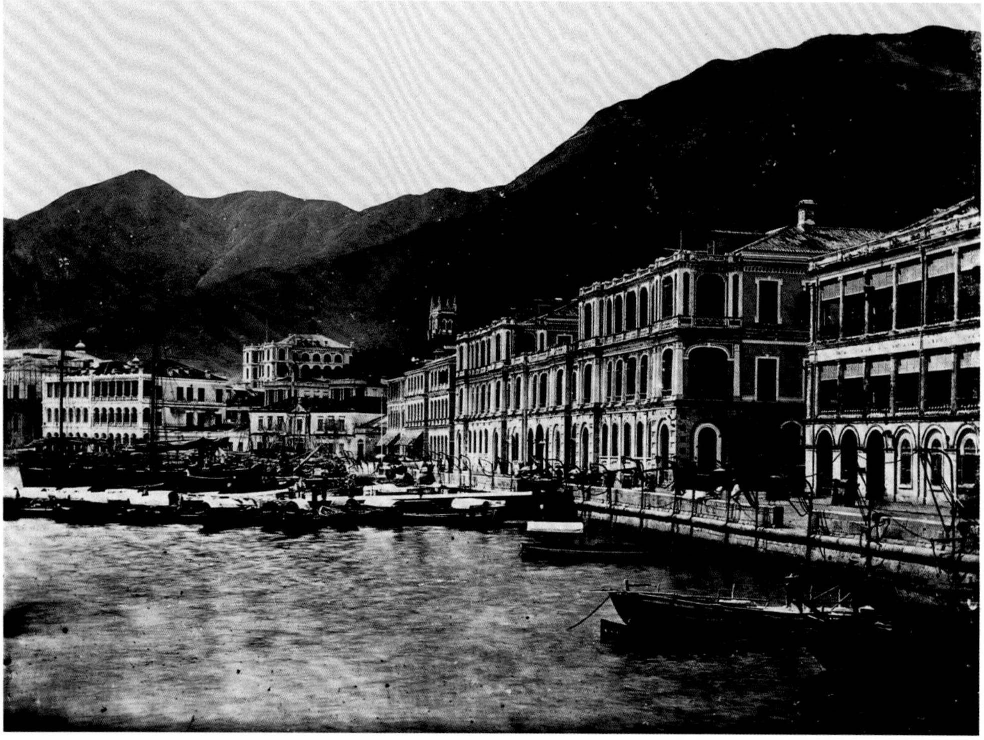

Fig. 1.1. J. Thomson, View Along Waterfront Road (now Des Voeux Road), Hong Kong Island, 1868. © Wellcome Collection, London (18693i).

Hong Kong's early urban history—comprising then just the island—has been written in several ways, from studies on land conveyancing and its civil and commercial administration to the growing influence of Chinese elites. Yet it is odd that this, one of our major world cities, lacks a coherent study of how the settlement, then a colony, was precariously established and *physically* developed in the mid-nineteenth century. We still do not systematically understand how the place transformed, from what Britain's then foreign secretary, Lord Palmerston, would famously denounce as a 'barren Island with hardly a House upon it', into a fully functioning city.[1]

In reading through a range of source material it is evident that the beginnings of settler life in the colony of Hong Kong in the early 1840s was anything but smooth. It was pockmarked by a variety of traumas, both human and natural, with, at times, the natural upheavals inadvertently amplified by the manufactured. As with many other locations across both tropical and subtropical regions settled on by European colonists, Hong Kong's early foreign population had to deal with the consequences of an aggressive climate: typhoons and tempestuous rains, scorching hot and humid days, combined with unexpected fires that swept through the early bamboo, matting, and timber city like a match to tinder. Among the manufactured shocks were the personal attacks on the early settlers from local brigands, highway robbers, and sea-faring pirates, and the occasional night attacks on warehouses and homes—the culprits escaping by slipping across the harbour into Chinese territory and outside of the town's fledgling jurisdiction. In contrast, British colonial justice was often meted out to both the deserving and undeserving harshly, peremptorily, and with blatant racial bias. As familiar history recounts, the new inhabitants fell victim to petty politics, the small, island-locked government intent upon demonstrating its new presence, issuing ordinance after ordinance as if to amplify its sense of self-importance, but with the effect of stifling the spirits of those optimistically engaged in commerce.

One of the most frightening and significant traumas to affect the fledgeling city was the emergence of wave upon sudden wave of human sickness. It would shape the reactionary strategy of settlers in the planning and construction of their settlement and its infrastructure and provide a symbolic imprint that carried several other manufactured traumas in its wake. 'Frightening' because these fevers struck, at first unexpectedly, in different positions across the city and sometimes in a brutal manner. The small group of medical professionals upon the island developed several theories to explain these deadly fevers and to support their uncertain countermeasures. In this pre-bacteriological world, the locus of the malignancy was thought to reside in the elements: in water; in rank vegetation; from within decayed rock; the misalignment of strange electromagnetic forces; or from the rays of the sun at its zenith, and the subsequent exuding of airborne contamination. There was ultimately no escape from the 'miasma' except by collective action in order to reform the city itself.

Hong Kongers' perceptions of their colony in the face of these threats to their well-being and, conversely, how remote outside audiences perceived the territory acted as significant pressures, agents of transformation. We must examine these in concert if a meaningful study is to be made on how the city developed and established an initial physical and behavioural pattern. This book examines, in detail, the first nine years of Hong Kong's development, presenting it as a sequence of related events, their causes and reactions, that provided the city with its 'accidental' urban grammar that would serve as its future template.

Malaria as Miasma

It is not the intention to pin an entire city creation story and its urban morphology upon the presence of malaria. One may look at the urban and architectural 'birth' of colonial Hong Kong through the lens of its economic and mercantile ambitions, of its rapid multi-ethnic immigration and the attendant threats to its peace and security. Or one can examine it from a traditional historian's perspective, through its political and local government development and its relations with Qing Dynasty China. Nevertheless, of all the underlying motifs that could be called upon to explain the decision-making processes that contributed to its physical development, contemporary concerns of *health* and *well-being* form the most natural glue. More than any other theme, these overarch and tie the disparate storylines, making collective sense of both the perceptions and responses of the early colonists towards the shaping of both space and discourse. Of these concerns, nothing so preyed upon the mind than that fatal ailment that seemed to arrive and depart within the warmer months of each year, yet whose manifestation, location, and virulence seemed to escape preparation. European settlers even gave the worst outbreak the name of the island itself, the 'Hongkong Fever', in 1843.

In addition, while many case studies of settlements around the world analyse the urban effects of disease upon changes to various governmental hygiene policies; upon the development of housing and construction; and the formation of sanitation infrastructure within cities and towns across the nineteenth century in both the tropical and temperate spheres and across colonies and metropoles; few can be said to offer as dramatic a study as that of the beginnings of colonial Hong Kong. Despite a significant Chinese population along the southern part of the island, new settlers perceived the stretch of coastal land to the north as a tabula rasa, a blank slate. Upon this, colonists vigorously interrogated their first impressions at a fundamental level, of topography and basic shelter, in response to sickness. Malaria, quite literally, operated as a transforming force upon the colony's genesis story.

The name malaria, derived from the Italian *mal'aria*, in turn derived from the Latin *malus aria*, 'bad' or 'evil air', betrayed a general belief that the disease was airborne, certainly up until the 1880s. The dominant view among most medical professionals in Europe during the 1840s was that of 'miasma theory' and 'contagion theory'. As Roy Porter neatly puts it: 'If it arose from the bodies of the sick, it would be called contagion;

if from marshes and standing water, miasma.'[2] 'Germ theory' would only be postulated within medical circles from about the mid-1860s.[3] In his report for the Hong Kong government's annual Blue Book to parliament in 1850, the Colonial Surgeon William Morrison pondered:

> The exact operation of those subtle atmospherical influences called malaria on the human body is one of the great mysteries which will only be revealed when we are able to solve the rationale of those laws of attraction and repulsion by which form is given to matter, and millions of worlds are permitted to revolve in space without danger of collision.[4]

Therefore, an obvious question arises: *Was the 'Hongkong Fever' actually malaria?* This present study does not attempt to answer this question from a current understanding, in part because what we now consider to be 'malaria' cannot be presumed to match what was then understood to be the same disease. The problem is essentially one of defining. 'Miasma theory' is a branch of disease aetiology (causation). From western antiquity up to the latter half of the nineteenth century, it was a generally held belief that disease could be caused by 'gases given off by putrefying decomposing organic matter, rotting flesh and vegetables'.[5] Before the development of the microscope and a more significant focus upon pathogenesis (the mechanism by which an aetiological factor causes a disease), the inability to map the changes in cells and tissues within the human body inevitably resulted in a focus upon the external. European doctors within the armed services in the 1840s were united by a belief that fevers arising from the (euphemistically named) China Expedition, military excursions often upon or by land that was marshy or surrounded by paddy, were caused by malaria.

> . . . The prevailing Diseases in the Naval Forces in China have been Remittent, and Intermittent Fevers, Acute Dysentery, and occasional Cases of Cholera.
>
> Now the Remittent and Intermittent Fevers, and in some degree the Dysentery are known to arise from Malaria, or Marsh Miasma . . .[6]

Malaria's invisible operations could only be identified through association with various symptoms. For example, one writer, evidently a doctor—since he signed himself anonymously as *Medicus*—wrote to the local Hong Kong press in 1844, enclosing his thoughts upon the nature of malaria and protections required.

> This, like heat, is an invisible, mysterious agent, but very deleterious to the human constitution. We cannot explain its modus operandi, and how much less do we know the laws which regulate its production, diffusion, and influence; and yet we are fully assured that such a poison is eliminated, from the earth's surface, at certain seasons and places, and that when it comes into contact with our bodies, that we are seized with fever, dysentery, and other disorders, which destroy myriads of people every year, especially in the tropics.[7]

Malaria was, therefore, thought of as an external agent that brought about fever, but not the fever itself. This aspect is important to note. Until we get to germ theory and the concept of infection, malaria was considered as a miasma or vapour: a nebulous, gaseous phenomenon that sickened or weakened the human constitution to the point where fever was an outcome. In this regard, one can consider that Hong Kong, as with other stations on the China coast, became a theatre for malaria and the fevers they induced—according, that is, to the paradigm of medicine at that time. That the fevers themselves were caused by malaria as we now know it—the protozoan (single-cell) parasitic organism *Plasmodium*, propagated by the female *Anopheles* mosquito (the 'vector')—seems highly plausible in most cases but not necessarily certain in all. The records used to determine this are obscured by the theoretical position with which contemporary medicine understood the cause.[8] The answer, then, to the question is both 'yes, certainly' to the old understanding of the disease and 'yes, probably' to our current understanding. This book is principally interested in the first reply, as herein lay the observations, opinions, and responses that shaped the outcomes which significantly contributed to the physical development of 1840s Hong Kong. In other words, this account focuses upon the *built environment* of the early colony and how perceptions shaped reality. Arthur Starling has attempted to do what this book has not—to diagnose, from a modern medical standpoint, the disease behind the 'Hongkong Fever'. Yet he too has concluded that 'it is not certain from the available accounts of Hong Kong fever, whether it was one disease or several . . . but most certainly, malaria would have been at least the most important of those diseases'.[9]

Causes and effects, however, are not quite so straightforward. Some historians of medicine, such as Randall M. Packard, have asserted that epidemics of malaria and their patterns of transmission have, in the past, arisen from dramatic shifts within an environment. Often, these result from complex human factors, making predicting malarial outbreaks difficult while also accounting for its opportunism and resilience. Packard argues that three essential ingredients are needed for an epidemic to occur: the local presence of malaria-transmitting mosquitoes; an environmental change that favours the breeding of these mosquitoes, essentially changes which disrupt the original flow and distribution of water; and the introduction of a new, large human population, particularly one comprising of malaria carriers or 'immunologically naïve' individuals.[10] Early colonial Hong Kong provided all three of these factors, making the argument for malaria particularly convincing. Settlers began the disruption by constructing the main coastal carriageway, the Queen's Road, blocking nullahs (streams), churning up earth, and thereby providing numerous pockets of stagnant water for mosquitoes to breed in, increasing the problem through widespread pits created from the excavation of land for construction. Contrary to previous historical accounts, it seems from military statistics that malaria was unwittingly *brought* to the island by sick troops of the British armed forces, the healthier members of whom proved both 'immunologically naïve' and therefore particularly susceptible to the first attacks across the years 1841 and 1842. As the colonial medical historian Mark Harrison asserts, 'War favours the spread of malaria in several ways. The movement of large numbers of troops and civilians introduces parasites and vectors into areas formerly free of them; the destruction of dams and levees cause low-lying areas to be flooded, providing ideal breeding grounds for mosquitoes.'[11] Due to both rampant city-building and the settlement as a military depot for sick soldiers, by early 1843, the disease had infected a critical mass of people. This number all but ensured the city-wide epidemic that would take place later that year. But, as this book will chart, indeterminacy as to the sources of malaria or 'marsh miasma'—this mysterious agency of fevers, diarrhoea, and dysentery—lent, by its very elusiveness to ascribable causes, certain pliability to political manipulation by special interest groups and personal agendas.

Miasmata, as a sickening force arising from a natural landscape, though first extending back as a recorded idea to Hippocrates (460–377 BCE), had also more recently captured the imagination of the Romantic Movement in quite a significant way. It could show the hand of God at work in the humbling of arrogant humanity in the quest to conquer and control nature. It could also play into the hands of a growing lobby of protesters writing in the early nineteenth century about the inherent dangers of the British military forces enduring tropical climates in which the European constitution was irreconcilably ill-suited. Francis Danby's painting *The Upas, or Poison-Tree, in the Island of Java*, is a startling example of the emotional and religious impact of exotic 'miasmatical' tropics on the minds of the early nineteenth-century British (**fig. 1.2**).

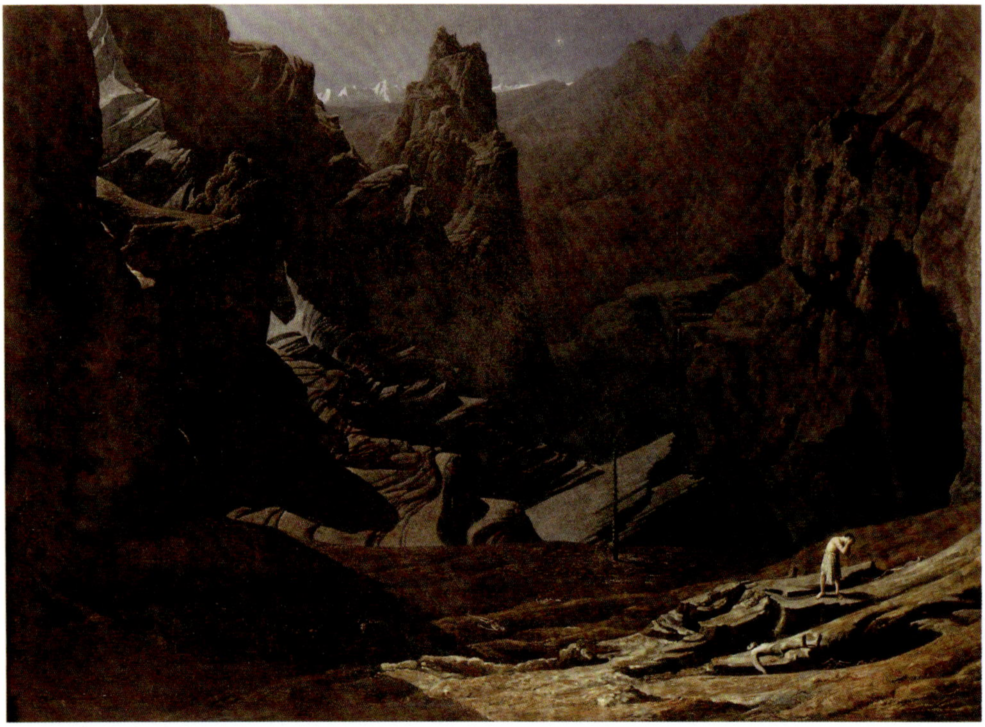

Fig. 1.2. F. Danby, *The Upas, or Poison Tree, in the Island of Java*, ca. 1820. Oil on canvas. © The Victoria and Albert Museum, London.

Danby's preferred subject matter was of an apocalyptic and biblical kind. Painted in 1819 and exhibited in London in 1820, it won his election into the Royal Academy. The 'tree', a single thin spike, protrudes from an utterly desolate landscape, the surface sickened by its toxic presence. Bodies are strewn in the right foreground with the last, grief-stricken survivor (evidently a pale European) trapped yet futilely attempting to shield himself from its malignancy. This painting gripped the British imagination and, contrary to what might be supposed, it was not seen as an allegory. The tree, or at least the deadly landscape of Java, was actually thought to exist. The London *Literary Gazette*, reprinted locally for Hong Kong's nervous readers in December 1846, would record, twenty-six years after Danby's painting, an incredibly similar description of a supposed real environment.

> THE VALLEY OF DEATH. The following is a probable explanation of the origin of the upas tree story: 'A real valley of death exists in Java; it is termed the Valley of

> Poison and is filled to a considerable height with carbonic acid gas, which is exhaled from crevices in the ground. If a man or any animal enter it, he cannot return; and he is not sensible of his danger until he feels himself sinking under the poisonous influence of the atmosphere which surrounds him. . . . Birds which fly into this atmosphere drop down dead; and a living fowl thrown into it dies before it reaches the bottom, which is strewed with the carcasses of various animals that have perished in the deleterious gas.'[12]

Hong Kong Island may not have seemed similarly marked out as a place of death. At least, not at first. But following their occupation in 1841, this would quickly change for the new colonists. Soon, after successive years of repeated outbreaks of malaria upon barracked troops, military cartographers were violently inscribing on surveys the positions of ridges and furrows upon and against which they built—the furrows increasingly recognised as locations of miasma, the ridges acting as barriers to wholesome ventilation (**fig. 1.3**). Such ventilation-craft in the analysis of topography was essential to military security and troop survival. This government map was drawn just as the Hongkong Fever abated. And if the graphic violence was not clear enough, the military draughtsman added, 'The land rises abruptly from the North Shore, in steep ridges and deep ravines—terminating in a lofty ridge extending from East to West. . . . The shaded portion shews the formation of the land in the Military Cantonment.'[13]

One may say that this book is partly a study in 'medical topography'. This branch of medicine came into its own in the early nineteenth century in British India, as developed by the Presidency Surgeon of Bengal Sir James Ranald Martin in his influential work *Notes on the Medical Topography of Calcutta* published in 1837. It was, as it sounded, the mapping and surveying of geographical terrain under the belief that certain areas possessed an inherent, malignant effect upon human health. Like Montesquieu before him, Martin believed that our environment and climate directly affected our communal character and, consequently, the nature of our political institutions.[14] This belief of climate and terrain effects was compelling during the centuries of European expansion and global colonisation, from the seventeenth to the nineteenth centuries. As David Arnold writes, prior to the nineteenth century, data was presented 'in the form of narratives, describing the epidemics that had afflicted a territory over a period of years, especially in relation to climate and seasons, but with only an impressionistic notion of the numbers and type of fatalities that had occurred'.[15]

During the 1820s to 1840s, a change occurred in mapping disease, emphasising statistical forms of measurement and, therefore, generating the illusion of diagnostic accuracy upon an indeterminate phenomenon. Gone, too, were the shaded hatchings of ridges and furrows of hillsides and mountains, their emotional charge dissipated by the flattened empiricism of contour lines. The first of these contoured surveys to be published of a sovereign territory, we will find, was of Hong Kong Island. 'The general effect', Arnold writes, 'as far as the early nineteenth century was concerned was to give a statistical and scientific specificity to the hitherto generalised dangers of tropical climates and to encourage measures to combat them'.[16]

'Systematic bedside observation' and the 'statistical analysis of cases' became a hallmark of the British East India Company's 'experimental and empirical' medical approach within their eighteenth-century hospitals in India.[17] The high number of military casualties, particularly through disease, afforded test subjects for British surgeons and doctors working in tropical environments. This allowed them the opportunity to innovate, for instance, with economic mass remedies, and to theorise.[18] The medical attendants of the troops stationed in early Hong Kong could be said to be disciples of this distinctly 'tropical' school of thought. Arnold alludes to a parallel development—the use of medical geographical and topographical surveys (that is, the inclusion of *height* measurement and landscape features), 'giving expression to perceptions of the particular local causes of disease through the impact of climate, vegetation and physical topography'.[19] These were the reinforcing tools of adventurers within the tropics brought up on a diet of Montesquieu, Hume, and Falconer, sharing their beliefs about the effects upon the human and natural worlds through the exertions of climate and geography.[20] As will be shown, statistics and topographical surveying played a crucial role in the medical mapping of Hong Kong and consequently influenced the decision-making of the civil and military wings of government in planning and building the colony.

▶ **Fig. 1.3.** Surveyor General's Dept., 'Plan of Victoria, Hong Kong', with Cantonment Hill (now Admiralty) (detail), 12 May 1845. Ink and watercolour. © The National Archives, Kew (WO 78/479).

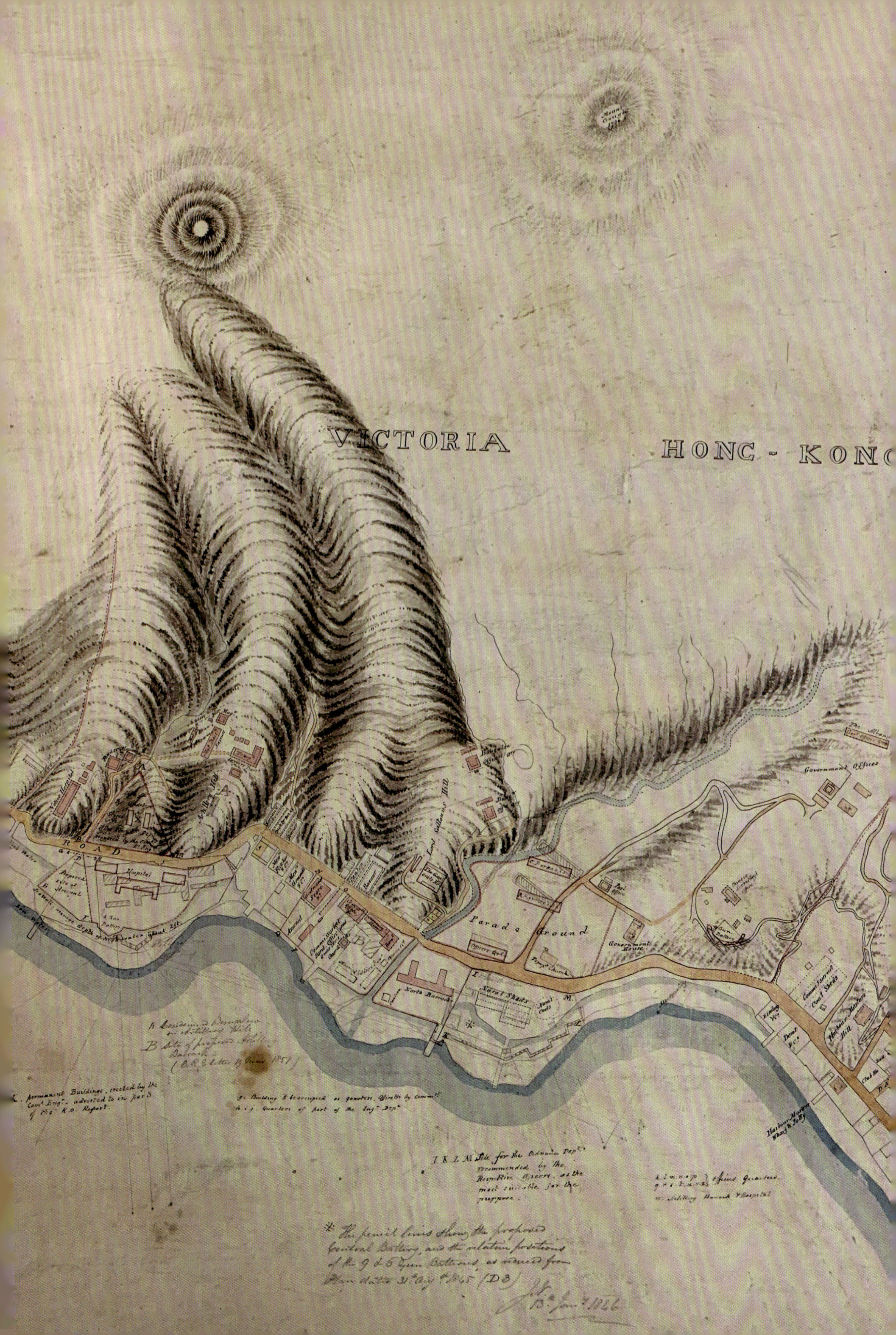

VICTORIA
HONG - KONG
ROAD
Parade Ground
Government House
Government Offices
North Barrack
Naval Shed
Dent & Co.
Harbour Masters Wharf & Jetty
I. K. L. M. Site for the Ordnance Dept. recommended by the Respective Officers, as the most suitable for the purpose.
* The pencil lines show the proposed Central Battery, and the relative positions of the 9 & 6 Gun Batteries, as reduced from Plan dated 31st Aug. 1845 (D3)
1846

Urbanisation and Its Discontents

Malaria is not an exclusively tropical disease. But it was thought by European colonists as a malignant emergent property of tropical peoples, climate, and context, and so, easily framed as such. Contemporaries considered its mode as environmental rather than parasitic. Therefore, as perceived by western medics of the time, the pathogenesis of most diseases was intensely spatial. Physicians, not architects or planners, became, as Michel Foucault puts it, 'the first managers of collective space'.[21] Developments in medical theory profoundly affected the perception and shaping of the built environment and cities by the early nineteenth century, especially within tropical colonies. Foucault identified four lenses through which European doctors viewed the transmission of diseases. The first was by combining local conditions and seasonal variations (regional climate, geology, humidity). The second was either between human and human (densities of populations and classes of people); between humans and natural substances (through sewage, gases, water); between humans and animals (stables and abattoirs); or between the living and the dead (cemeteries). The third was related to where one resided (buildings, foundations, ventilation). And the fourth concerned human displacement (migration, movement of soldiers, disease propagation).[22] This book shows that all these factors in synthesis played a fundamental role in the initial settlement, perceptions of the epidemic, and subsequent reactions and development of Hong Kong. This work, then, is principally an architectural, urban, and landscape history of the colony, as affected by medical inquiry, military- and civil-settler sentiment, and their combinative political consequences.

Since my earlier work on this subject, scholars have made new inroads that have connected and widened the research fields of architecture, urbanism, landscape, and colonialism, with a heightened degree of spatial and material understanding.[23] Though this book may be considered a monograph across a tight historical timeframe, it is important to consider the broader themes through which these events may be viewed. For instance, as Jiat-Hwee Chang has exposed, the metrics and discourse which bind the term 'tropical architecture' and its genealogy—a term which he has extended back from the mid-twentieth century and into the nineteenth—does not equally frame its antithesis, 'temperate architecture', revealing asymmetric power relations between the west and non-west.[24] There was no such category as temperate architecture because it meant western architecture. Rather this term was replaced by finer-grained cultural, stylistic, and national categories (such as English Baroque, French Neoclassicism, and Italian Mannerism). Tropical architecture, on the other hand, was approached by western contemporaries without such distinctive niceties. Instead, stripped of any cultural and historical attributes, considered autochthonous, its form and applications were thought entirely responsive to external factors rather than the artistic choices of local builders. By extension of prejudice, those local builders were thought to lack the sophistication to produce works of genuine architecture; they were merely reactive. And so, Hong Kong's 'infancy' (as several contemporaries termed it) was saddled with the inability to fashion itself into a respectable city as it lurched from crisis to crisis, with malaria playing a symbolic and amplified role in the futility of planning and constructing the beleaguered colony. It may have been the environmental inadequacy of an indigenous 'mat-shed' as an army barracks, or the misalignment of windows on a 'knock-off' of a classical façade for a public official's residence, or the damp walls of a hastily constructed speculative development, all examples we will encounter. Nevertheless, whether by form or through practice, all sat under the same condemnatory rubric of inescapably 'tropical' architecture or architecture devoid of culture. To be forced to build reactively implied that one could not plan to civilise.

Irrespective of the overt racism, such condemnation of early Hong Kong architecture by European visitors to the colony attempted to conceal obvious hypocrisy. The mat-shed, the godown (or warehouse), and the market shophouse were non-descript precisely as intended by the western client as they were also products of craft by the Chinese builder. Modern imperialism and its economic logic, as exercised within frontier territories, demanded that the bulk of its architecture conform to simple templates, easily reproducible buildings, to a 'grey architecture' as G. A. Bremner defines it.[25] Hong Kong's early architectural assemblage was necessary to knit it quickly and more efficiently into wider networks of commerce and militarism, allowing its facilities to adapt as needed to shifting and unforeseen demands and risks. As Bremner later describes in his study on Jardine Matheson & Co., this grey architecture must be considered a kind of 'facilities infrastructure', recognisable and standardised to generate a familiarity of use by its transient patrons and confidence in its extendibility.[26] It also aligned with the forming of facilities enclaves, a peculiar urban phenomenon of early military and commercial life upon the island.

As of going to print, Cole Roskam is close to completing a remarkably ambitious study of the urban and architectural history of Hong Kong, spanning from the 1840s to the present day. Presently entitled *Hong Kong: Uncertain City*, it extends and amplifies the thesis that crisis and precarity, rather than retardants, were essential, propulsive forces that continually shaped the city of Hong Kong across its nearly two centuries of urban development. The book examines the evolving environment within which Hong Kong's architecture played a dynamically participatory role. Historians and critics have often argued that the territory's urban language contributed to a derived city, absorbing and replicating aspects and appearances of both east and west. Instead, the research determines how, because of Hong Kong's unique conditions, the built environment responded, often in blunt terms, as a legible critique of its particular relations to such generative crises and that we must examine its architectural history from the ground up.[27]

Before the city, with all its uncertainties, could gain a foothold on the island, colonists had to establish its legitimacy. Maxime Decaudin, a historian of landscape, has recently explored in his doctoral work how the as-found 'barrenness' of the island had first to be agreed upon as an accepted environmental discourse to justify colonisation, both in terms of the rights to urbanise and to distinguish the British as good stewards compared to the indigenous population. As Robert Peckham has observed earlier, in botanical literature, Europeans initially regarded Hong Kong as a 'fallen world'. In these colonial narratives, a tense ambiguity arose of inherent degradation of the island's geology, on the one hand, against those claiming human causes: that it had been the 'reckless' indigenous population who had stripped life-saving vegetative cover from the mountainside surface. Subsequently, colonists could blame native inhabitants for malaria and justify European preeminence once they could formulate a connection between vegetation and miasma, yet protection by tree cover.[28] It helped that extended urbanisation forced some indigenous people out of their cultivated lands to cut down and sell vegetation from nearby hills, merely reinforcing such a narrative. In contrast, schemes for (re)afforestation would portray colonial good governance.[29] Moreover, by playing upon the claims that careful modern management of the island's 'natural' landscape had devolved into the capable hands of colonists, officials could simultaneously justify the expansionary tactics of urban development with island-wide tree planting as a combined project.

An interwoven understanding of landscapes, cities, and sickness, provoked by the global pandemic, has been explored in a spate of recent studies, amplifying modern urbanism's malignant relationship with contagious diseases and their propagation. Such studies include, by way of example, Mohammad Gharipour and Caitlin DeClercq's edited volume *Epidemic Urbanism* (2021). Thirty-six geographically divergent historical accounts serve to remind the reader that the communication of disease across modern history reveals the vulnerable extent of a city's globality as well as its social inequalities.[30] Sara Jensen Carr's work, *The Topography of Wellness* (2021), focuses upon how architects, landscape designers, and urban planners responded to disease outbreaks across America's urban landscape, in turn producing unexpected consequences.[31] Nida Rehman's doctoral work at the University of Cambridge, 'Epidemiological Landscapes' (2020), demonstrates how urbanism and its politics persists in shaping the landscape of mosquito-borne epidemic diseases.[32] Though miasmas have long been discounted as a mode of malaria transmission, a mid-nineteenth-century physician in Hong Kong could be just as attuned and responsive to the variety of urban factors contributing to the disease as a modern epidemiologist is in postcolonial Lahore. Insect-to-human-spreading epidemic diseases are shaped by the physical, economic, political, and social geographies that bind both species together. If anything, the topographical tropes of ditches, waterways, and damp soils from pre-bacteriological medicine became sharpened loci of eradication once the insect vector and its breeding grounds were identified.[33]

Epidemiology and urbanism have grown significantly through recent Hong Kong historical studies, especially concerning the plague epidemic at the end of the century. As just one example, Cecilia L. Chu's detailed work on late-nineteenth- and early-twentieth-century housing speculation and its relations to disease (among other aspects) highlight the connection between the colony's first urban renewal project at Tai Ping Shan and the 1894 bubonic plague.[34] In her recent book, Chu amplifies the precarity and class manufacture of such urbanism and its amplification of a transient pathology of the colony. This structure is made apparent by the contradictory logic of a colonial-sanctioned 'speculative landscape', one in which Chinese investment is both encouraged yet kept segregated within Hong Kong's geographically stratified property market.[35]

In uncanny anticipation of the Covid pandemic, *Contagious Cities*, a 2019 Hong Kong art and heritage exhibition at Tai Kwun Contemporary (at the old prison site) and supported by the Wellcome Trust, explored Hong Kong's long relationship with pandemics and how they have significantly shaped the city's development physically, socially, and culturally.[36] Artworks evoked the complex psychological and trepidatious urban daily existence living through an epidemic.

Nevertheless, despite renewed and remarkable interest in the subject, surprisingly little has been added to Hong Kong's establishment history and its founding epidemic story of urban transformation across the early 1840s. One exception is Ria Sinha's *longue durée* essay study of malaria across Hong Kong's entire colonial history. 'Fatal Island' (2018) demonstrates the disease's outsized importance in the most significant episodes of the colony's growth.[37] Though briefly touching upon the early period, Sinha emphasises the enigmatic quality of malaria through the nineteenth century and how speculations as to the source of its emanations continued to provide an underlying fear as the city grew in numbers and extent. The *Hongkong Fever* was as much a convenient label of concealment as it was of identification. It could address the symptoms while absorbing the ambiguous cause, allowing other diseases exhibiting similar symptoms to be confounded with it. This uncertainty as to source led to landscape-altering projects which, though intended to dissipate the city's chief malady, merely refuelled it. Perhaps the most significant example was the expansive afforestation programme of the 1870s. Here, the concealing of the island's barren granite rock, long considered a potential source of the disease, was replaced with abundant vegetation and shade for many more mosquitoes to breed within.[38]

Every doctor had his theory as to malaria's source, from atmospheric disturbances through electrical storms to stagnant pools of water. But it was 'ground miasma', the fear of gases rising from disturbed soil or broken rock, that most influenced the first urban development of the city of Hong Kong since it was the most ambiguous and least understood of the various medical hypotheses. It is hard to imagine now, but each stage in Hong Kong's early city growth was accompanied by uncertainty and hesitancy as to whether that step would trigger another outbreak. It was a fearful factor of urban change that only in the last century or so we can comfortably dismiss.

Hongkongraphia

Much of the material used for this study comprises primary sources. Textually these include contemporary sources such as local and central government records, medical reports, personal diaries, published newspaper and journal accounts, advertisements, and the like. Visual materials play an intrinsic role, revealing settlers' ideological, perceptual, and even psycho-spatial anxieties. These materials consist of military and naval surveys, maps, prints, personal sketches, trade paintings, and construction drawings. This forensic approach has been taken because scant research exists regarding the founding period of Hong Kong's colonial development concerning the physical growth pattern of the city of Victoria—the name given to the urban settlement stretching along the northern shore facing the peninsular of Kowloon. Of course, many secondary sources have played a guiding or contextualising role in shaping this book, though I shall discuss only a pertinent few.

My initial investigations as an architectural historian were focused, rather obviously, on those agents who built the colony: on military engineers, private speculators, government contractors, and Chinese builders. John Weiler's unpublished doctoral thesis on the Royal Engineers as 'army architects' serving Britain's global imperial enterprise was especially formative.[39] However, during my early research, I chanced upon the transcript of an 1845 medical lecture given by Hong Kong Colonial Surgeon Dr. Francis Dill, suggesting that there were strong views within the medical fraternity of the time as to *safe* and *unsafe* forms and methods of building.[40] His lecture at a meeting of the first medical society to be formed on the island, the China Medico Chirurgical Society, recounted the terrible years suffered by all in Hong Kong during 1843 and 1844. Hong Kong had undergone the trauma of repeated attacks of 'miasmatic vapour', sometimes also called 'malaria'.[41] He made a critical connection between poor construction and sickness, and implied that better dwellings could mitigate against the harmful effect of the 'rays of the sun, sleeping under the direct rays of the moon, and the exposure to the night dews'.[42] Health issues, particularly of what was understood to be malaria, began to take on a central organising role in my research (and a life of its own), tying together various processes of urban and architectural development. It linked almost every aspect of material culture in the story of the colony's establishment: a mapping of the island, the means of construction, governance and taxation, and even the habits and views of the European and Chinese inhabitants.

For written documentation related to governmental correspondence, I principally concentrate upon the British Colonial Office (CO) and War Office (WO) and, to a lesser degree, Admiralty (ADM) and Foreign Office (FO) papers, the originals of which now reside at The National Archives at Kew. Counterpart copies and many local government papers in Hong Kong have been lost or destroyed during WWII. These include colonial dispatches and internal memos, government reports, legislative records, and official ordinances. The second primary source of written documentation has been local newspapers, in forms such as articles, contemporary advertisements, and foreign news extracts. This 'public' medium has proved an essential foil for government correspondence, often triangulating shared events and offering differing reactions and approaches to official pronouncements. Documentary evidence from some quarters has, understandably, been fragmentary. For instance, it took a while for Hong Kong to standardise its reporting on economic matters. In addition, funding sources shifted after the ratification of the Treaty of Nanking (Nanjing) in late 1842, from the 'military chest' to voted sums from parliament. This shift had a profound effect upon government expenditure, changing the relations of power and, therefore, physical influence between the military and civilian wings of government upon shaping the island colony. It would take a few more years for the civil administration of Hong Kong to become financially self-supporting and, with this, begin to enjoy greater freedom and speed in investment upon its public works. Eventually, there would be no need for delay in waiting for approval from London or the crafting of tortuous local government justifications.

There is evidence from newspaper sources that the daguerreotype (an early photographic technique) was in use in Hong Kong from the early 1840s.[43] However, no photographs seem to exist depicting Hong Kong until the late 1850s and are therefore unable to support this period of investigation. For drawn sources, I have relied entirely upon hand-produced documents: maps, land surveys, and architectural drawings, principally from The National Archives at Kew, London, and China Trade paintings from several repositories and directions, but most especially from the Hong Kong Museum of Art, Hong Kong, and the Peabody Essex Museum at Salem, Massachusetts.

In addition, the present research draws across five other archival repositories. Within Hong Kong, the University of Hong Kong's 'Special Collections' (particularly the Morrison Collection's original newspapers such as the *Canton Register*) and its extensive microfilm and microfiche collections are of considerable importance, as, of course, is the Hong Kong SAR government's Public Records Office (HKPRO). In London, the British Library has supplied my research with a range of nineteenth-century publications, such as the *Professional Papers* of the Royal Engineers, while the stuffed shelves of the Royal Institute of British Architects (RIBA) Library brim with such specialist architectural British journals as *The Builder* from the period of the 1840s, offering insightful early Victorian commentary on British and British colonial matters related to the built environment. The library of the Corps of the Royal Engineers adjacent to their museum and barracks at Chatham, Kent, have provided me with a wealth of further published and unpublished materials on their significant constructions across the island. Meanwhile, the substantial Jardine Matheson Archives at The Department of Manuscripts and University Archives,

Cambridge University Library has shed valuable light on the complex desires and fears of an elite merchant house deliberating whether to invest in or abandon Hong Kong.

In addition to these primary sources, other documents need to be briefly acknowledged. First, one must mention the charming and informative set of letters at the HKPRO by the cartographer Lieutenant Thomas Bernard Collinson of the Royal Engineers to his parents and sister in Gateshead, northern England. The young Collinson has emerged as one of the central figures in the story of the construction of colonial Hong Kong.[44] Also valuable have been the richly illustrated diaries of Edward Cree, a surgeon of the Royal Navy and a future deputy inspector-general of hospitals and fleets, now kept at the Caird Library and Archive, National Maritime Museum (NMM), Greenwich, London. Cree, like Collinson, was in his twenties when he visited Hong Kong. But he acquired a different perspective to his friend Collinson due to the spread pattern of his visits. The latter remained in Hong Kong for about three years (1843 to 1846), while the former, as was the norm with naval personnel, made repeated forays to the island over an extended period, beginning at its inception as a British settlement in 1841.[45]

It would be useful to provide an outline of the various contemporary Hong Kong–based (and Macau-based) newspapers and their political allegiances to familiarise the reader with the complex terrain of relative bias among the colonial broadsheets of the time. When one considers the limited readership available, Hong Kong was blessed with a surprisingly large number of newspapers, albeit all in English. Literate Chinese would have to wait until 1853 for the monthly periodical the *Xia'er guanzhen* (*The Chinese Serial*), a journal published by the London Missionary Society.[46] Meanwhile, the only Chinese-language notices in circulation across the 1840s concerned government pronouncements and shipping advertisements, often carried by the English press. Otherwise, all communications by the colonial government to the Chinese population were via intermediary officials and police, community leaders, compradors, and through hastily pasted bill stickers (wall notices), the latter as depicted by the artist Edward Ashworth in one of his recently discovered watercolour views of Hong Kong in 1844 (see **fig. 4.4**).[47] This voracious English reading culture, together with its linguistic hegemony, most certainly originated in Calcutta as earlier carried into Macau via the major trading houses or foreign 'hongs'. Calcutta was, after all, 'a city with a very vigorous printing industry'.[48] No less than five English-language newspapers were in circulation during the years 1841 to 1849 within Hong Kong, though not all were in existence at the same time.[49] The *Canton*

Press and the *Canton Register* were the earliest, and in 1841 both had forsaken Canton (Guangzhou) and were operating from the relative safety of Macau. The *Canton Register* was run by John Slade and owned by James Matheson, then head of the principal hong on the island, Jardine Matheson, and may be seen as a mouthpiece of mercantile interests. However, it appears to be the case that Matheson did not involve himself very much in influencing the opinions of his editor. The *Register* relocated to Hong Kong in 1843, changing its name to the *Hongkong Register.* The *Canton Press* remained in Macau, eventually folding in March 1844. The short-lived *Hongkong Eastern Globe* ran for just a few months in 1843, and we know very little about it.

In the meantime, the *Hongkong Gazette*, the colony's short-lived government newspaper, was established in May 1841, just in time for the first land sales. The new *Friend of China* soon joined it, and both quickly merged to become the *Friend of China and Hongkong Gazette.* This newspaper moved its operations from Macau to Hong Kong in 1842, becoming the first newspaper established on the island. Following a transfer of editorship to John Carr in early 1844, it shifted its attack towards the government and subsequently lost its gazetted status. It would become the Hong Kong government's most vicious critic. The new 'organ of government' (a derogatory term much used at the time) was briefly held by the *Hongkong Register* only to be forfeited once again and won by a new newspaper, the *China Mail*, in early 1845. Edited by Andrew Shortrede, the *China Mail* remained relatively subdued in tone towards the local government than its incendiary contemporaries and outlasted its competitors by several decades. Its survival contradicted a generally held opinion that having government backing was the kiss of death to a newspaper's longevity and the amassing of a popular readership. Apart from the *Eastern Globe*, with no archival copies in existence, this book weaves across all four newspapers starting from early 1841 and attempts to reflect the spectrum of divergent opinions surrounding colonial Hong Kong's city formation.

The historiography of Hong Kong is a small but concentrated field. Along the way, I have read my Tarrant, Eitel, Sayer, and Endacott, and of recent vintage, my Smith, Sinn, Chan, Welsh, Tsai, Munn, and Carroll, to name some of the more significant historians to address this early period.[50] Tarrant, the only eyewitness in this group, wrote the first 'history' of the colony. Well, not quite. An earlier account of the settlement comes from Lieutenant John Ouchterlony of the Madras Engineers and the island's first chief military builder. Yet, despite his significant role, the only image we have of Hong Kong in his

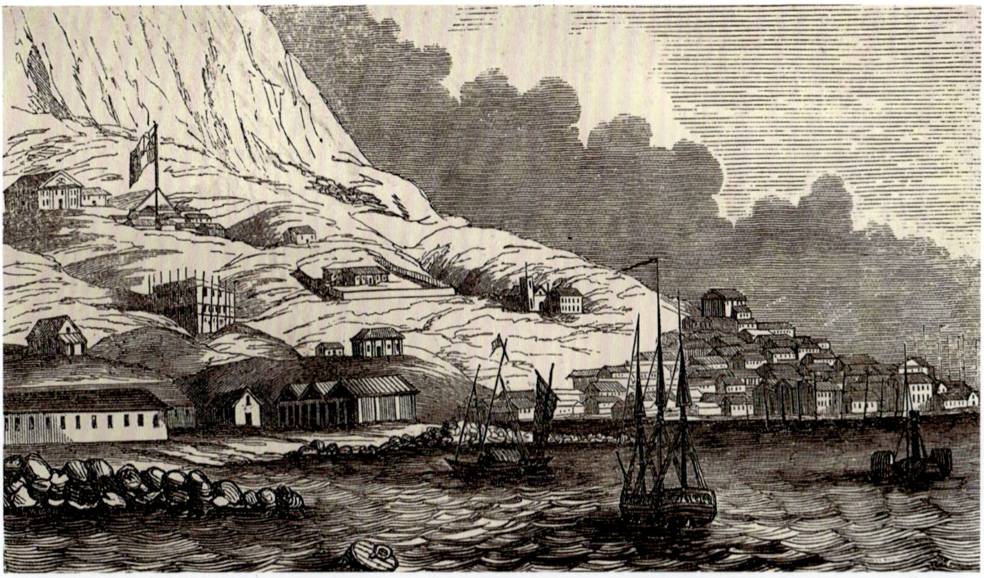

Fig. 1.4. Lt. J. Ouchterlony, 'Hong Kong' (frontispiece), *The Chinese War, London*, 1844.

1844 memoir on the First Anglo-Chinese War—though considered significant enough to grace it as a frontispiece—is a naïvely drawn and liberally scaled attempt to depict the locations of major constructed works across the settlement (**fig. 1.4**). It is as if he had not even visited the place let alone helped to build it. The mast and outsized flag of the harbour master are wrongly placed above the magistrate's prison, godowns (warehouses) are imprecisely oriented, and cartoonish houses are constructed with insufficient scaffolding. It suggests that Ouchterlony saw the colony in figurative terms, more of a process than a place, as a drama rather than a destination.[51]

Considering his tour of duty, Ouchterlony's account of the development of Hong Kong in his war memoir is surprisingly slim yet characterised by the giddiness of rapid development across the first year of colonisation.[52] At the other end of the spectrum regarding type and time, three works of fiction, historical novels, have tapped into this same disorientation—of Hong Kong as a process. These works, each in their turn, have vividly conveyed the dizzyingly rapid and raw growth of the city that must have been experienced by settlers, priming the imagination of modern readers for almost the last sixty years. The first novel is the now-familiar narrative of James Clavell's classic work

Tai-Pan (1966), which in the mid-1960s introduced readers to the turbulent world of colonial politics and the opium trade on the 1840s South China coast.[53] It is a thinly-veiled, romanticised account of the actual British mercantile house of Jardine Matheson & Co. and James Matheson's (Dirk Struan's) early ambitions to gain a foothold in Hong Kong during the initial stages of colonial settlement. It is one of the first fictional works to attempt anything like a cohesive portrayal of the landscape of Hong Kong as the city and colony rapidly emerged, and numerous parts of the island are used as backdrops to the storyline, particularly Happy Valley and East Point. Clavell, though, is often more interested in dialogue than description.

The second work, published precisely two decades later, is by the Anglo-Chinese author Timothy Mo and entitled *An Insular Possession* (1986). With a somewhat more sophisticated descriptive approach, Mo relies on primary research, much from newspaper sources, interspersing these within the dialogue as article cuttings under fictitious newspaper titles. He also provides the reader with a sense of the shock of first settling in Hong Kong and the rapid pace of development.

> Gideon gapes. He had expected the beautiful anchorage of Hong Kong again, of course. But the extent of development on shore is extraordinary. He was prepared for nothing more than the 'jumble of wild ravines' and a desert shore, with perhaps a handful of tents and a few sailors and Chinese. Yet this is like strolling through a large fair in some populous town. Where he and Walter walk, on a foreshore extended by wholesale flattening of the hillocks and rocks above the beach, they mix in a crowd of sailors in best white ducks, Irish soldiers in red, coolies, hucksters, fishermen, lascars, mountebanks, laundry-girls, fruit-sellers, boothmen, and barbers. The square of Canton was nothing to this. Like white pepper-pots to the East are the tents of the military lines, but these are outnumbered now by the ugly mat-shed constructions: wooden huts some 100 feet long, with chinks in the walls crudely plastered in mud, or often not at all, and rude grass-weave roofs. They can glimpse through the crowds the men lying on their palliasses inside or smoking while they clean their accoutrements.[54]

This evocative and realistic depiction of life onshore during the first months of 1841 appears as if it belonged in the diary of naval surgeon Edward Cree, as captured in his rough, on-the-spot watercolours of that year (see **fig. 2.8**). Although, as will be seen, the harsh and uncertain reality of the early colony was even more frightening than Mo paints in his work of historical fiction.

Amitav Ghosh provides the third, most recent fictional narrative to continue the trope of Hong Kong as a barren, sickly, and forlorn island suddenly transformed into a goldrush town of colonial opportunity. Among the final portions of his last book in the *Ibis* trilogy on the India–China opium trade, *Flood of Fire* (2015), he describes

> Soon some of the new arrivals began to move ashore, building huts and shacks, settling where they could. The beach where Paulette's daily climb began did not long remain deserted. A shack appeared at its far edge one day and within a week a hamlet seemed to have sprouted around it.
>
> . . . For centuries Red Incense Burner Hill [Hong Kong] had been considered a place of misery and misfortune—insalubrious, racked by disease and lashed by devastating typhoons. In the past, mainland people had gone to great lengths to avoid Hong Kong; the inhabitants had been objects of pity because they were condemned to eke out an existence on a barren, ill-starred island.
>
> Now suddenly it was as if the island had been transformed into a lodestar. The old-time islanders had begun to fear that their land, their homes, would be expropriated by the British.[55]

Ghosh implies plausibly that the First Opium War (1839–1842), a war run by merchants that brought about the possession of Hong Kong, was managed through bribery and corruption of the British army and navy. Land was always the focus. The military protected traders' interests, ensuring that the choicest plots went to the leading British hongs, while installing a trade-friendly local civil administration to oversee the process.

Speaking of land, among the many secondary sources on the early colony relied upon, the present author owes a particular debt of gratitude to the late Professor Dafydd Emrys Evans. He stands out in his attempts to produce a connective narrative, piecing together the earliest physical events in the formation of the settlement and linking these events in a causal sequence. Evans was founding Dean of the Faculty of Law at The University of Hong Kong, teaching there from the late 1960s to the 1980s. He had ambitions to produce a thorough study of land administration, the leasing and conveyancing of land in the 1840s as a mechanism to investigate the politics and conflicts of the first inhabitants. Sadly, such an ambition was never fully realised. However, he did produce several fascinating studies. These vignettes include 'Hong Kong's First Government House' (1968), an attempt to pinpoint the location of the governor's first 'bungalow' residence from a confusing and conflicting array of primary and historiographical material;[56] 'Chinatown in Hong Kong: The Beginnings of Taipingshan' (1970), demonstrating the chain of events in the renting of land before and following the ratification of the Treaty of Nanking and how this propagated the forced eviction and resettlement of the Chinese inhabitants within the small city;[57] also, 'Jardine, Matheson & Company's First Site in Hong Kong' (1968), which correctly argued that the foremost British hong first established its commercial interests within the area now called 'Admiralty' alongside the future 'Central' district and not yet at East Point, and by inference was a significant catalyst in that location.[58]

However, it is a lengthier paper entitled 'The Foundations of Hong Kong: A Chapter of Accidents' (1975), which proved to be Evans's most important piece of scholarship in the genesis story of colonial Hong Kong.[59] His underlying thesis was that the history of these first years could be divided into three sections: Hong Kong under Captain Charles Elliot's brief administration (1841), under Sir Henry Pottinger before the ratification of the Treaty of Nanking, and therefore before confirmation of crown sovereignty of the island (1841–1843), and events after 1843. From the first surge of opportunism and haphazard land-grabbing (1841) to inadequate governance amidst an uncertain future (1841–1843) to a state of inability by the government to adapt to changing commercial pressure following this, Evans argues that the government seemed consistently out of step with both individual commercial interests and, conversely, with the reining in of these interests collectively for the sake of a coherent urban plan for the city. It was, quite simply, a wasted opportunity. The present book builds upon this tactic and content. Yet, when one adds to this political stew an alarming uncertainty as to one's very survival; a Russian roulette of land selection based upon uncertain notions of the relative locations of healthiness; the equally uncertain suppositions as to why one year should prove more fatal than the preceding or succeeding; and the various theories of miasma prevailing upon residents; then it makes it, perhaps, less surprising that the colony stumbled so blindly in the attempt to find an equitable balance between these various interest groups.

Synopsis

Complexities arising from the interdisciplinary nature of the study have suggested that the simplest solution is to position each chapter chronologically. Nevertheless, making one's life simpler is not the driving force behind this chronological approach. It is an essential argument of the book that the year-by-year unfolding of events within the new island colony was a relentless educational process for the inhabitants. Malaria is presented as a harsh teacher, repeatedly thrusting itself upon the community and causing society to progress on several fronts: physically, politically, and socially. In addition, this account is as much about the *building* of the island city of Hong Kong itself as it is about the perceptions of malaria and the concerns of well-being that generated it. Conversely, the word 'construction' in the title must be seen to represent not just the physical making of the city but also its communal imaginary and conceptual formation. Therefore, with the reader's indulgence, the lens will move at times off medical and onto urban analysis, essentially a transition from *malaria* into *making*, hoping that both can be seen to influence each other within the broader context.

Chapter Two explores the development of Hong Kong after its unofficial declaration as a British colony in late January 1841. This includes the subsequent two years of rampant development upon the northern shore of the island, up to the initial signing of the Treaty of Nanking. A driving argument is that the first, crude steps towards shaping a habitable environment were largely imported: the know-how, the labour force, the materials, and even the very disease of which the island would, unfairly, be attributed as initially generating.

Chapter Three concentrates upon 1843—the year of triumphant, permanent possession by the British Crown and the year of the worst outbreak of fever the colonial island settlement had yet suffered. Through the trauma of the experience, a forensic concern for topography determined the future decisions of all elite sections of the colonial community: the military, the merchants, and the government. Military officers and civilians tested a set of approaches as to how and where to build, frustrating the government's ambitions for a linear, mercantile waterfront and the proposed move of the city's centre eastwards.

Chapters Four and Five may be seen as a couplet—encompassing four distinct yet interrelated themes—in examining the three years following 1843 and the story of a city and island colony's determination to rebuild and expand. Brenda Yeoh asserts that often for colonial histories 'the tendency is to emphasise the influence of the colonising culture in space-making processes at the expense of the colonised, who usually remain as locally abundant but faceless units of labour ministering to the coloniser's

Notes

1 Lord Palmerston to Captain Elliot R.N., 21 Apr. 1841, as quoted in Hosea Ballou Morse, 'Appendix G', *The International Relations of the Chinese Empire, Vol. I: The Period of Conflict, 1834–1860* (London: Longmans, Green, and Co., 1910), 642. The description of Hong Kong Island as a 'barren rock' is a common misquotation.

2 Roy Porter, 'Public Medicine', *The Greatest Benefit to Mankind: A Medical History of Humanity from Antiquity to the Present* (London: Harper Collins, 1997), 262.

3 In Britain, this arose autonomously from advances within veterinary medical research. See Michael Worboys, *Spreading Germs: Disease Theories and Medical Practice in Britain, 1865–1900* (Cambridge: Cambridge University Press, 2000), 16.

4 The National Archives, Kew [hereafter NA]; Colonial Office [hereafter CO] 133/7: 95a, William Morrison, 'Colonial Surgeon's Report for 1850', *Hong Kong Blue Book*: 1850, Mar. 1851.

5 Porter, *The Greatest Benefit*, 411.

6 NA; Admiralty [hereafter ADM] 1/5530, Inspector-General of Naval Hospitals and Fleets to The Secretary of the Admiralty, 26 Oct. 1843.

7 'Medicus', *Friend of China*, 22 June 1844.

8 This cautious view is supported by the medical historian Randall M. Packard: 'Constructing a global historical narrative for malaria is also difficult because, for much of the period covered [prehistory to the late nineteenth century] . . . there was no knowledge of the role of the malaria parasite in the transmission of the disease and thus no basis on which to make a definitive diagnosis of malaria. Without such evidence, we must rely on contemporary descriptions of symptoms to identify the disease.' See Randall M. Packard, *The Making of a Tropical Disease: A Short History of Malaria* (Baltimore: Johns Hopkins University Press, 2007), 17.

9 Arthur E. Starling, et al., eds., *Plague, SARS, and the Story of Medicine in Hong Kong* (Hong Kong: Hong Kong University Press, 2006), 297.

10 Packard, *The Making of a Tropical Disease*, 7–8.

11 Mark Harrison, *Disease and the Modern World: 1500 to the Present Day* (Cambridge: Polity Press, 2004), 157.

12 *Literary Gazette* (extract undated), as reprinted in the *Hongkong Register*, 22 Dec. 1846.

13 NA; War Office [hereafter WO] 78/479, 'Plan of Victoria, Hong Kong, Copied from the Surveyor General's Dept. to accompany the Report of the Respective Officers', 12 July 1845.

14 Mark Harrison, 'Tropical Medicine in nineteenth-century India', *British Journal for the History of Science*, vol. 25, no. 3 (Sept. 1992): 310.

15 David Arnold, 'Introduction: Tropical Medicine Before Manson', in David Arnold, ed., *Warm Climates and Western Medicine: The Emergence of Tropical Medicine, 1500–1900* (Amsterdam: Editions Rodopi, 1996), 9.

16 Ibid.

17 Mark Harrison, 'Disease and Medicine in the Armies of British India, 1750–1830: The Treatment of Fevers and the Emergence of Tropical Therapeutics', in Geoffrey L. Hudson, ed., *British Military and Naval Medicine, 1600–1830*, Clio Medica, vol. 81, Amsterdam (New York: Rodopi, 2007), 89.

18 Ibid., 88–90.

19 Ibid.

20 Ibid.

21 Michel Foucault, 'The Eye of Power', in Colin Gordon, ed., *Power/Knowledge, Selected Interviews & other Writings, 1972–1977* (New York: Pantheon, 1980), 151; see also Jiat-Hwee Chang, *A Genealogy of Tropical Architecture: Colonial Networks, Nature and Technoscience* (Abingdon, Oxon: Routledge, 2016), 3.

22 Foucault, 'The Eye of Power', 150–151. I elaborate on some of the categories.

23 Portions of Chapter Three 'A Town Redrawn, 1843–1844' have previously been published in Christopher Cowell, 'The Hong Kong Fever of 1843: Collective Trauma and the Reconfiguring of Colonial Space', *Modern Asian Studies*, vol. 47, no. 2 (Mar. 2013): 329–364, in particular, parts of subchapters 'The "Hongkong Fever"', 'The Valley Experiment', 'A Link between Buildings and Miasma', and 'A Battle for the Centre'.

24 Chang, *A Genealogy of Tropical Architecture*, 5–6.

25 G. A. Bremner, Johan Lagae, and Mercedes Volait, 'Intersecting Interests: Developments in Networks and Flows of Information and Expertise in Architectural History', *Fabrications*, vol. 26, no. 2 (2016): 236.

26 G. A. Bremner, 'Tides that Bind: Waterborne Trade and the Infrastructure Networks of Jardine Matheson & Co., *Perspecta*, vol. 52 (2019): 31–47.

27 Cole Roskam, *Hong Kong: Uncertain City* (Hong Kong: University of Hong Kong Press, anticipated release in 2024).

28 Maxime Decaudin, '"A Barren Rock": An Environmental History of the Landscapes of the British Colonization of Hong Kong, 1794–1898', PhD diss., Centre André-Chastel, Université Paris-Sorbonne, 2021; Robert Peckham, 'Hygienic Nature: Afforestation and the Greening of Colonial Hong Kong', *Modern Asian Studies*, vol. 49, no. 4 (2015): 1193, 1203.

29 Maxime Decaudin, 'Founding the Barren Rock: Landscape Transformations and Discourses in Nineteenth-Century Colonial Hong Kong', *Journal of the LUCAS Graduate Conference* (2019): 58.

30 Mohammad Gharipour and Caitlin DeClercq, eds., *Epidemic Urbanism: Contagious Diseases in Global Cities* (Chicago: University of Chicago Press, 2021).

31 Sara Jensen Carr, *The Topography of Wellness: How Health and Disease Shaped the American Landscape* (Charlottesville, VA: University of Virginia Press, 2021).

32 Nida Rehman, 'Epidemiological Landscapes: The Spaces and Politics of Mosquito Control in Lahore', PhD diss., University of Cambridge, 2020. https://doi.org/10.17863/CAM.62263

33 Ibid., 75.

34 Cecilia L. Chu, 'Contagious City: The Bubonic Plague and the First Urban Renewal Scheme in Hong Kong', *HKIA Journal*, vol. 76 (2020): 25–29.

35 Cecilia L. Chu, *Building Colonial Hong Kong: Speculative Development and Segregation in the City* (London: Routledge, 2022).

36 *Contagious Cities: Far Away Too Close*, Tai Kwun Contemporary, 26 Jan.–21 Apr. 2019.

37 Ria Sinha, 'Fatal Island: Malaria in Hong Kong', *Journal of the Royal Asiatic Society Hong Kong Branch* [formerly *Journal of the Hong Kong Branch of the Royal Asiatic Society*, or JHKBRAS], vol. 58 (2018): 55–80.

38 Ibid., 60, 64.

39 John Michael Weiler, 'Army Architects: The Royal Engineers and the Development of Building Technology in the Nineteenth Century', PhD diss., University of York, 1987. Weiler did, however, publish a valuable article synthesising part of the thesis. See John Weiler, 'Colonial Connections: Royal Engineers and Building Technology Transfer in the Nineteenth Century', *Construction History*, vol. 12 (1996): 3–18.

40 William Tarrant, *Hongkong Part 1, 1839–1844* (Canton: Friend of China, 1861), 65–77.

41 Ibid., 65.

42 Ibid.

43 The earliest mention of the use of a daguerreotype in Hong Kong is found in an advertisement announcing the opening of a portrait studio in the *China Mail*, dated 6 Mar. 1845.

44 Hong Kong Public Records Office [hereafter HKPRO]; file: HKMS 140-1-1, 'Transcripts of Correspondence of Lieut. Thomas Bernard Collinson R.E., Dec. 1838–29 Mar. 1846' [hereafter 'Transcripts'].

45 Edward Cree, *Naval Surgeon: The Voyages of Dr. Edward H. Cree, Royal Navy, as Related in His Private Journals, 1837–1856*, ed. Michael Levien (New York: E. P. Dutton, 1982).

46 The *Xia'er guanzhen* stopped publication in 1856, just three years later. See Zhuo Nansheng, *Zhongguo jindai baoye fazhan shi 1815–1874* (*The Development of Chinese Newspapers in the Modern Period, 1815–1874*) (Taipei: Zhengzhong shuju, 1998), 78–101; as also noted in Elizabeth Sinn, 'Beyond "Tianxia": The "Zhongwai Xinwen Qiribao" (Hong Kong 1871–1872) and the Construction of a Transnational Chinese Community', *China Review*, vol. 4, no. 1 (Spring 2004): 93–95; and Elizabeth Sinn, *Pacific Crossing: California Gold, Chinese Migration, and the Making of Hong Kong* (Hong Kong: Hong Kong University Press, 2013), 344.

47 For a rare glimpse of Chinese bill stickers in Hong Kong in the early 1840s, see Christopher Cowell, *Edward Ashworth, Artist & Architect: Fourteen Watercolour Studies of Hong Kong & Macau, 1844–46* (Sydney: Hordern House, 2014), Catalogue no. 3, 'Chinam's Hong'.

48 P. J. Marshall, 'The White Town of Calcutta under the Rule of the East India Company', *Modern Asian Studies*, vol. 34, no. 2 (May 2000): 324.

49 Apart from personal contact with the newspapers themselves, an excellent general guide to aid the researcher remains Frank H. H. King, ed., and Prescott Clarke, *A Research Guide to China-Coast Newspapers, 1822–1911* (Cambridge, MA: Harvard University Press), 1965.

50 The histories I refer to, in order of publication, are: William Tarrant, *Hongkong Part 1, 1839–1844* (Canton: Friend of China, 1861); E. J. Eitel, *Europe in China: The History of Hong Kong from the Beginning to the Year 1882* (Hong Kong: Kelly and Walsh / London: Luzac & Co., 1895); G. R. Sayer, *Hong Kong 1841–1862: Birth, Adolescence, and Coming of Age* (London: Oxford University Press, 1937); G. B. Endacott, *A History of Hong Kong* (London: Oxford University Press, 1958); G. B. Endacott, *A Biographical Sketch-book of Early Hong Kong* (Singapore: Eastern Universities Press, 1962); G. R. Sayer, *Hong Kong 1862–1919: Years of Discretion* (Hong Kong: Hong Kong University Press, 1975); Carl T. Smith, *Chinese Christians: Elites, Middlemen, and the Church in Hong Kong* (Hong Kong: Oxford University Press, 1985); Elizabeth Sinn, *Power and Charity: The Early History of the Tung Wah Hospital, Hong Kong* (Hong Kong: Oxford University Press, 1989); Chan Wai Kwan, *The Making of Hong Kong Society: Three Studies of Class Formation in Early Hong Kong* (Oxford: Clarendon Press, 1991); Frank Welsh, *A History of Hong Kong* (London: Harper Collins, 1993); Jung-Fang Tsai, Hong Kong in Chinese History (New York: Columbia University Press, 1993); Christopher Munn, *Anglo-China: Chinese People and British Rule in Hong Kong 1841–1880* (Richmond, Surrey: Curzon, 2001); and John M. Carroll, *Edge of Empires: Chinese Elites and British Colonials in Hong Kong* (Cambridge, MA: Harvard University Press, 2005).

51 Lt. John Ouchterlony, *The Chinese War: An Account of All Operations of the British Forces from the Commencement to the Treaty of Nanking* (London: Saunders and Otley, 1844).

52 Ibid., 216–217.

53 James Clavell, *Tai-Pan* (New York: Dell Publishing, 1966).

54 Timothy Mo, *An Insular Possession* (London: Chatto & Windus, 1986), 512.

55 Amitav Ghosh, *Flood of Fire* (London: John Murray, 2015), 480–481.

56 Dafydd M. E. Evans, 'Hong Kong's First Government House', *Journal of the Hong Kong Branch of the Royal Asiatic Society* [hereafter *JHKBRAS*], vol. 8 (Hong Kong, 1968): 156–160.

57 Dafydd M. E. Evans, 'Chinatown in Hong Kong: The Beginnings of Taipingshan', *JHKBRAS*, vol. 10 (Hong Kong, 1970): 69–78.

58 Dafydd M. E. Evans, 'Jardine, Matheson & Company's First Site in Hong Kong', *JHKBRAS*, vol. 8 (Hong Kong, 1968): 149–153.

59 Dafydd M. E. Evans, 'The Foundations of Hong Kong: A Chapter of Accidents', in Marjorie Topley, ed., *Hong Kong: The Interaction of Traditions and Life in the Towns* (Hong Kong: Hong Kong Branch of the Royal Asiatic Society, 1975), 11–41.

60 Brenda S. A. Yeoh, *Contesting Space in Colonial Singapore: Power Relations and the Urban Built Environment* (Kuala Lumpur: Oxford University Press, 1996), 6.

61 The present title is a play on that famous axiom of the Modern Movement in architecture 'form follows function', a phrase coined by the Chicago-based architect Louis Sullivan in his essay 'The Tall Office Building Artistically Considered', *Lippincott's Magazine* (March 1896), 408, though the actual phrase is 'form ever follows function'.

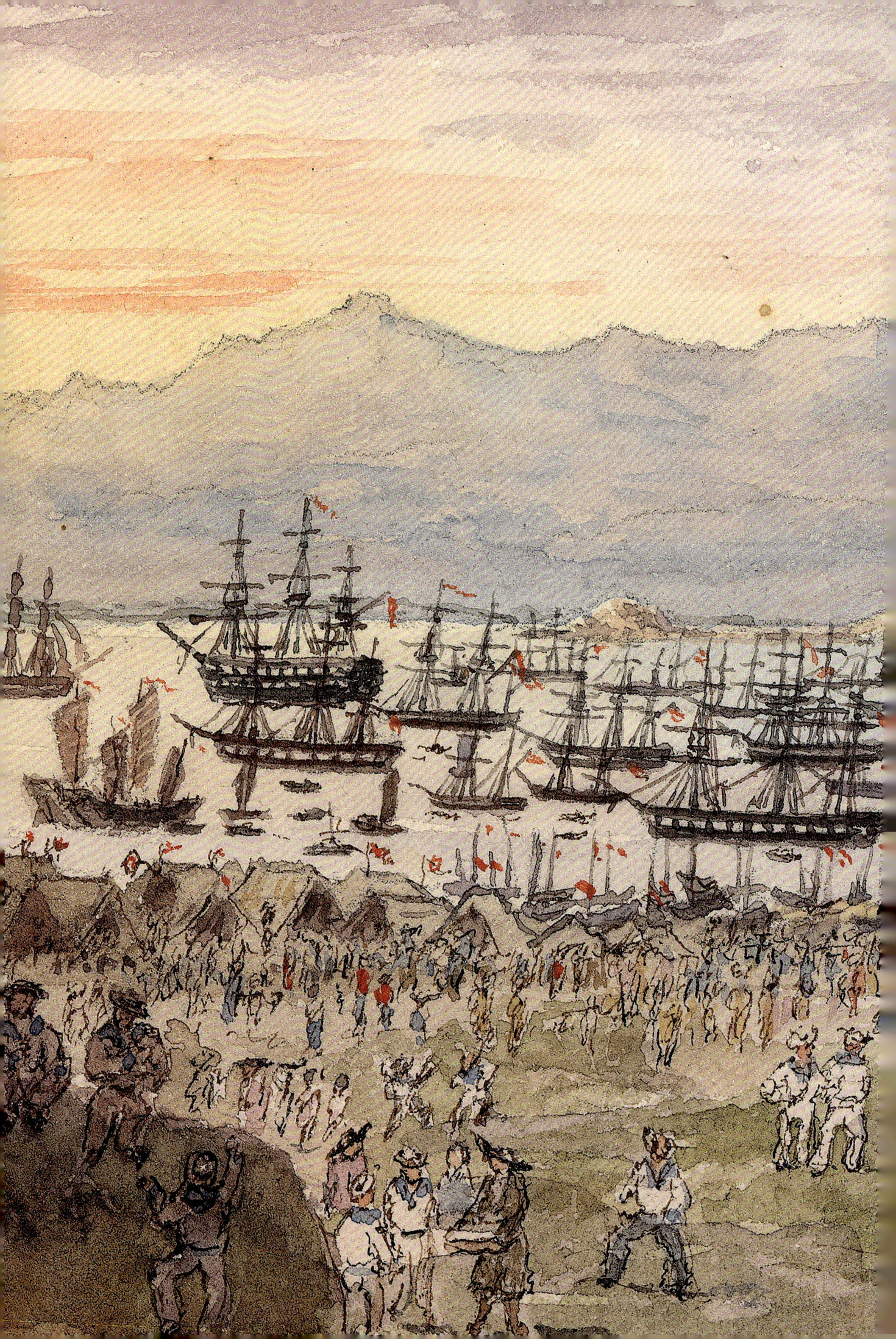

CHAPTER 2

An Island Reclaimed, 1841–1842

> No sooner, also, did the Chinese population of the island perceive that the English were no longer averse to invest capital in the soil, than the example was eagerly imitated, and with such extraordinary celerity were these building operations carried on, that, in the course of two months, the native town, Victoria, which had before presented to the eye scarcely anything but streets and rows of houses, formed of the most crazy, perishable, and inflammable materials, now boasted at least a hundred brick tenements, besides a spacious and commodious market-place . . . a stone jail, a wide, excellent road, drains, and bridges, wherever necessary, and an official residence for the presiding magistrate.
>
> —Lieutenant John Ouchterlony (comparing 1842 with 1841), *The Chinese War*, 1844.

It began almost as soon as the Union flag was planted. During the cold weeks of early 1841, under the pretext of an unratified treaty with China, British army surveyors hastily set out crude peg markers upon the undulating ground. Their hold was uncertain, their occupation likely temporary, as were the rapid and speculative claims made upon the staked-out ground by civilians and merchants that hung about the military. Yet, by avarice or compulsion, with such a scarcity of plots, diverse interests quickly conjoined into some ill-fitting alignment one might vaguely call a town. By the close of 1842, circumstances and sentiments had improved. At the end stage of the First Anglo-Chinese War (or First Opium War, 1839–1842), British troops returned from Nanking (Nanjing) with the promise of a permanent settlement in their grasp and the near certain guarantee of sovereignty of the island under British rule.

These first few years forged the principal elements that comprised the substance of the new colony: its name; its studied hydrography and geology; the crafting of physical infrastructure—roads, gullies, drainage—and the associated social and economic world that this infrastructure influenced; the earliest building typologies—such as warehouse and market construction—and its social imprint upon the patterns of colonial living; the little-islander enclave identity; the ill-contrived selling of land and its long-term repercussions; the methods of speedy speculation; the fears of climate and topography upon the human constitution; and the eventual horrors of inexplicable fever against a newly formed metropolis where geographical position and building style exerted the beginnings of a terrain-based vocabulary of control and morality. It is in understanding the relationship of these causes and effects, these conditions and manifestations, that we may begin to understand the processes that physically shaped early Hong Kong.

From Water to Rock

Before 'Hong Kong' became an island, it was water; a patch of water, to be precise. The inlet was situated on the southwest side of the island and located between the tiny southern islet of Ap Lei Chau and a natural bay. A straggle of fishing villages clustered against the northern slopes of this small harbour whose trade included the exporting of incense trees (*aquilaria sinensis* or *pak muk heung*) culled some distance northwards upon the foothills of the mainland. The smell of these trees led the bay to be named Heung Gong or 'Fragrant Harbour', in turn giving the name to an adjoining settlement.[1] For the indigenous Chinese, who clung to this south-westerly edge of the island, the comings and goings of the first British enquirers seemed harmless enough. For a few decades these Europeans had filled their vessels with water from a nearby mountain waterfall. The puzzling foreigners eventually hoisted their flag somewhere distant over the mountains along the gloomier and nastier northern shore. For the fishermen, it first seemed a remote and curious affair, since it was common knowledge that the northern side lacked the benefits of a south-westerly breeze to counteract the heat. It was also common knowledge that among the granite island's countless crevices, left untended, was gathered pools of stagnant water thick with vegetation. After the seasonal monsoons, the baleful presence of these features caused, in some, fits of fever and even death. At least, this became the established myth during the first years of colonial urban development, as if reminding the British that they had chosen poorly.

Before becoming hydrographer to the Admiralty, Alexander Dalrymple, then working for the British East India Company, provided the first relatively accurate chart of the region of coastline that included Hong Kong (**fig. 2.1**) considered part of a cluster known as the Ladrones Islands or the 'Islands of Thieves'. Published in 1792 but from observations made in 1764, this chart was one of more than one thousand prepared by Dalrymple over ten years mapping the coasts of Asia and displays the white heat of discovery.[2] As if ignoring all previously received information from earlier nautical maps, he etched in on a blank surface where ascertainable, empirical data directly observed. Coastal edges are fragmentary, islands and mainland alike acting as corridors between the nautical soundings. He labelled Hong Kong as 'Fanchin Chow', its outline incomplete. Ironically, it was left unfinished along the very edge that would secure its future within British interests; its magnificent deep-water harbour to the north went unrecorded and presumably remained undiscovered.[3] By the time hydrographers Daniel Ross and Philip Maughan, lieutenants of the Bombay Marine, completed the charts in 1810, Hong Kong was filled in and, for the first time, in its recognisable form (**fig. 2.2**).[4]

Confusion was common in the European labelling of the names of various islands and coastal locations. Imperial Chinese maps had earlier labelled Hong Kong 'Hung Heung Lo Shan' 紅香爐山 (Red Incense Burner Mountain). This was inadvertently blended on later editions of Ross and Maughan's map into 'Hung Gong' 紅江 (Red River), a sound-meaning confusion with the small southwest bay that was 'corrected' into its ultimate form 'Hong Kong' 香港, the name the British believed the island to be called when they had asked the south-westerly locals. Hong Kong, then, was *their* mistaken name for the island, *their* invention. This phonetic misstep of Ross and Maughan in labelling reveals that the conflation of the name of the village with a name for the island must have come about from spoken and not written dialogue between the Chinese and the foreign sailors when the locals were imprecisely asked 'What is the name of this place?'. The British would soon discover that water would not just provide them with a place name but would affect their very chances of survival and that of the new colony.

Clarke Abel, Fellow of the Linnean Society, chief medical officer and naturalist to the embassy of Lord Amherst to China, published an early description of this now-familiar southwest side of the island. Awaiting news of the emperor's receptivity to their mission, Abel's party had agreed to rendezvous with a portion of the embassy in early July 1816 on Lamma Island, from which they could spend a day and a night on Hong Kong to fill their vessels. 'As seen from the ship', Abel recalled as he neared, 'this island was chiefly remarkable for its high conical mountains, rising to the centre, and for a beautiful cascade which rolled

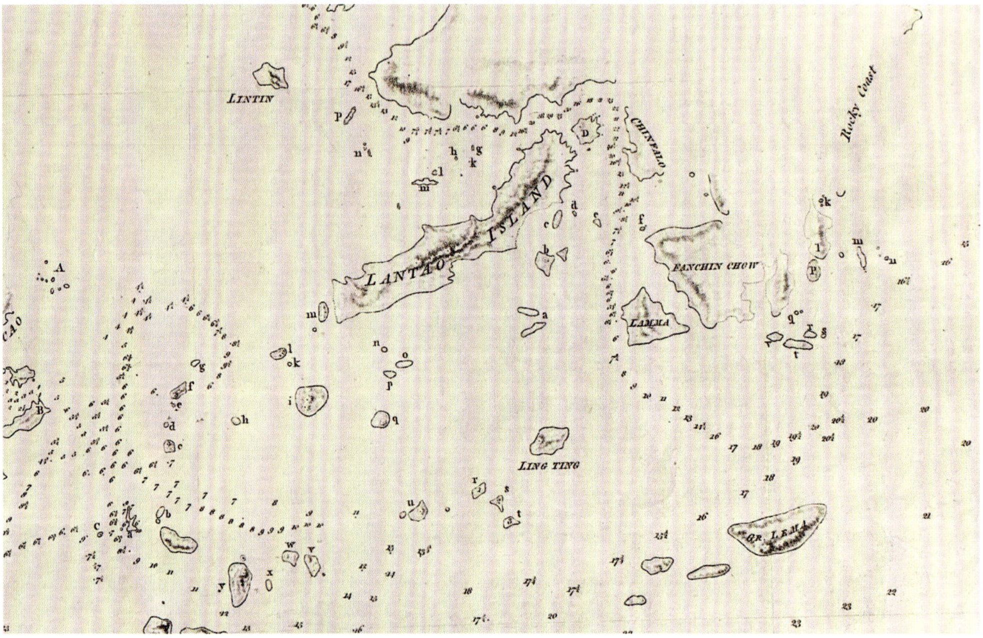

Fig. 2.1. A. Dalrymple, *A Chart of Part of the Coast of China* (detail), 1760–1770. Engraving. © The National Archives, Kew (ADM 352/412).

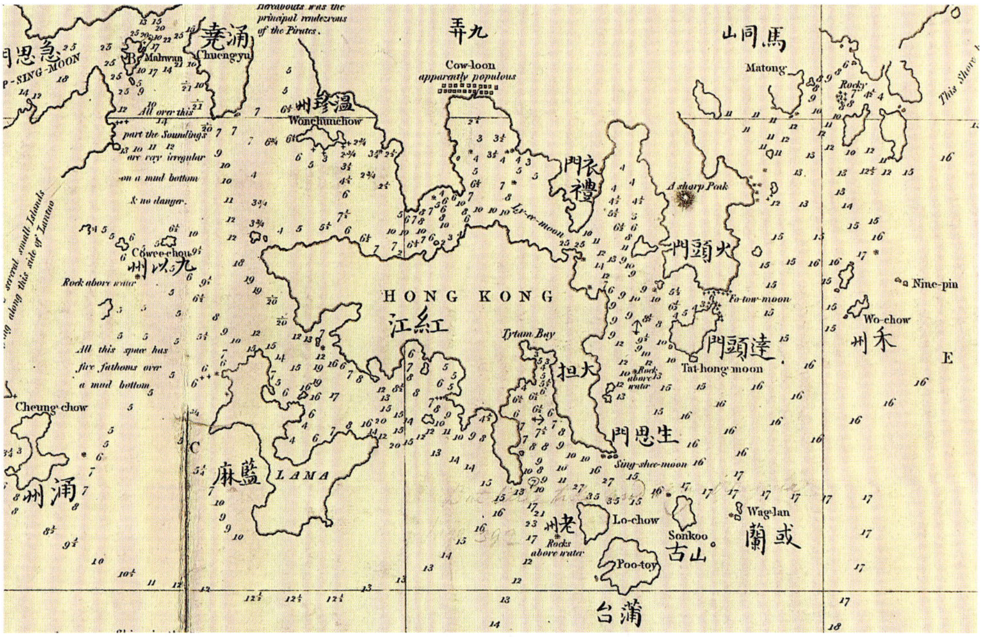

Fig. 2.2. D. Ross and P. Maughan, *The Macao Roads* (detail), 1810. Engraving. © United Kingdom Hydrographic Office Archive (SVY/A/y13Bb4).

over a fine blue rock into the sea' (**fig. 2.3**).[5] If Captain Ross had been the first to measure the height of the island's tallest peak, probably by triangulation, (under)estimating it as one thousand and five hundred feet above sea level, Abel was among the first to climb it. So, taking advantage of his vessel's watering stop, the naturalist decided to follow the stream leading from the waterfall as high as it would take him. The geologist in Abel was elated, while the botanist in him felt thwarted. 'The general surface of the mountain, and indeed of every part of the island of Hong-kong that I was able to visit, is remarkably barren, although in the distance it appears fertile, from a fern . . . which supplies the place of other plants.' By the morning of the next day, he had concluded that Hong Kong's 'scenery is composed of barren rocks, deep ravines, and mountain-torrents, but presents few characters of a very picturesque description. Of its inhabitants none were seen but some poor and weather-beaten fishermen, spreading their nets, and during the produce of their toils on the rocks which supported their miserable mud-huts'. The northern side of Hong Kong Island remained unexplored but was 'represented by my naval friends as affording admirable shelter for ships of any burden'.[6]

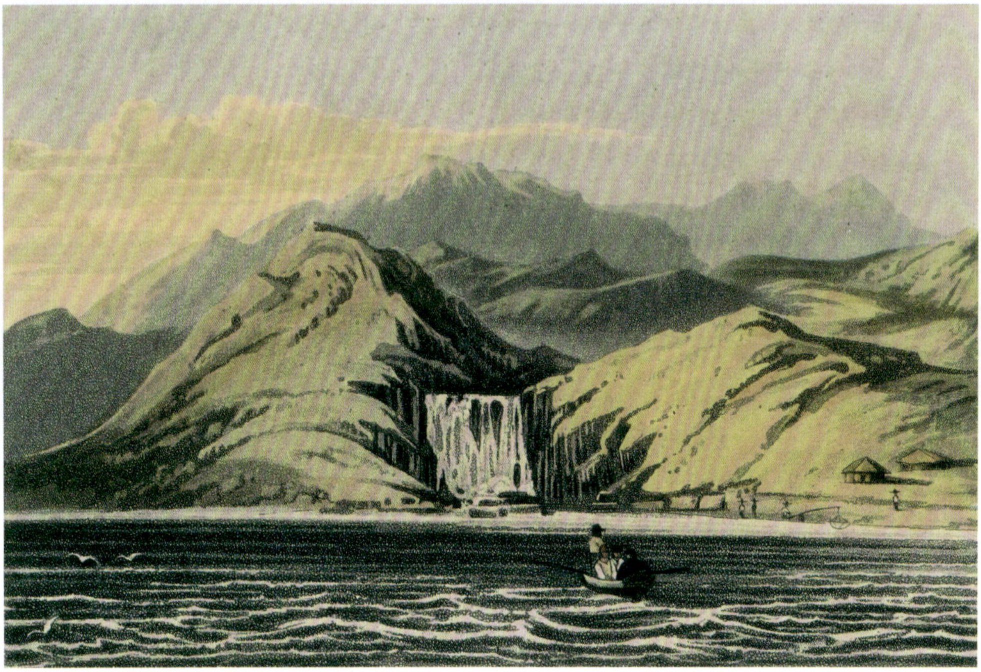

Fig. 2.3. Anon. (C. Abel?), T. Fielding (engraver), 'The Waterfall, at Hong Cong', 1816. Aquatint. © Hong Kong Museum of Art Collection (AH1964.0362).

Hong Kong Island, together with the peninsular of Kowloon, was then loosely populated by three main ethnic groups. The first of these inhabitants, the Punti 本地 ('aborigines'), drifted down from the neighbouring Tungkoon District in stages between the Tang and Ming Dynasties. They chopped down most of the forests for timber and tilled all the available arable land. On Hong Kong Island, they settled in the natural valley locations, notably that of Wong Nai Chung ('Yellow Muddy Stream') Valley, more familiarly known in English as Happy Valley. Here, they built the village of Kwantailou, adjacent to the future 'East Point' (now absorbed into Causeway Bay). On the east and south sides of the island, the Punti formed fishing villages at Shek O and Chek Chue (Stanley).[7]

After the Punti had occupied the best locations, they were followed by the Hakka 客家 ('strangers', literally 'guest family'). A long history of conflict lay between both—the names Hakka and Punti having been given by each as a term of derision for the other. The Hakka migrated down from the northeast of Guangdong Province, inserting themselves in the remaining, lower-grade land between the Punti settlements. Experienced at using neglected sites, they began working actively in transforming their landscapes, from swampy ground reclamation to the cutting of terraces for crop growing on steep hillsides. Consequently, the Hakka became proficient carpenters and cutters and dressers of stone, opening numerous granite quarries. Hakka villages on Hong Kong Island included Tung Lo Wan (Causeway Bay), Tai Tam Tuk (Tai Tam village), Sai Wan or 'Sywan' (now Chai Wan), Hok Tsui (Cape D'Aguilar), Wong Ma Kok (on the Stanley Peninsula), and Heung Kong Tsai ('Little Hong Kong', Aberdeen). These were in addition to their four hamlet-quarries, including Tsat Tsz Mui (east North Point, near Quarry Bay) and A Kung Ngam (northwest of the island in northeast Shau Kei Wan).[8] Late-nineteenth-century historian and long-time resident of Hong Kong, E. J. Eitel, recounts that the British found in the Hakka natural allies in helping construct Hong Kong. The Hakka became the 'purveyors, commissariat and transport coolies of the foreigners, whilst the fishing population provided boatmen and pilots for the foreign trade'.[9]

Finally, the third group of Chinese settled in the region. These were the Hoklo 福佬 (Fujian person) which the Hakka write as 學老 ('knowledge aged'). The bolder Hoklo were generally feared by the other settlers. Their outward trades were sea-faring and fishing, but the Hoklo supplemented their income through smuggling and piracy along the

China coast. Hong Kong Island provided just one of several convenient bases.[10] The most infamous smuggler, the pirate Cheung Po Tsai 張保仔 (Cheung Po the Kid), believed to have used Hong Kong as his headquarters for four years from 1806 to 1810. Victoria Peak (Tai Ping Shan) formed his fortified lookout and was used in conjunction with a chain of neighbouring islands including Cheung Chau.[11] Hong Kong's naturally dramatic topography was a feature that the British would quickly take advantage of both for surveillance and attaining status in the early development of their city.

Added to this mix was the Tanka 蜑家 people, a name that conveyed their low status within Chinese society. These boat people, forbidden since 1730 by Imperial decree from settling on shore, shuttled across the coast in their small barges and narrowboats and clustered in heavily populated regions of South China.[12] The Tanka acted from the earliest times of the various East India companies present in Canton (Guangzhou) as suppliers and pilots to the foreign merchants. Despite the decrees of treason held over them, they remained steadfast in their loyalty, if only for this vital line of income. They formed part of a crucial supply chain for British military forces during the First Opium War and eagerly accompanied them in the establishment of Hong Kong.

Sojourners to the island, especially those who had emotionally prepared themselves for a long-term stay, were dismayed by the landscape before them, much as Clarke Abel had been back in 1816. One explorer in 1845 observed that 'the surface of Hongkong is exceedingly uneven, rising into numerous ridges and peaks, and having only a few narrow patches of level and arable land'. However, he noted optimistically, 'in the ravines, there are streams of excellent and never-failing water'.[13] One gets a sense of this geological drama in the method of rendering the island in the first detailed hydrographical chart of the soundings around it, Commander ('Captain') Sir Edward Belcher's nautical chart of 1841 (**fig. 2.4**). The explorer noted that the rocky terrain was composed of trap (large columnar and stepped masses of rock), granite as often split protuberances, and hornblende (a dark crystalline amphibole). The granite was 'found in large round masses' ideal in-situ material for constructing a sturdy city. 'Much of the soil along the ridges', the observer continued, 'is mere disintegrated rock, and in some places the strata of new earth are as distinctly seen as they could have been when solid rock'.[14] This 'disintegrated rock' would later be imbued with imageries of disease—'decayed' granite, accused by some, such as the future colonial treasurer, Robert Montgomery Martin, of generating or being a receptacle of miasma.

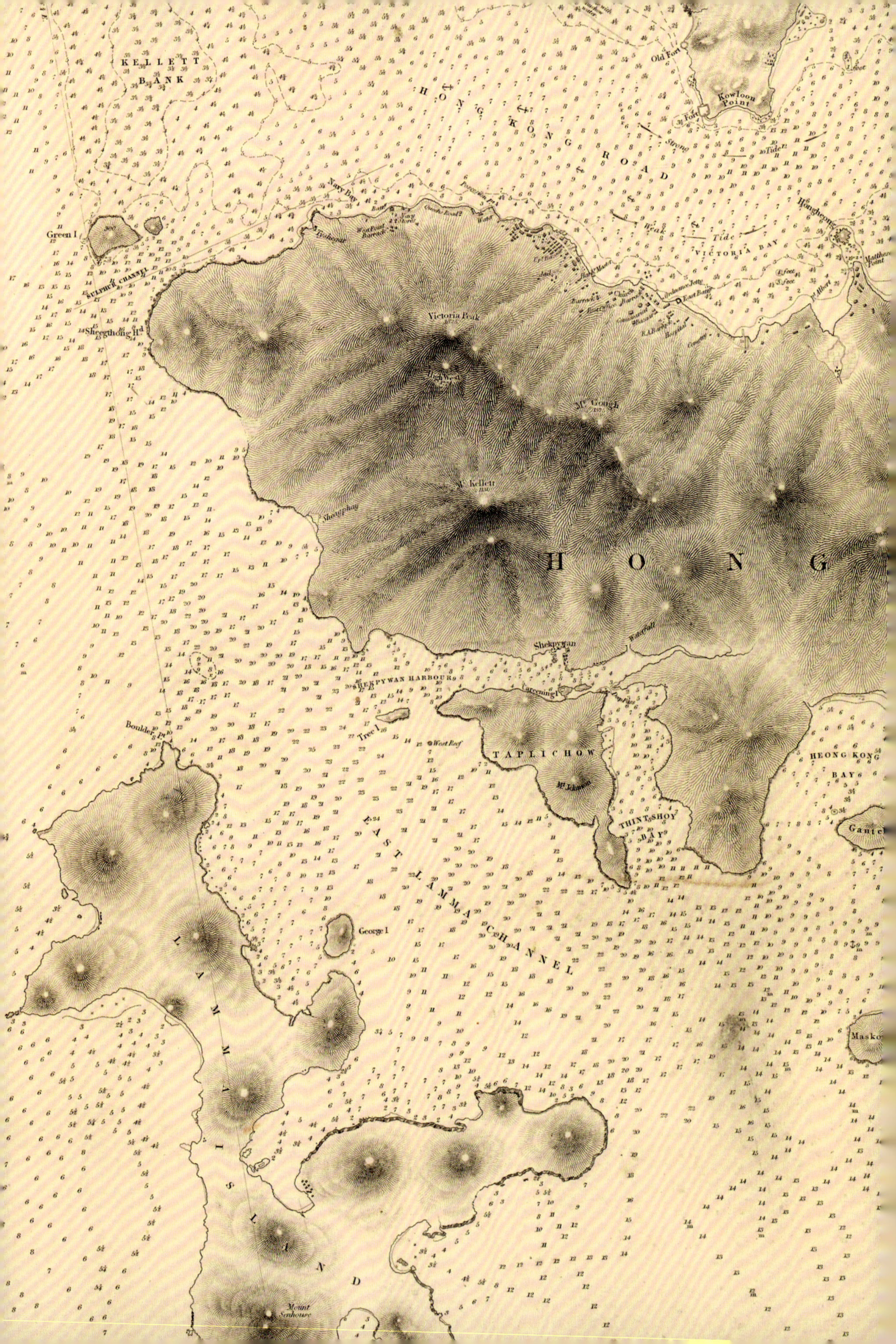
KELLETT BANK
HONG KONG ROAD
Old Fort
Kowloon Point
VICTORIA BAY
Green I.
SULPHUR CHANNEL
Victoria Peak
Mt. Gough
Mt. Kellett
HONG
Shekpywan
SHEKPYWAN HARBOUR
Tree I.
West Reef
TAPLICHOW
THINT SHOY BAY
HEONG KONG BAY
Boulder Pt.
EAST LAMMA CHANNEL
George I.
LAMMA ISLAND
Mount Senhouse

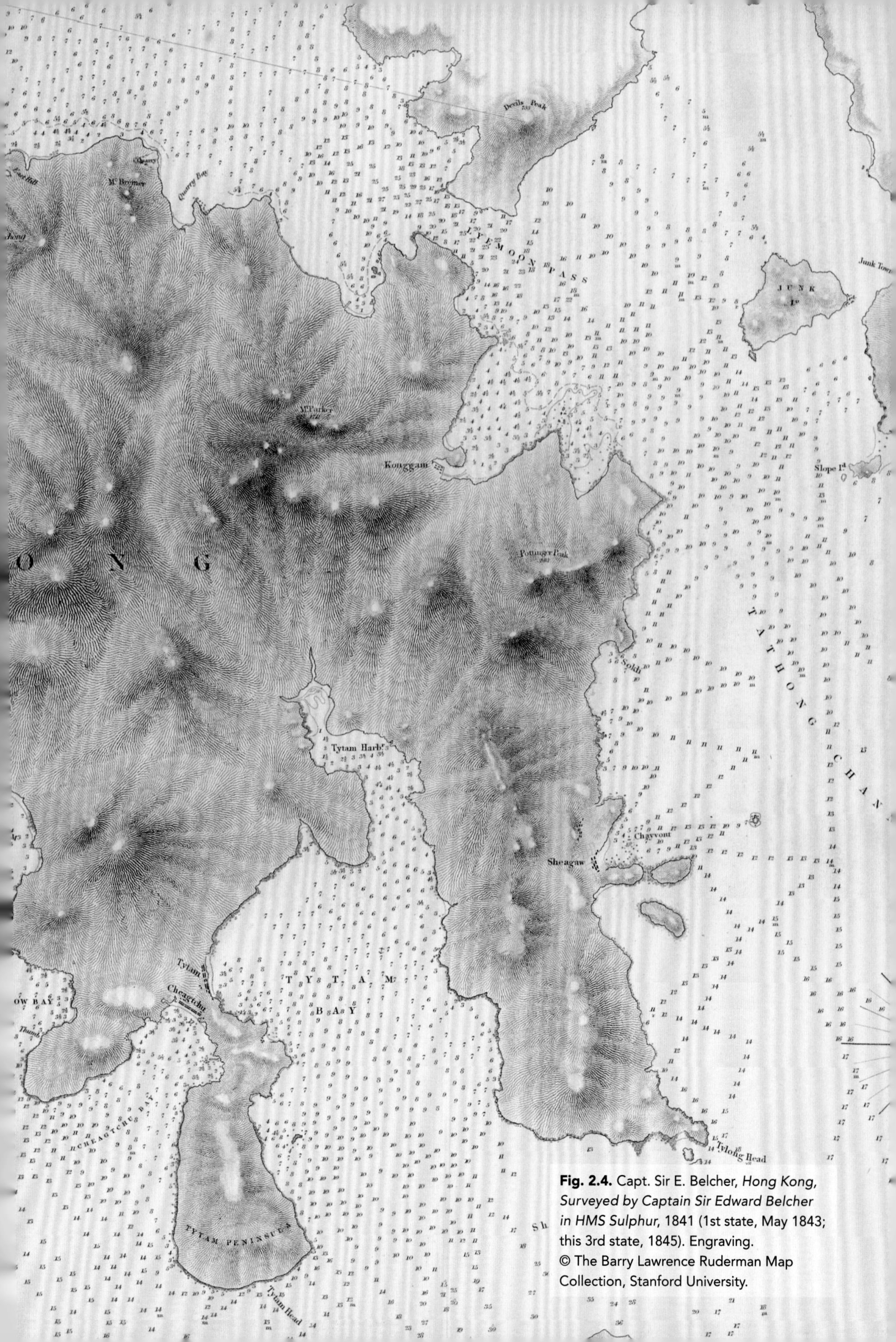

Fig. 2.4. Capt. Sir E. Belcher, *Hong Kong, Surveyed by Captain Sir Edward Belcher in HMS Sulphur*, 1841 (1st state, May 1843; this 3rd state, 1845). Engraving. © The Barry Lawrence Ruderman Map Collection, Stanford University.

Roads and Their By-Products

The British military planted their flag along the northern shore at Possession Point (now in Sheung Wan) on 26 January 1841. This promontory was certainly proclamatory but entirely unsuitable for habitation. Its position signified a claim to the island while serving as an entry marker for the strip of land behind it, acknowledging the general direction of ships arriving from the west into the harbour. Army tents had to be pitched at a distance 'inside' to its east, along an area soon known as Tai Ping Shan, where the land was relatively level and low-lying, between which was a spring of 'good water'.[15] Proof of this can be seen on Captain Belcher's rare earliest published version of May 1843 (not shown) of his nautical map of the island surveyed in 1841 and in the work of the watercolourist John Collins who offers us the first glimpse of a colonial settlement pattern on Hong Kong Island mere days after the flag was hoisted (**fig. 2.5**). Since traders and camp followers immediately congregated there to serve the troops, it was later designated the first Chinese enclave and named Lower Bazaar.

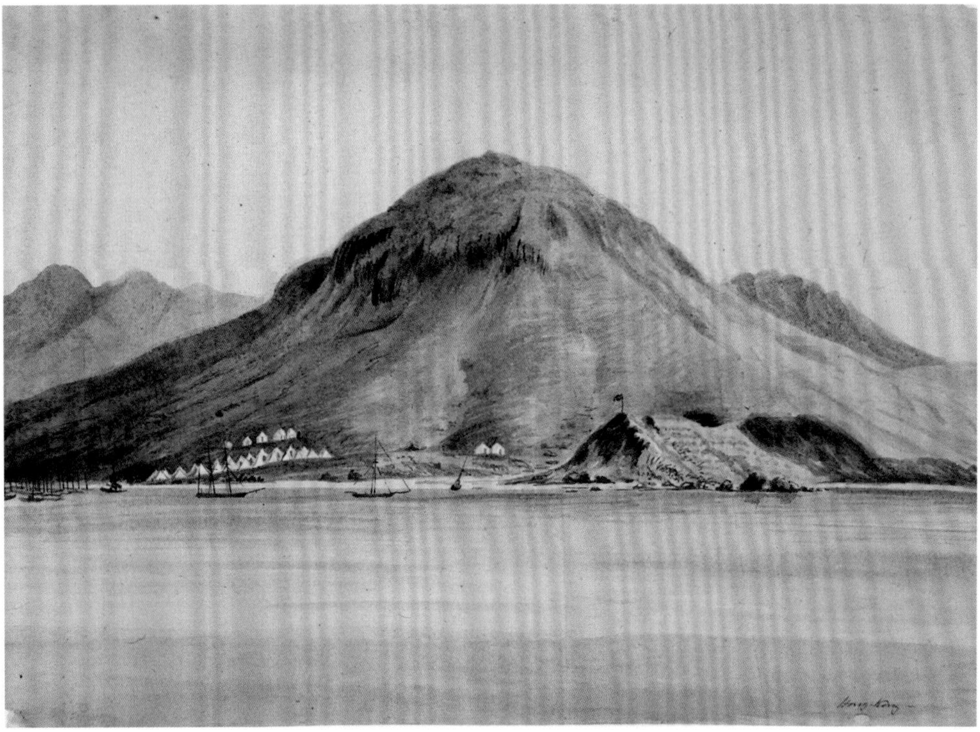

Fig. 2.5. J. H. Collins, 'Hong Kong', late January 1841. Ink and grey wash.
© Hong Kong Museum of Art Collection (AH1976.0019).

But it was not just about finding level ground. Army engineers were able to extend a short length of coastal road further eastwards across a stretch later known as the Central District up to Admiralty.[16] Granite rock, the sloping roots of mountains, would prove an unforgiving surface upon which to carve a necessary coastal carriageway along the island's northern contour. It impeded this first road's initial length, forcibly breaking it into pieces, thereby hemming the positions of building development and dictating their density. Studying road provision as early Hong Kong grew reveals a rudimentary pattern and logic of infrastructure for the movement of people and the establishment of the framework of the city. But roads also became a nefarious tool of governance, used both by the military and civilian government to measure its own progress and as a yardstick waved by its detractors. Road construction required large, organised gangs of labour—the most visible manifestation of British intent to claim the terrain, dominate the Chinese, and use the criminally convicted. Roads meant the taming of land and the conquest of space. They converted the terrain they passed into commodifiable parcels of investment. Roads also provided an easy highway for criminals at night. They were feared to cause the festering of harmful materials as the earth was churned in the digging of foundations, presenting in their excavated states a need for drainage, sewerage, and maintenance—for fear that these very same roads might become the arteries of contagion.

The island had long been riddled with rudimentary paths marked by the movement of local villagers between settlements, particularly along the south side of the island. Some of these descended upon the north side and across to isolated hamlets. One significant route, described as a 'bridle path' by the first western explorers, followed a line high above the coastline from the future area of West Point to the hamlet adjacent to what would become East Point (from Shek Tong Tsui or Belcher's Point to Wong Nai Chung or Happy Valley). This rough, rocky path was thought to be used by the crewmen of trading junks to track their passage using a towing line attached to the foremast. Its crenelated passage against the undulations and indentations caused by the descending ridges of the island, as seen from the mainland opposite, caused locals to name it Kwantailou (or 'petticoat string road'). It was the name also given to the Punti village by which its path ended.[17] Interestingly, the Hakka had applied this name to the entire northern side of the island, acknowledging the volatile topography that would exert such a constraining force at every step of the early colony's growth, both in road construction and land allocation.

The first European settlers would soon ask themselves if this uneven terrain, with its pockets of stagnant water, played a key role in the sicknesses that began endangering their lives.

Dr. Duncan McPherson of the 37th Madras Native Infantry, among the earliest physicians to live on the island, described the shoreline as he first saw it in 1841:

> Its northern side is formed by a connected ridge of mountains, the highest of which is about 2,000 feet above the sea. Except in a few spots, these mountains are barren and uncultivated; formed by black projecting masses of granite, the intervals giving shelter to herbage and brush-wood. There are no trees of any size, and, unlike the generality of mountain districts, it possesses but a few valleys, and these not of any extent. The mountains, for the most part, fall perpendicularly into the sea, thus leaving but little space for building at their base.[18]

One of the few significant level spaces apart from the flat terrain of the Wong Nai Chung Valley to the east, discounted due to its more exposed conditions, was the land below what would be named 'Cantonment Hill' (now Admiralty). The first view of this is again by Collins, painted slightly later than his grey wash, possibly in February 1841, the white peaks of the conical tents dotting the shoreline and lower hillside. Also discernible is that pre-colonial pathway, the Kwantailou, winding itself up one side of the mountain ridge (**fig. 2.6**).

This narrow stretch of shore, southwest of the mainland peninsular, was situated under the lee of Kowloon and relatively protected from the north-easterly winter monsoon—a phenomenon the military would have experienced in the first cold months of arriving at Hong Kong. Had the plenipotentiary and chief superintendent of trade, Captain Charles Elliot, claimed the island at a different and warmer time of the year, they may have occupied an entirely different part of the coast. Accordingly, the first stretch of road to be constructed by the Madras Engineers, in earnest from about May 1841, was a hastily cut passage from their settlement straddling the Albany Nullah (immediately west of Cantonment Hill) and its gently sloping banks to an area approximately at the junction of the future Wellington Street in Central.[19] The engineers intended to extend the passage to the second military installation a mile further westward at West Point. But for the present, they found it convenient to use this stretch when Elliot instructed them to propose and survey appropriate parcels of land for public auction in June 1841.

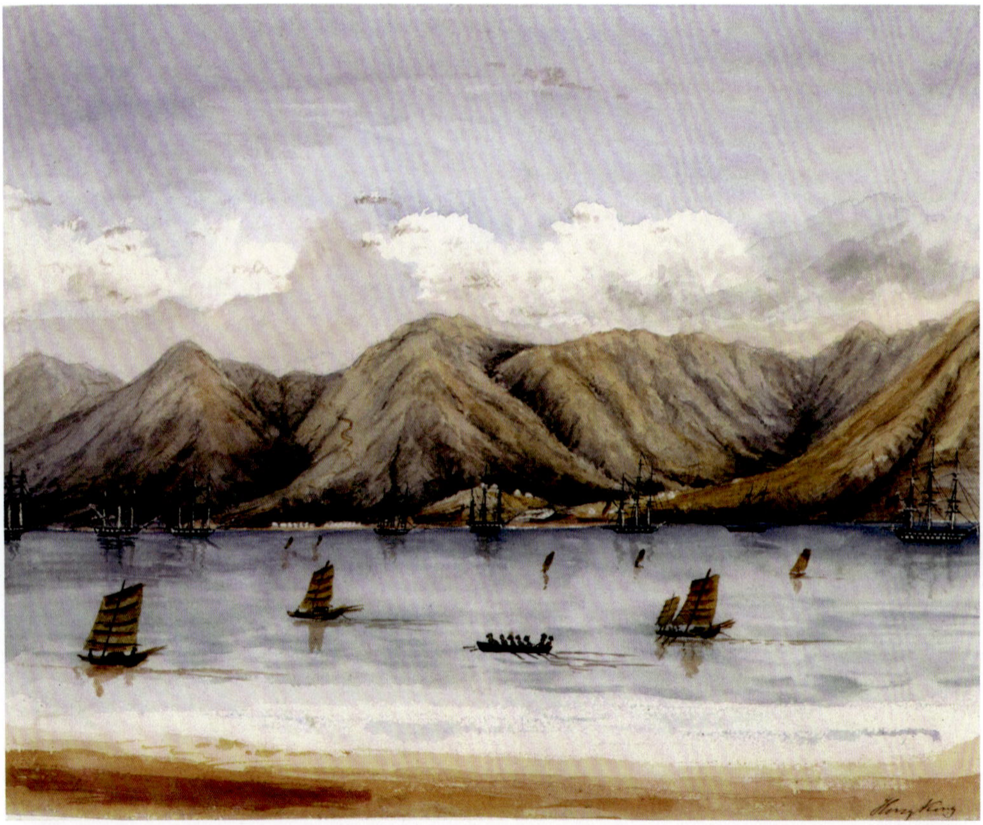

Fig. 2.6. J. H. Collins, 'Hong Kong', 1841. Watercolour. © Hong Kong Museum of Art Collection (AH1976.0015).

The military engineers also surveyed and subsequently extended the road along the length of shoreline stretching from their camp to Hospital Hill in the east (the future Seaman's Hospital, now site of the Ruttonjee Hospital), after which there was an insurmountable obstruction of rock to negotiate.[20] This road was initially given the name Victoria Avenue, but, concerned not to compete with the town's new name (quickly changed from Queenstown to Victoria), the colonists renamed it The Queen's Road by the beginning of August.[21] The corps of engineers employed a Chinese workforce in the labour-intensive task of road construction and rudimentary land levelling. This labour appears to have been easily procured, despite an imperial decree forbidding the Chinese to offer any assistance to the British in developing their new possession. In late June, the deputy superintendent of trade, Alexander Robert Johnston, was commissioned by

Captain Elliot to command the government of Hong Kong on his behalf while absent. Johnston eagerly took it upon himself to supervise the Chinese workforce, and by 1842 the results were manifestly apparent.[22] Johnston quickly realized that governing was as much a performative act as actual. The two-storey house that he built for himself on the ridge west of Cantonment Hill perched impressively upon the hillside situated so as to easily surveil the first stretches of roadwork (**figs. 2.7** and **2.20**). As the Reverend James Legge would later recall, Johnston's house rose 'as conspicuous as are now Messrs. Heard and Co's Offices, which have been manufactured from it'.[23] The house sat close to the apex of a triangular complex of government buildings, framed by two roads meeting at an upper point. From there a bridlepath was created linking the civil government to the magistracy and prison along the other ridge, bypassing the city below.

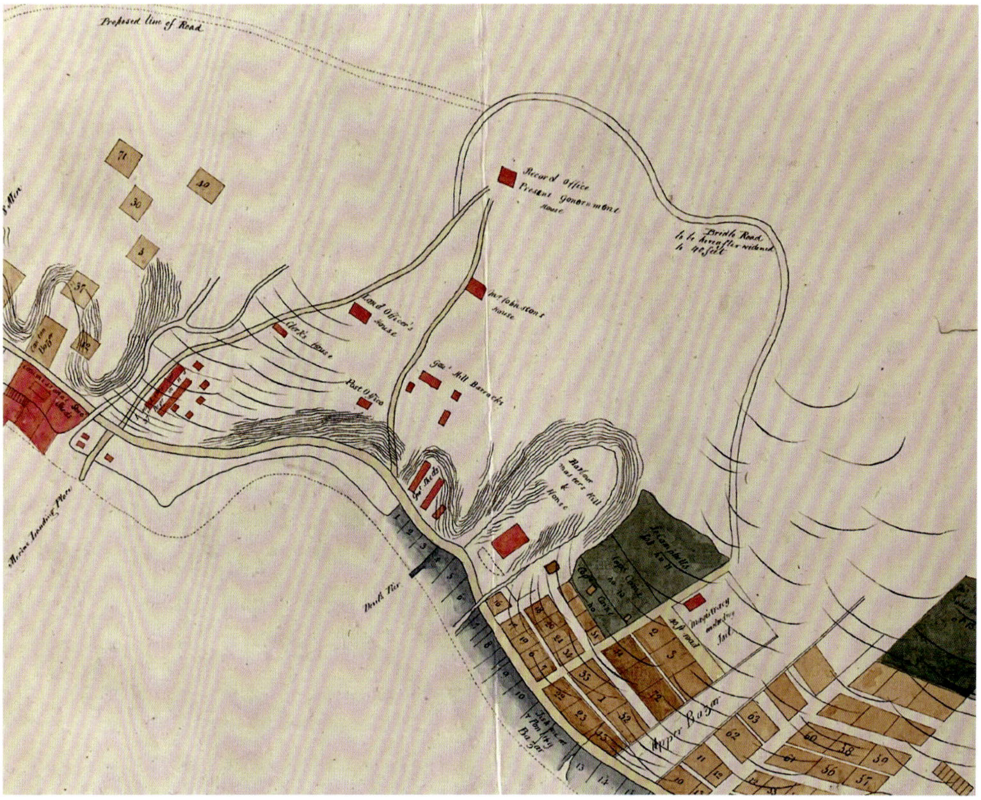

Fig. 2.7. Anon. (attrib. to Lt. E. W. Sargent), Mr. Johnston's House and Government Buildings on 'Pottinger's Map' (detail), 1842. Ink and watercolour. © The National Archives, Kew (FO 925/2427).

Johnston was among the first individuals to use height as a technique of prestige and power, recognizing that governing required the most proclamatory of terrain, despite the trade-off in difficulty of access. During the construction boom of 1841 to 1843, while Johnston remained acting governor to the peripatetic plenipotentiary of trade, Sir Henry Pottinger, 'coolie' labour could be purchased easily at the miserable rate of a single dollar per day for seven to eight men. 'Work away while we can draw on the Canton ransom money', he was known to repeat.[24] These coins were Spanish silver dollars, a long-standing currency acceptable in the China trade. Hong Kong would only begin to mint coinage in the 1860s. Unlike Pottinger, Johnston had no qualms about pouring capital into construction projects to accelerate development. Though officially commenced in May 1841 'under the superintendence of the corps of engineers', speculative road construction had, in fact, begun much earlier. The civilian government would soon oversee the building of roads, placing the military in a subordinate, supervisory role. This transfer of control was due to the inevitable vicissitudes of military personnel, including a significant departure of troops for the northern expedition with Pottinger in late August 1841.[25] Their fluctuation in number was the cause of some anxiety for those involved in the civil works. Nevertheless, from the beginning, most projects were procured through private contracts with Chinese contractors. These new relationships had teething problems which merely fed latent prejudices. From the perspective of the British, local contractors had little experience with this kind of work or familiarity with the standards demanded by the settlers in both construction and the honouring of written agreements. 'There was', complained William Tarrant the colony's inspector of roads, 'hardly one agreement which did not break down before its fulfilment'.[26] One example Tarrant could cite from personal experience involved a contract to cut a much-anticipated passage, known as 'The Gap', through the mountainside east of the city, needed to connect Wan Chai through into the Wong Nai Chung Valley. The contract was signed by the bid winner at 'the absurdly low sum' of $2,600 with a promise to finish the work by an equally ambitious time. Unfortunately, as Tarrant complained, the work cost three to four times the agreed amount and took 'as many years as stipulated months'.[27] Still unfinished, the road pass was inaugurated in June 1843 by a celebratory carriage trip through its narrow crevasse by the future first governor, Henry Pottinger, and the imperial commissioner, Qiying. 'No means, we are sure', wrote Tarrant, 'could have been better adapted to impress on the Tartar magnate the energy and determination of Englishmen to drive through every obstacle than the spectacle of this deep cutting in so comparatively short a period'.[28]

In December 1841, and with somewhat cooler weather accompanying him, John Slade, editor of the *Canton Register*, decided to take a trip across to Hong Kong Island to examine the colony's state of progress. The Queen's Road astonished him.

> This road is an excellent carriage road nearly from the hill on which the British flag was first hoisted in January last, to the eastward, for about five miles, when it becomes impracticable for safe riding in a carriage.
>
> . . . The making of this road could have been accomplished only by great labour and perseverance, for in many places, the bases of the granite hills run down to the water's edge. Below this, most of the land allotments lie.[29]

Slade counted 'upwards of twenty brick habitations on various elevated sites' already sprouting above and to the south of the road. Deputy-Governor Johnston, though, 'still resides in a boarded and matted house'. What also struck Slade was his observation that the making of the road and the removal of rock and soil that this entailed by thousands of workmen had inadvertently provided new land. 'Chinese labourers excavating the bases of the hills, digging out the stones, and carrying them and the earth down to the water's edge, [are] filling up the shallows for the purpose of forming foundations for houses and quays.'[30] This unexpected benefit would have enormous consequences in the developmental logic of Hong Kong's future urbanism. Almost as a by-product, the construction of the Queen's Road generated the first informal stretches of land reclamation. It was a principle quickly seized upon by marine-lot owners. Another perhaps more surprising outcome due to the new roads and paths that cut into and climbed the hillsides, was the rapid and regular clearing of fern and grassy scrub that covered the island. Locals could now reach these materials with relative ease, stripping the already treeless hillsides of low-cover vegetation. The Chinese brought these down the mountainsides in large bundles to sell to native vessels docking at Hong Kong for boat repairs. The toxins released in the burning grasses smoked out and killed the wood-boring insects that had eaten into their hulls.[31]

By February 1842, the Queen's Road had become part of a more extensive, interlinked system. This system included widening original Chinese tracks into bridal paths such as the mountainous route leading from the Wong Nai Chung Valley in the north over and across into the south, via Tsin Shui Wan (Repulse Bay) and on to the village of Chek Chue (Stanley). Another widened path was constructed to link two significant British military encampments together, one situated in an area northeast called Sai Wan (a corruption of Shai Wan, or more accurately, Chai Wan) and over the mountains past Tai Tam Bay to the barracks at Chek Chue. The network now running from the town through the Wong Nai Chung Gap was described by the *Canton Press* as 'a work of great labor, for during its whole extent of about 8 or 9 miles, it is cut into the sides of hills, or leads over ravines, and manifests considerable engineering skill, not however wholly ascribable to the English engineer as some part of it had already been made by the Chinese'.[32]

Naval Surgeon Edward Hodges Cree was one of the earliest amateur artists to capture the settlement of Victoria at Hong Kong in his watercolours. His initial arrival, at the age of twenty-seven, was in early April 1841 with some members of the 18th Regiment aboard *HMS Rattlesnake.* It was to be the first of many visits to the island stretching over several years. That month and into the next, interrupted by short, recreational excursions to the mainland, 'well armed' with both rifles and 'ham sandwiches, sausages, and ale which we enjoyed under a banyan tree surrounded by a gaping crowd of natives', he witnessed the setting up of the island's first town.[33]

> *Mon. 19 April* Dined with the 18th officers. Afterwards went over to Hong Kong, where the people all living under canvas. A great influx of natives—all the ruffians from Canton—have erected huts and shanties, where are drinking booths and gambling booths and every kind of debauchery.
>
> *Fri. 30 April* On the shore with Bull and his wife to see the new village which is springing up rapidly in Hong Kong and roads are being constructed. Thousands of Chinese labourers are being employed.[34]

The 'new village' was the kernel out of which would grow the city of Victoria. Cree was not exaggerating, it seems. He accompanied his diary with detailed yet evocative watercolours. One of these, painted the very day of this second entry, shows Hong Kong from a unique vantage point, the first in-situ illustration that we know of (**fig. 2.8**).

Superimposed onto a massive granite boulder, Cree entitled his view 'Victoria, Hong Kong, before the town was built', suggesting that this inscription was added in hindsight. Instead of a typical trade-painting view from water to land we look in reverse, from the foot of Cantonment Hill along and across to the shoreline. In the waning light of early

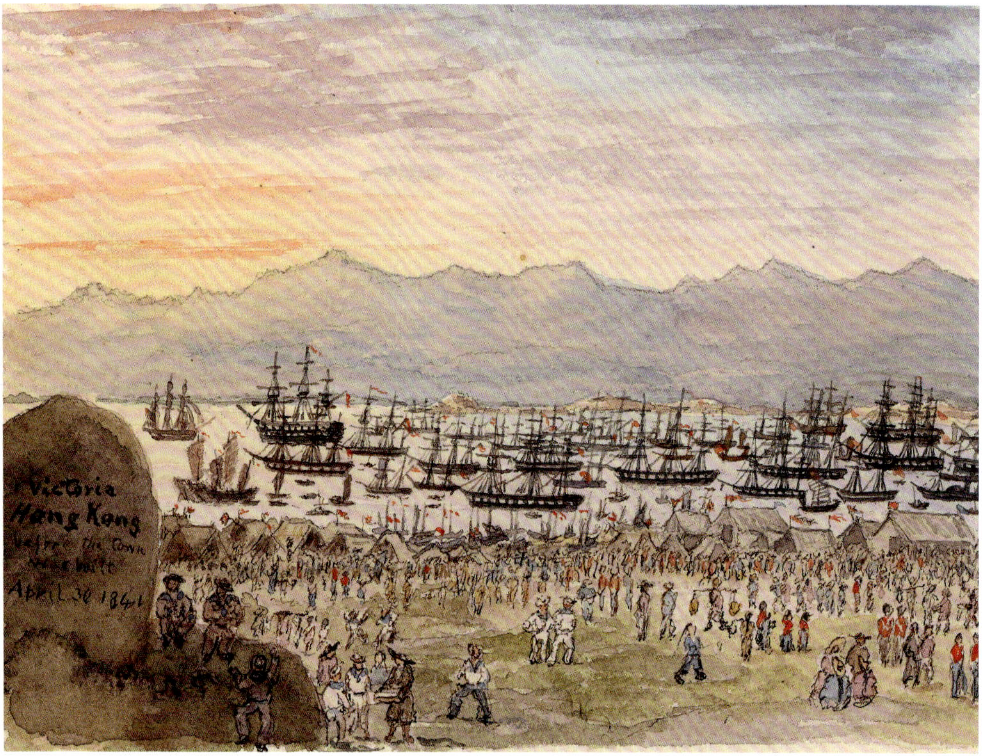

Fig. 2.8. Dr. E. Cree, 'Victoria, Hong Kong, Before the Town Was Built', 30 April 1841. Watercolour. © National Maritime Museum, Greenwich, London (CRJ/5).

evening, beyond the thrusting boulders, on recently flattened land, a multitude of people mill about. Soldiers in red tunics and sailors in white ducks and blue neckerchiefs appear to mingle freely with Chinese labourers. A clutch of canvas tents can be seen in the mid-ground to the left. Along the beach, extensive rows of mat-sheds march uninterruptedly across. Mat-sheds would spring up everywhere, adapted to all purposes. These were skeletons of lashed bamboo, covered in palm leaves the Chinese called *kwai*.[35] The rows of sheds would form the urban seeds of native commerce and Hong Kong's first market bazaars. Finally, Cree filled the painting's horizon with an insect-like swarm of ships. Life here in early 1841 teemed more upon water than on land.[36]

Of course, with the thousands of Chinese came the attendant hawkers and sellers to support such an endeavour. It had about it 'the air of a Gold Rush town'.[37] As the *Canton Register* recorded,

> Vast numbers of natives are now employed at an extremely high rate of wages, in making roads on Hongkong. . . . it is said that even a slap-bang shop has been opened, where, at the sign of the government arms, swinging in glory to the breeze . . . may be seen the following bland invitation, to be chanted to the tune of rich and rare: Victoria sausages rich and good, Prince Albert's black-puddings, an excellent food.[38]

Out of this hubbub and commotion arose a string of bazaars, permanent market structures. Initially, these were of the type shown in Cree's sketch: a long line of sellers' stalls skirting the street edges, small ad-hoc possessions built by the Chinese out of matting and bamboo. But soon, this lucrative business potential was picked up by Europeans on-the-ground, men such as Lieutenant John Ouchterlony of the Madras Engineers, constructor turned investor and the island's chief military engineer. Spotting the opportunity first-hand, he borrowed two thousand dollars from his powerful friend, the trader Alexander Matheson. He purchased a plot below Cantonment Hill close by the ordnance stores, catering to Indian troops.[39] These entrepreneurs consolidated the sellers' stalls into large, covered enclosures, privately constructed markets with the spaces divided into units and rented out. Partly this evolution was a result of the newly created roads that had to remain unhindered once widened, their sides cleared for the June 1841 land auction. Such consolidation by private European enterprise, of course, served the government's desire to eradicate the many unregulated Chinese constructions dotting the roadside. Soon, the dominant pattern adopted for bazaars were specially designed stalls with alleyways open to the main street and strategically inserted into locations where there was maximum growth potential, such as the base of ravines between the ridges of hills (**fig. 2.9**).

One of the first bazaars built was by Captain William Morgan, agent to Jardine Matheson, in 1842. Alexander Matheson saw this as an essential toehold in local commercial investment, suggesting to his Parsee trading partner Jamsetjee Jejeebhoy in Bombay that 'We shall invest $30,000 for you at Hongkong in the mode that may appear to us most profitable, which we think will be a range of shops for Chinamen.'[40] It was one of two bazaars located within what would become the military cantonment district along the Queen's Road, north of Cantonment Hill and west of Ha Wan (later named Wan Chai) and close by the early colonial cemetery. Nuzzling against the hillside and built over a nullah (or watercourse) the Morgan's Bazaar soon merged with its nearby competitor, Ouchterlony's Bazaar, to form the Morgan's & Ouchterlony's Bazaar. By 1845, now within the new militarized zone, the bazaar had been built as two rows of shophouses of a 'Singapore-frame' construction, bisected by a short avenue (**fig. 2.10**).

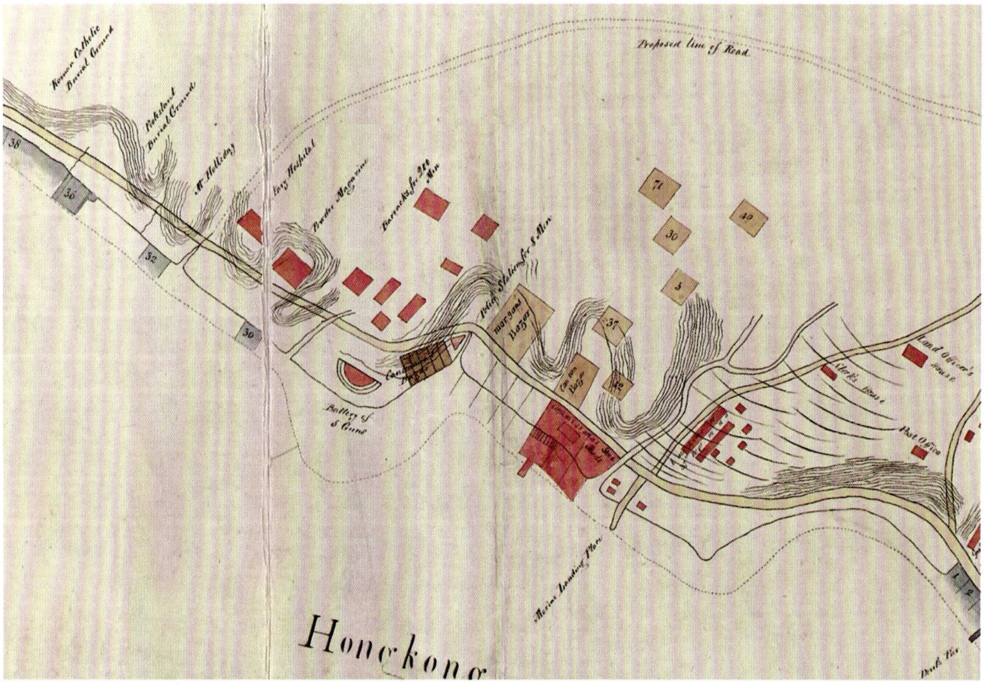

Fig. 2.9. Anon. (attrib. to Lt. E. W. Sargent), The Bazaars by Cantonment Hill on 'Pottinger's Map' (detail), 1842. Ink and watercolour. © The National Archives, Kew (FO 925/2427).

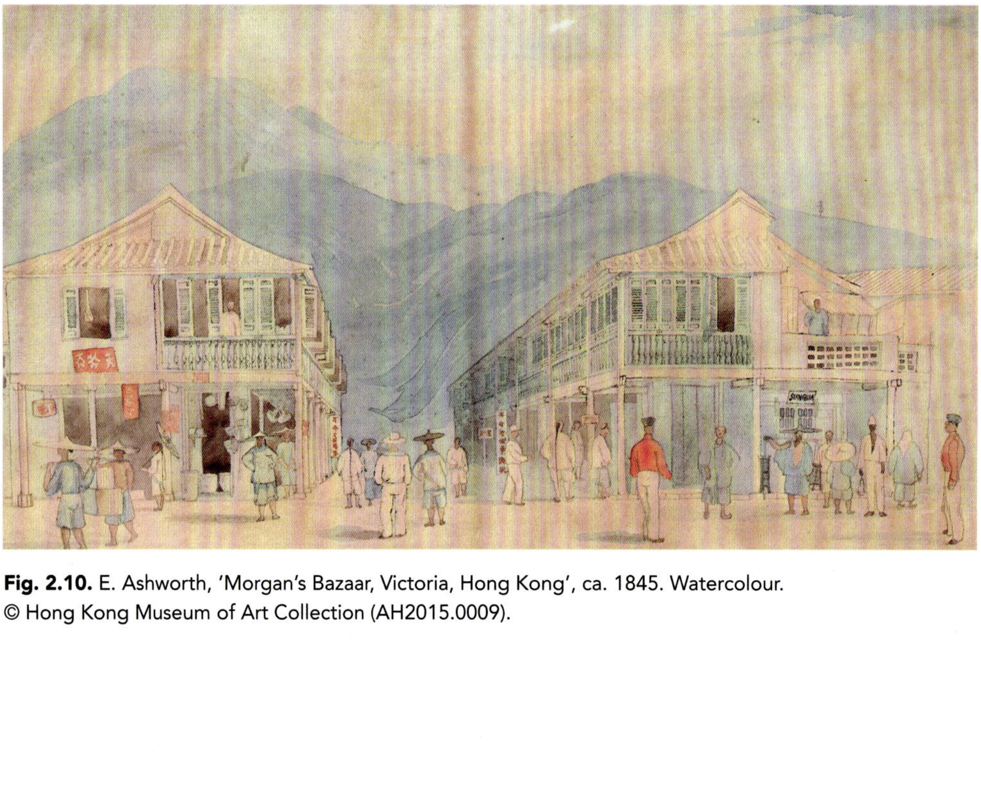

Fig. 2.10. E. Ashworth, 'Morgan's Bazaar, Victoria, Hong Kong', ca. 1845. Watercolour. © Hong Kong Museum of Art Collection (AH2015.0009).

The Morgan's Bazaar had a direct competitor in the Canton Bazaar built only a few dozen yards to the west (see **fig. 3.19**). Given the early importance of this stretch of land to the armed services, both marts thrived by catering to British and South Asian soldiers (or 'sepoy') within the East India Company's armed forces and sailors of the Royal Navy. The visiting English architect Edward Ashworth drew this rare view of an early bazaar. He had been attracted by the boom in construction following the January 1844 land auction and spent two years in the city seeking building commissions. More will be spoken of him later. We see that the street clientele has not much evolved since Cree's early sketch. A soldier conspicuously walks about under the sun's baking heat in his red tunic, sailors in white ducks haggle by a shopfront with Chinese sellers, while others enjoy the shade of the long verandas. These timber-covered ways were the first arcades of Hong Kong, soon to be a prominent grammatical feature of its subsequent granite architecture. Hong Kong's bazaars would become essential test cases for advances in building safety as these, for the first few years, were the densest locations for the growing mass of the colony's population. By 1844, writers could still be read complaining in the broadsheets about the roads in front of the Canton, Malcolm's, and Morgan's bazaars remaining 'so impracticable'.[41] It was not just the human crush. Fires repeatedly broke out. The paranoia of Hong Kongers would be reflected by spurious and unfounded claims of agent-provocateurs sent from the mainland to staunch the city's local economy. The most likely reasons, of course, were a combination of flammability, density, and risk. Unsurprisingly, the first government ordinances regarding hygiene and safety had these premises in mind.

Executive paranoia in unregulated market-selling also brought about the first government-run market. 'Malcolm's Bazaar' referred to Lieutenant-Colonel George Malcolm, the secretary of legation and acting colonial secretary. While Malcolm was unknotting the already intricate land ownership legacies across the northern stretch of the island in mid-1842, he decided upon a central market space that would help eradicate hawkers. These were Chinese street sellers that he considered were impeding traffic movement, or, in his words, 'country people [who] came over and exposed their goods for sale along the principal roads and thoroughfares'.[42] Malcolm chose a marine plot along the Queen's Road suitably close to the foot of the Upper Bazaar—two parallel streets of shophouses and Hong Kong's centre of legalised Chinese trade. The Central Market, established in May 1842, was the British colonial government's first significant intervention into Chinese practices on the island. But this intervention was also indirect. By corralling hawkers into a well-regulated space and establishing careful rules in the management and selling of goods, the daily running of the market could be left to Chinese overseers controlled by a Chinese superintendent. Hong Kong's Central Market may be considered the first public organization run by Chinese elites in the colony, predating the City Temple (1843) and Man Mo Temple (1847). The colonial authority feared street hawkers as loci of petty crime, their stalls clustered with vagabonds and itinerant labourers. They were considered sites of illegal gambling and alcohol selling, sources of loud commotion, and their street cries disturbed the public peace. Conversely, hawkers were recognized to be particularly vulnerable to extortion, racketeering and bribe paying, and attacks by drunken European army and naval personnel.[43] With one stroke, the government believed that architecture could reduce this perceived urban and social evil while also providing the means to control and regulate the local market economy centrally.

Storehouse Hong Kong

If investors imagined Hong Kong's crude bazaar markets to be the first temples of local commerce, warehouses were their international repositories. Foremost, Hong Kong was a vital dumping ground for a broader global trade. Hong Kong Island was ceded to the British under the unratified Treaty of Chuanbi (or Chuenpi) in 1841—though it was not Captain Elliot's first choice. Chuanbi, an island near Humen, was principally desired, as were more trading ports further north along the China coast. Writing from Macau to his business partner William Jardine, now back in Britain, James Matheson, merchant of the most potent Canton trading house of 'Jardine Matheson & Co.', expressed his regret at this lost opportunity.

> On the whole, the prospect before us is to my mind far from satisfactory. Equal privilege and security for good treatment at places of trade in China are what I should have most desired; but I fear these will be in some measure, lost sight for the bait of a possession on the borders only of the Empire.[44]

Notwithstanding his private misgivings to Jardine, Matheson would be quick to spin the positive attributes of possessing a base within this forlorn 'border' territory to his business associates. Writing the next day to Jejeebhoy in Bombay, he appeared to confide that

> I learn confidentially from Captain Elliot that Ki Shen [the imperial commissioner] has agreed to our having an outside possession of our own, but objects to cede Chuenpee in lieu of which Captain Elliot has proposed Hong Kong, one of the finest harbours in the world; and I have little doubt it will be granted. But as there are no warehouses or facilities there for carrying on this season's business it is probable it will have to be conducted as before at Canton for this year only, till we have time to make warehouses &c at the new settlement.[45]

James Matheson was the first to realise that, despite the likely impermanence of Hong Kong as a British possession, it could serve as a convenient port of unlading. A place to deposit goods quickly and easily into land-bound storage facilities made sound fiscal sense. The overheads on keeping opium and cotton in Bombay-rented vessels, let alone the penalties of demurrage, while Canton maintained its ban, was a constant worry. For those firms rich enough to maintain their own fleet, such as Jardine Matheson, the issue was still one of poor use of a valuable resource. Irrespective of sales on the Chinese side, India's supply and transfer pattern had to be maintained.

Of course, there was Lintin Island or the 'Solitary Nail', a three-mile-wide island crowned by a single peak. Lying about twenty miles west-northwest of Hong Kong, this had been used for decades as an exchange station for the Country Trade—swapping opium into shorter-draught vessels before entering the shallower, silted waters of the Pearl River estuary to its immediate west. Lintin grew in importance as one of the only storage sites for opium during the blockade—nimble 'crabs' and other local craft willingly ignoring the Imperial prohibition to aid the drug's distribution through Whampoa (Huangpu).[46] Customised 'storeships' also anchored here, reflecting the belief among many traders that storage upon land put their goods at greater risk of theft than placed offshore. Though for lower-value commodities such as cotton, this was less of a concern. As the war continued, exacerbated by a proclamation in 1840 by the Governor of Macau refusing British merchants the right to store goods there, it became clear that an alternate location to Lintin had to be sought.[47] Hong Kong was long known to opium traders as a haven from official scrutiny and a shelter from typhoons. By 1837, it had become a general rendezvous point for many vessel classes, including military craft, usually congregating among the seasonal shipping.[48] Captain Elliot almost certainly selected Hong Kong based upon this prior familiarity.

To entice his principal Bombay dealer to increase cotton supplies while also allaying his fears of storage safety, Matheson wrote to Jejeebhoy from Macau in late May 1841.

> We have requested Captains Morgan & Baxter to consult about the possibility of landing the *Bombay Castle*'s cotton at Hong Kong. On a well raised stone platform, well matted over—we think it would be safe under protection of the military stationed there, and it would give us an additional market for making small sales of the article. We have already commenced building a rough store house on Hong Kong.[49]

This 'rough store house' would prove to be the first sturdy, masonry building on the island.[50]

The construction was certainly illegal under British authority—the first land sale was to take place the following month. However, it was considered worth the risk. This location, at the base of Cantonment Hill, was invaluable to Matheson as it was under the surveillance of the military camp, offering the only police protection available. The military, therefore, shaped the pathology of terrain for those that followed by their very presence.

Some in retrospect believed that Elliot should have observed Matheson's maverick approach and sat back, allowing merchants to build as and where they wished entirely at their own risk since any official land sale was jeopardous without confirmation of British sovereignty.[51] However, it could well have been Matheson who persuaded Elliot to launch the land auction as this would ensure igniting a property market while providing investors with some rudimentary town layout. In the meantime, Matheson took the lead, using the work of the military to his advantage. He was, after all, closely tied to army officials such as Ouchterlony. Matheson could claim that he had created an enclave of stability and security from a blank and sterile canvas, promoting this impression to his distant agents and lenders, despite whatever doubts he privately held in the project.[52]

Jardine Matheson & Co. purchased the plot of land beneath their illegal structure in the June land auction, a bid that went unchallenged due either to fear of the firm or to an unusual display of gentlemanliness by rivals. The company then proceeded to improve upon it.[53] Thus Matheson could write one month later to Jejeebhoy:

> What is arriving &. [via the vessels] *Tweed*, *Asia*, *Julia*, in addition to the *Bombay Castle*'s is in the course of being securely and economically stored at Hong Kong, where we have 300 feet of sea frontage admirably situated between the Cantonments of the Sepoy & European troops. We have made considerable progress in building a large stone warehouse, but the cotton is for the present stored in mat sheds, which will be surrounded by a high stone wall, as a security against thieving & fire. We shall do all we can to encourage sales of cotton there by asking only moderate prices.[54]

Matheson was convinced that the remaining components needed to achieve success were 'thoroughly protected roads made and settlers encouraged' and was willing to spend twenty-thousand dollars in this conviction.[55] But he concealed from Jejeebhoy the state of the troops' health, an aspect causing growing concern throughout the settlement. He even found it hard to share this news with his old London-based partner William Jardine, until he felt sure that the army was moving towards recovery and able to provide a semblance of the 'protection' he was projecting.

> Our building at Hong Kong is going on apace, and we have now 8,000 bales [of] cotton stored there. The sickness of the troops is diminishing, but there will not be a move to the North till the arrival of the expected reinforcements from Bengal.[56]

There was no question yet of storing opium in this untested, walled enclave. On 21 July, Hong Kong was struck by a devastating typhoon, uprooting most of the mat-sheds and flattening many of the properties, most still under construction. Edward Cree recorded the devastating effects on the smaller vessels of the unfortunate Tanka community within the harbour (**fig. 2.11**). It was followed by another weaker storm five days later. The destruction was significant enough to reach the ears of the Emperor Daoguang, according to an apparent translation of a Canton public notice. In a fit of schadenfreude, the emperor thanked heaven for the destruction of the new colony.

> On the 4th day of the 6th moon . . . a typhoon commenced which forced the waves to run mountains high, and at the same time torrents of rain descended . . . of the barbarian banditti and native traitors the number drowned exceeds calculation; all the tents and mat-sheds were blown away by the wind, none were saved. The new built landing places were swept clean away, and nothing left but an empty space, and the sea was covered with floating corpses. Such is the report.
>
> I, the emperor, having turned over and looked at the rest, feel most grateful for heaven's favours; . . . long and much have they travelled in unrighteous paths; but at last, they must bow their heads to heaven's extermination.[57]

To paraphrase a well-known witticism, news of Hong Kong's demise was greatly exaggerated. It turned out that the level of damage reported was an embellishment crafted to please the emperor. Yet, the sombre Matheson felt compelled to write to Jejeebhoy on 7 August:

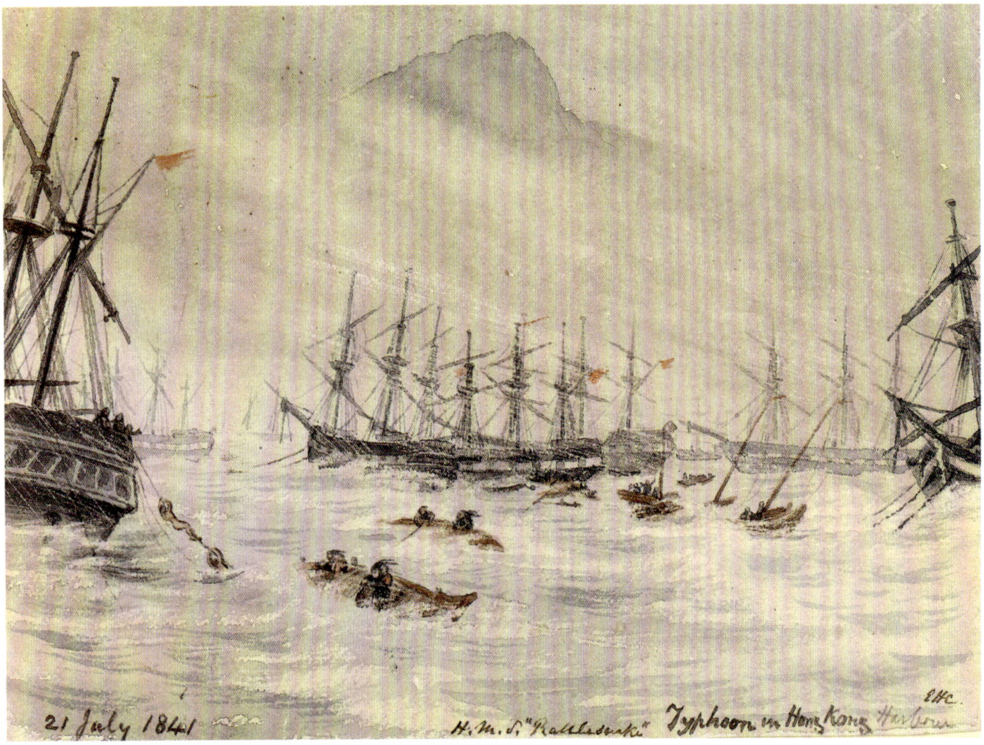

Fig. 2.11. Dr. E. Cree, 'Typhoon (in) Hong Kong (Harbour)', 21 July 1841. Watercolour. © National Maritime Museum, Greenwich, London (CRJ/5).

> We had the most disastrous typhoon ever thrown here, and another on the 26th. I refer you to the newspapers for an account of the heavy losses they occasioned . . . our mat warehouses with cotton at Hong Kong escaped with a slight exception occasioned not by the wind but by a torrent of water overflowing & spreading too near the foundation.[58]

Matheson would not forget this lesson. The flooding likely provided impetus for his subsequent strategy to diversify his storage locations. Through his agent Captain William Morgan, he had already purchased in the June auction, over a mile eastward, the spur of land and receding hillocks by the shores near the Wong Nai Chung Valley. It was higher and free of nullahs. In hindsight, it was a shrewd approach when considering the departure of 900 troops from the island two months later in August, leaving 'but poor protection for Hongkong'.[59] By the end of 1841, Alexander Matheson, James's nephew, had taken charge of affairs in Hong Kong. He was able to write to Jejeebhoy in January the following year, 'We secured three adjoining lots—& have built on the centre one—but contemplate establishing our chief seat of business elsewhere—on a point jutting out into the sea, some little distance from our present premises.'[60] The young Matheson was soon obliged to release these three lots below Cantonment Hill, including that 'rough store house' to the military, something he did graciously. Instead, he focused the company's investment interests almost entirely upon their new eastern enclave, an enclosed area known as East Point.

Even before the June land sale, Hong Kong found itself transformed into a commercial emporium, albeit a floating one. Apart from the usual Tanka craft constantly rubbing against merchant and military vessels, a few European brigs had become floating wholesalers and provisioners (**fig. 2.12**). These ships would have their masts dismantled and decks enclosed by a temporary roof structure, adopting a method used when docked at Whampoa in Canton.[61] Among these large ark-like vessels moored at Hong Kong was the brig *Governor Findlay* whose presence was first advertised to the buoyant community in the *Canton Register* in early May.

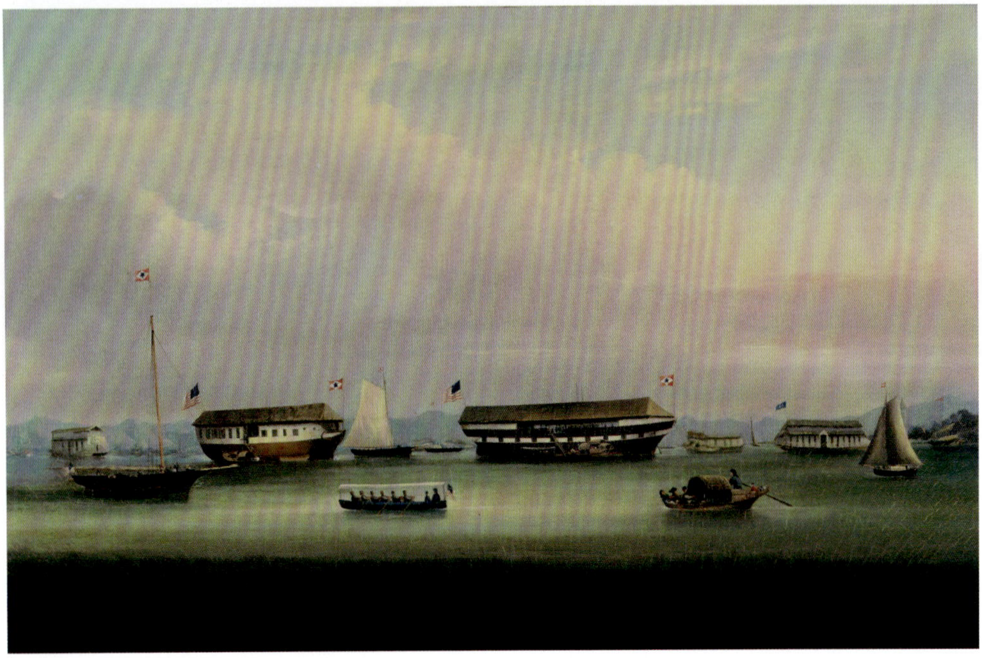

Fig. 2.12. Anon. (Chinese artist), Thomas Hunt's Provisioning Ship at Whampoa, ca. 1850. Oil on canvas. © Peabody Essex Museum, Salem (M246).

> FOR SALE—A rare selection of delicacies for the table, made up by the celebrated firm of PAYNE & Co. Calcutta: and expressly sent on by them for the use of their Friends from Bengal.[62]

The floating merchant's provisions included a dozen cases of chutney, essence of chillies, curry pastes and powders, lime juice and lemon syrup, plain and chilli vinegar, veal and mutton broths, and various meats 'in tin canisters'. These foodstuffs may have satiated the tastebuds of discerning Indian-army military officers busied on civil engineering works across the island, but many 'old China hands' were still unconvinced of Hong Kong as a viable place of residence and remained firmly in Macau. This, however, did not stop them from contributing to developing the settlement. Another vessel, the *General Wood*, owned by Jardine Matheson & Co. and overseen by their agent Morgan, acted as a floating lumber yard. They first advertised its wares in late August in response to the growing need for residential and commercial construction materials in the wake of land sales. Their ship offered 'a quantity of Timber and Planks fit for Ships and House building. Spars 70 to 90 feet by 20 to 27 inches and 50 to 60 feet by 11 to 20 inches, daily expected from Manila'.[63] Manila, a direct sailing 700 miles south-eastwards, was the primary source of this essential material since Hong Kong Island was virtually tree-barren. Timber of lower grade went into seawall construction in some early sporadic land reclamation and into bridges rapidly constructed to span the various nullahs and streams that ran down the mountainside. Still, for buildings themselves, teak and mahogany were the wood of choice. These were supplied by the firm of C. de Otadui—a Portuguese company working from Manila and Jardine Matheson's agent for several years in tropical hardwoods. They were not always the most reliable suppliers, but they were recommended to Ouchterlony in his capacity as military engineer of Hong Kong and consequently to Pottinger's government for various public-building works. There would always be a shortage of timber for the civil works, so getting adequate supplies in good time would form the critical path for planning any project.

After Manila, Singapore was the leading supplier of quality timber—especially in building frames for shophouses or *tong lau*. These were pre-jointed and easily assembled onto in-situ bases. In Hong Kong, this transpired to be a lower course of either brick or local granite.[64] For this construction type, the bazaar market buildings by Cantonment Hill lead the way.

The godown, a warehouse situated at a dockside, is thought to derive its name from the Portguese *gudão*, first used in the mid-sixteenth century, in turn a name borrowed from the Malay (*godong*) or perhaps of Tamil, Telugu, Kannada, or Malayalam origin, to mean a store or warehouse. Regardless, the godown serves as an excellent typology to trace rapidly changing materials and techniques used in constructing buildings during the first two years of Hong Kong's colonial existence. These were the earliest and most basic building type in the colony, generally the first substantial structures constructed, being funded by the wealthiest inhabitants for whom content security outweighed construction costs. Any contemporary reader of advertisements printed in Hong Kong newspapers through 1841 and into 1842 could not fail to notice the rapid development of one particular set of godowns. They were managed by Charles Vanbruggen Gillespie, an enterprising American merchant from Macau, who, unlike most other agents, lost little time in building upon his lot, at 46 Queen's Road.[65] This lot, no. 36 in the land sale purchased by Framjee Jamsetjee, Gillespie's Parsee business partner, stood at the eastern end of Ha Wan, by the foot of Hospital Hill. Meanwhile, the lack of a warehouse did not stop Gillespie continuing his business afloat in the harbour. Through July, he sold his usual diversity of goods from two ships: from champagne, sherry, sheathing copper, and nails from the brig *Jane* 'lying off Government quay' to pickles, Wilson's New York Wine Biscuit, and Russia duck from the ship *America* 'lying off the Mansion House'.[66] Yet as soon as early September, he could announce:

> NOTICE—Tea and other valuable merchandise received in double matted Godowns.[67]

Double-matted construction boasted better internal temperature conditions than single-matted though offering only modest security from theft. But like in the tale of The Three Little Pigs, this proved inadequate, so Gillespie was obliged to move on to brick construction. Four months later, in January 1842, he had rebuilt and extended the premises to offer:

> FOR SALE OR TO RENT—The Brick and Mat Godowns on lot No. 36 Queen's Road HOUWAN Bay Hongkong; the Brick building will be altered to a dwelling if desired. Apply to FRAMJEE JAMSETJEE—Macao or C. V. Gillespie.[68]

Godowns could, it seemed, be eminently adaptable to changing market circumstances. By February 1842 in total 'five or six substantial godowns, built of brick, with a foundation of granite' stretched across the town.[69] Unsatisfied with the security features of brick and unable to convince a buyer to alter the construction to a house, Gillespie soon tore down this second iteration. The final phase of his warehouse compound arose two months later, with some added marine features.

> NOTICE—The Granite Godown No. 46 Queen's Road, HOUWAN, will be completed and ready on the 1st proximo for the reception of Merchandise on rent at low rates; this Godown has a Stone Pier in front, 25 feet long, and is situated at a distance above high-water mark, with a double sea wall that will protect it against the rise of the sea usual in Typhoons.[70]

These granite godowns were two-storied, providing storage in both the lofts and the ground floor.[71] Yet, only half the original lot was used. Soon, under Gillespie's frenetic labour, an adjacent and extensive pair of godowns sitting at No. 47 Queen's Road sprung up. Built of granite 'and in the most substantial manner', they were boasted of being 'each capable of containing about 2,000 Bales of Cotton'.[72] Others followed, each as advertised expanding upon a favoured lexicon of sales phrases that reveal the psyche of the young merchant community on the island. Gillespie's 'extensive' and 'substantial' godowns were matched by his competitors 'spacious, dry and secure' warehouses (**fig. 2.13**).[73] After the malaria epidemic of the following year, in 1843, these sales phrases were adopted by investors to sell private dwellings. Terms such as 'commodious' captured the essence of what was thought to be beneficial for health and life.

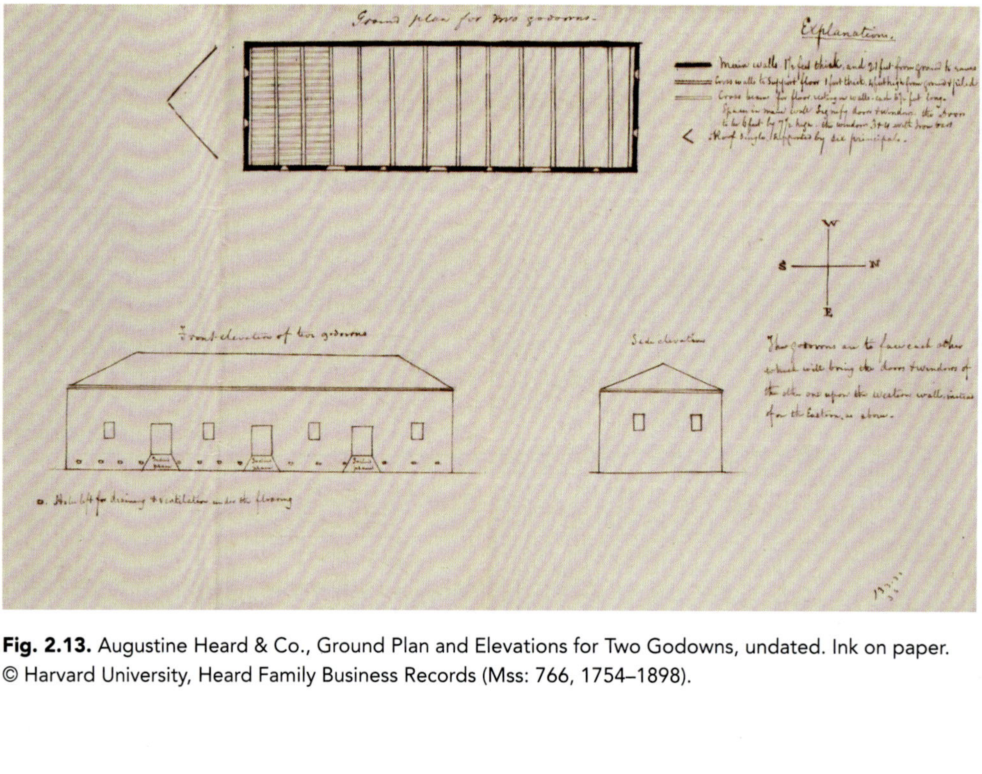

Fig. 2.13. Augustine Heard & Co., Ground Plan and Elevations for Two Godowns, undated. Ink on paper. © Harvard University, Heard Family Business Records (Mss: 766, 1754–1898).

Interior Worlds

European merchants were used to living within a small, protected enclave. The Thirteen Factories site at Canton had once constituted their entire world as they traded during the spring and summer months. It measured barely one-thousand feet wide by nine-hundred feet deep, from the public back street to the foot of the Pearl River; the factories themselves occupying about two-thirds of this space.[74] However, this boundary was imposed. It was an area of land that belonged to Cantonese Hong merchants who easily rented it to the coerced Europeans since imperial decree strictly restricted the foreigners' movements beyond this patch of ground. Repeated incendiary attacks over the years caused the site to be enclosed by high-level railings. Of course, no such policy restrictions existed in Hong Kong. Still, the shortage of level ground in Hong Kong, its inaccessibility, and the dangers of theft or molestation were confining, creating a similar effect. For instance, on purchasing East Point, Jardine Matheson immediately set about ringing it with a fence, then hired armed sepoys to patrol the perimeter. This act may have been the most famous early example of enclave mentality on the island, but it was certainly not the only one.[75]

There were other replicas of the 'Thirteen Factories' environment contrived in early Hong Kong. Spring Gardens, a short chain of factories-cum-residences alongside a quay in Ha Wan seemed almost a copy in miniature, a row of mansions, their porticoed façades facing a set of waterfront gardens. The enclave provided a sense of sanctuary sufficient for solitary European ladies to be seen safely walking their ornamental dogs (**fig. 2.14**). The district of 'Spring Gardens' borrowed its name neither from a garden nor a nearby spring but from a granite residence originally belonging to Turner & Co. (Lot no. 43 of June 1841), built in 1844. This building would later be known as 'Old Government House', becoming home to a governor for a short time.[76] The Scottish architect Murdoch Bruce drew a second view of this peculiar enclave, from above, by the hilltop house of the chief justice, John Hulme. Here we get a sense of how Hong Kong as a low-lying, linear coastal city almost came to pass, with mansion-factories along the quay strung together via the broken spine of the Queen's Road behind (**fig. 2.15**). If the perceived perils and divisive politics of malaria had not hampered this vision, these coastal enclaves could have eventually fused.

Reminiscing upon his first sight of Hong Kong in 1843, the Reverend James Legge recalled seeing at the western end of the town European properties raised above the Chinese amidst 'thread-like paths' spotted with Chinese houses and disrupted by

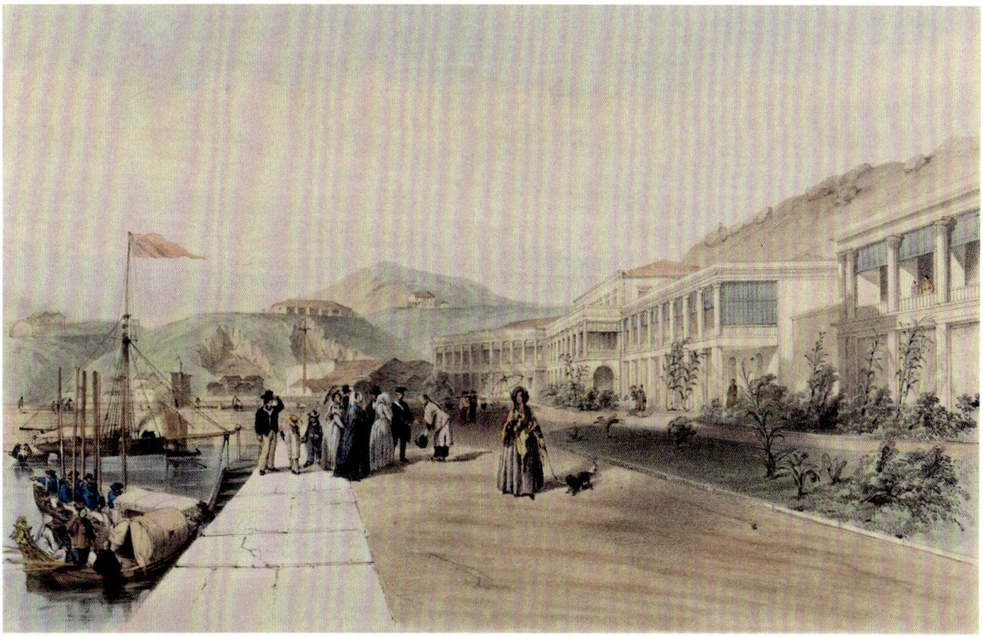

Fig. 2.14. M. Bruce, *View of Spring Gardens*, 1846. Coloured lithograph. © Hong Kong Museum of Art Collection (AH1964.0389.010).

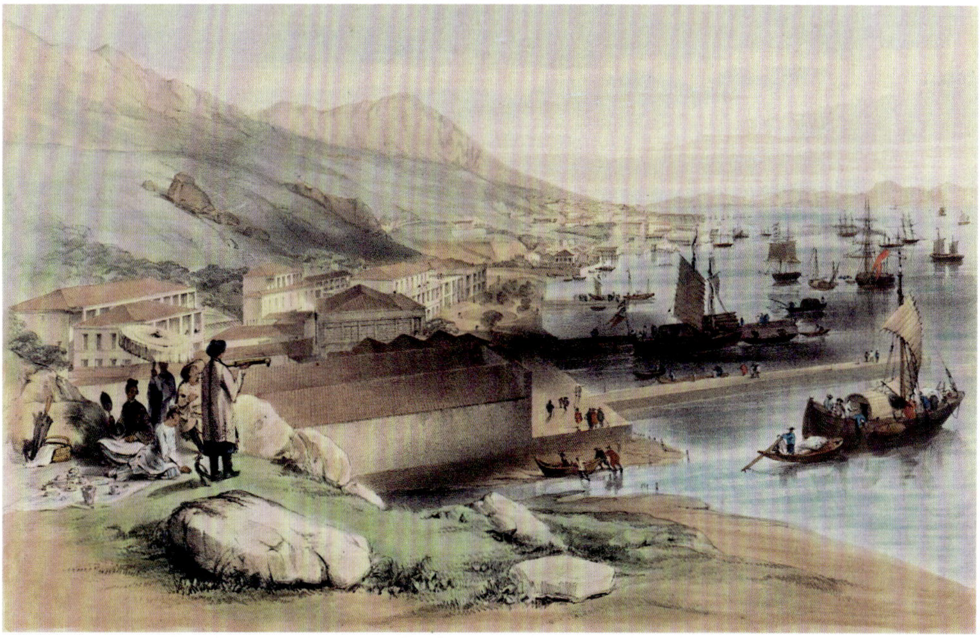

Fig. 2.15. M. Bruce, *View of Victoria Looking from the Garden of the Chief Justice*, 1846. Coloured lithograph. © Hong Kong Museum of Art Collection (AH1964.0389.011).

boulders. Most conspicuous among this cluster were the merchants Gibb, Livingston & Co. whose elevated enclave sat 'enclosed within a ring fence, and where partners and employees all managed to reside—with none of the massive godowns which now seem to serve as buttresses to the offices'.[77] Thus, a fitful urbanism was forming along the north shore of Hong Kong by late 1841. These were a series of interior worlds closed off from their neighbours, self-regulated cells loosely tied along straggling mud paths strewn with boulders and the occasional untraversable roots of mountains, their occupants waiting anxiously for breaches and the connecting roads to free them from boat dependency. 'As the *town* now stands', commented the editor of the *Canton Register* on his December visit, 'it is very much scattered over a space of about 3 or 4 miles, and the habitations on the slopes of the hills are approachable only by steep and zigzag ascents from the main road.'[78] The most elevated and prominent of these worlds to greet an arriving visitor to the island was the prison enclave and magistracy of Captain (later Major) William Caine, thought 'to be nearly as high above the sea as the Monte fort in Macao is'.[79] Below it was the three neat rows and twin streets of Chinese shophouses carved upon the ridge edge called 'Upper Bazaar'.[80] Beyond these, several isolated houses dotted this unnavigable cosmos, climbing upon the hillside, many lying half-constructed or left as empty shells. The official terms of the land auction compelled lot purchasers to construct a property within six months of purchase up to an agreed amount, or risk forfeiture.[81] The city of Victoria's extremities remained ghost-like for quite some time while many of the property owners remained comfortably at Macau or lived on vessels out in the harbour.

One writer concocted a new term to describe these land-locked inhabitants: 'Hongkonians'. *Hongkong and the Hongkonians* is the first published descriptive account or travelogue of the new city. The title given by this 'noble and distinguished author' parodied several works of a similar vein, sensationally promising 'to vie with Mrs. Trollope's "Paris and the Parisians", "Vienna and the Austrians", and Sir E. L. Bulwer's "Athens"'. But there is no trace of a book with this title, and no name ascribed to the author, merely two excerpts published in the *Canton Register* in December 1841 and January 1842.[82] The writing is excessive, self-congratulatory, often trite, and borrows tropes from other writers, paints overt allusions, and steals references. How much of it is an eye-witness account and how much is a literary construction remains a fascinating point of debate.[83] But what the text does is convey a disturbing sense of how much the new city was seen by contemporaries as a vacant location requiring borrowed parts cribbed from other places. And yet, in the process of 'becoming', how ungainly and ill-fitting these parts seemed to European inhabitants as they were assembled. The writer's florid journey, as much fancied as partaken, traverses the town, concentrating upon the various interiors and their inhabitants—as if a *flâneur* prying into the private worlds of soldiers, fishermen, and gamblers to assemble and make sense of this newly formed society. What exactly, the writer implies, does it mean to be 'of Hong Kong'?

Attempting to comprehend the community as a totality was geographically futile, the author argued. 'As to its length or breadth, or, in fact, any analysis of its dimensions I cannot speak from personal experience; being one of those who live in anxious expectation of seeing one or more tunnels cut through the hills which intersect the settlement and pause in further discovery till such expectations be realised.'[84] The hilly island, 'this tumorous propensity of soil', lacked classical pretensions. 'Dido built Carthage on a bull's hide—we have never heard that anything in Hongkong was fabricated—[in] so fashion.' Hastily constructed mat-sheds for soldiers, here the modest quarters of regimental officers, were described in *Hongkonians* as 'simple and unpretending to a degree—delightfully accessible to wind and shower in the sultry season, and admirably adapted to shake off inertness and indolence during the wintry months'. Despite this romanticised notion of simplicity, the structures would soon be despised for their poor conditions and blamed as a factor in the coming epidemic. These mat-sheds were the product of local methods of building. The Chinese troops themselves occupied such structures in front of the European factories during their blockade of Canton.[85] For an army accustomed to tents, especially the British troops of the Chusan (Zhoushan) campaign of July 1840, mat-sheds were seen as a considerable improvement. Their white conical tents had proved a disaster. Unable to be adequately pitched on the uneven ground, they contributed to the exposure of men to the sun. Consequently, one year after embarkation from Calcutta, five hundred men had died from fever.[86] Roadside market stalls had been covered in simple palm leaves, but they went through a necessary metamorphosis for military residences. The *kwai* leaves were now skilfully woven together against bamboo strips into boarding that could be positioned as operable doors and windows. Some other building types, such as warehouses, extended this further, as we have seen with Gillespie's godowns, using a double layering of boarding and even constructing internal rooms made entirely of brick for added security and stability.[87]

Upon entering the shared accommodation of one officer's 'stoutly-built bamboo house—well boarded and leaved', the voyeur of *Hongkonians* described the surroundings:

The interior measured twelve feet by six, with 'two cots comfortably fitted up with mosquitoe curtains'. Mosquitoes were a nuisance but had another forty years of unattributable freedom before modern medicine would link them decisively to malaria. As with all servicemen forced to travel frequently, the inhabitant carried his portable environment of small possessions with him—an eclectic mélange of the utilitarian and the personal. This officer's inner world revolved around

> A table, in one corner, strewed with books and papers of all sizes and colors, denoting business—a second less ambitious table in the centre of the room, on which stood a half-emptied bottle, a square cheroot-box, and a phial of quinine—denoting the relaxation of leisure hours—a chest of drawers groaning with accessories of furniture of every description, from a Shakespeare to a tooth-brush, denoting comfort—and a wash-hand stand formed by two cross sticks and a centre-piece, denoting the luxuries of the toiled. Altogether, there was a 'je ne sais quoi' about the apartment which it were vain for me to describe further than it was perfectly 'Hongkonian'.[88]

Each portable possession is decoded for the reader: business, leisure, comfort, necessity, yet all collided together into a culturally indecipherable whole. To be a Hongkonian meant to be incongruent, a work in progress, an assemblage of borrowed parts each created to address discreet needs but lacking a coherent placed-ness.

By the time the young Royal Engineer and surveyor Lieutenant Thomas Bernard Collinson arrived on the island in late 1843, army officers were living in dry and secure civilian lodgings billeted out to them. Despite this, the Hongkonian interior lifestyle with its eclectic features lingered on. In a letter to his mother dated November 1845, Collinson charmingly captured his own domestic interior in an enclosed sketch to allay her maternal fears. 'Da Costa & I are still living together in Grant's Bungalow—which is known in official documents by the title of Letter G. You have had the view from it & of it, & now there is the view in it' (**fig. 2.16**).[89]

Collinson—known as Bernard or 'Ber' to his family—plundered some of his naval brother's possessions to deck out his accommodation. 'I ransacked Dick's drawers to furnish it handsomely; but I am afraid it will disappoint some of the grandchildren if they have been reading Aladdin lately.' For, instead of an excitedly expected 'oriental' interior, he drew for his family one of recognisable European features. A long, high-ceilinged space with several glazed doors along one length and one at the end frame the ridges of the town beyond.

The room is sparsely filled with elegant furniture. A light woven-cane recliner or chaise longue—the only object betraying the sub-tropical climate—lies by a cloth-covered table in the centre, strewn with books. A writer's bureau sits by the window near the end. A Roman-styled padded armchair and a low sofa to the left frame the doorway to a room beyond. A Doric-pilastered stove and mantelpiece can be seen on the far left, and to the far right a table of knick-knacks described as 'the museum, as you may see by the bit of coral that hides half of Otterburn tower'.[90] Apart from the medieval Northumberland tower, a number of other framed paintings girdle the walls over windows and furniture, like postcard mementoes of distant visits—all probably the handiwork of Collinson himself. For officers, at least, living standards had improved dramatically since 1841.

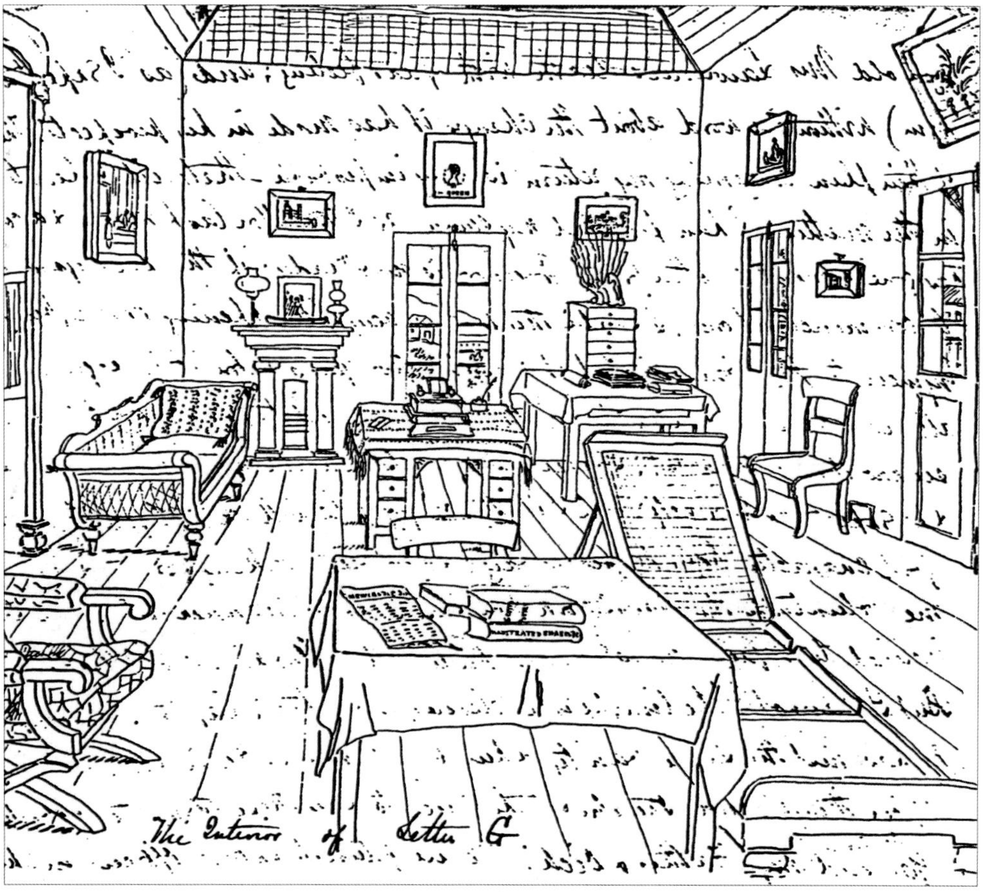

Fig. 2.16. Lt. T. B. Collinson, 'The Interior of Letter G', Hong Kong, 23 November 1845. Ink on paper. © Hong Kong Public Records Office, 'Transcripts' (HKMS 140-1-1).

In the first busy months of construction in late 1841, there was already the semblance of a vital town. The Chinese lots that Johnston established at the then western fringes of the intended civic plan, the Upper and Lower Bazaars, generated a natural gravity, tugging the city's future development in their direction. In his next instalment, the writer of *Hongkong and the Hongkonians* scanned this exuberant yet gritty panorama. If a Hongkonian's interior world was indecipherable, the exterior expressions of this new society were considered hardly more coherent, giving the city's first streetscape a strange interiority of its own. Here race and profession are crudely painted in, from the tailor to the prostitute, an incongruous London of the East laid out in its most basic components, as the writer attempted to construct a kaleidoscope of class and service.

> The shops on either side of the grand road present an animated scene of bustle and activity. On the brow of the hill stands the phlegmatic Sheik Modeen, with well-trimmed hooka and affable mien, mutely inviting the passers-by to purchase of his stock lately arrived from Macao: opposite is the smiling Chunqua, who is an English tailor of the first class, though of Chinese extraction. Here is the newly built hotel, the 'Victoria', insinuating to the stray visitor from its neat and refreshing aspect—here, the celebrated Chinese physician whose skill in herbs and pharmacy is only equalled by his urbanity and politeness—here is the cook-shop, where you may dine cheaper than in Gracechurch street and Bucklersbury, though not quite at the low rates of Holborn Hill—and there is the abode of the fallen of the fair sex—beautiful, but full of wickedness.[91]

From the veranda of that single hotel, with a commanding view of 'the shops, harbour, shipping, inhabitants, and ambitious "lots" beneath', the writer tauntingly recalled a passage from Lord Byron's narrative poem Childe Harold's Pilgrimage.

> —Stood in Venice on the Bridge of Sighs;
> A palace and a prison on each hand.[92]

Hong Kong residents would need no further clues to know that the 'prison' was Caine's domineering magistracy and jail complex teetering above the city. But what of the palace? The 'palace', we soon learn, belonged to Loo Aqui, Tanka trader and long-time provisioner to the British in Canton, now turned Hong Kong gambling boss. Given preferential treatment by the British to purchase a large plot along the Lower Bazaar he constructed 'a long building, built after the approved Hongkonian style of architecture.

Venetian in its moist exterior—in the interior, decidedly Attic'.[93] Aqui's large gambling house was 'Hongkonian' precisely because of its dyslexic attitude between the inside and out. Once inside, it offered the disorientated patron a maelstrom of pleasurable possibilities. 'Aqui has a mart for all; his stock exchange is a continual vortex of business and locomotion. It is difficult, where such chaos of excitement exists, to fix the eye upon any one solitary object.'[94]

It seems that the combinative effect of this portrayal was to convey the impression to the reader that Hong Kong was like a growing infant, still a clumsy, unformed juvenile with all 'the smell of the nursery'. It was merely a derivative product of imperial need, mistaking the playground for independence, more of a child than a Childe Harold.

> Although deeply interesting to watch the progress of a child of civilisation . . . yet we *will* affirm that if old England acts the wet nurse to so many, there is no knowing but that some of those new big boys, whose bulk her breasts have served to develop, may be smitten with the growing and infectious spirit of ingratitude . . . and forget the hand that fostered them in pursuit after the mistaken independence of a play-ground![95]

And so, the writer of this strange 'book' *Hongkong and the Hongkonians*, the first supposedly published account of the city of Hong Kong, reveals their hand at last. All these vignettes, all the plasterboard orientalism and borrowed scenery, served the purpose of ridicule and warning. Such a colony was a necessary parasite attached to the British imperial body. It lacked internal coherence, as it ought; its only logic was to serve at the empire's pleasure so long as it served its purpose. But Hong Kong betrayed signs that it would outgrow this purpose and need for support. Within just a year, the city was producing signs of a coherent character. It was this that the writer feared. Hong Kong might last.

'The Best Site for an English Town'

Though the Hong Kong settlement garnered detractors entirely opposed to the project, many colonists merely opposed its location. Several settlers and visitors were drawn to what they considered some much-preferred land opposite, along the northern peninsula, in Chinese territory. Why, they argued, could we not renegotiate with China or simply take the opposite piece of land and incorporate it into the colony? After all, it was the deep-water harbour and not the island that was the reason for moving here in the first place. In May 1841, an anonymous writer to the *Canton Register*, a disgruntled resident with evident military knowledge named 'Epsilon', argued: 'Yet, by much the most convenient portion of the passage, either for anchorage of ships or for building on the shore approximating to them is on the northern continental side.'[96] Epsilon's concerns centred upon security and defence. Preliminary military investigations into defending the northern shore of Hong Kong Island were shown to be costly. 'I have been informed that a military survey of the point and bight in question has been made, and the engineers declare that the making it effectually defensible would cost a sum far beyond the worth of affairs at issue.'[97] The editor of the *Canton Register* agreed. 'The engineer's estimate for fortifying Hong Kong against all enemies amounts to £500,000.'[98] Two months later, after the first land auction, security concerns were amplified by many who noted that the city, to secure available level ground, tended to sprawl along the shoreline. It was complained to extend 'to the length of three miles . . . in a country surrounded by enemies and guarded by a feeble garrison'.[99] Epsilon proposed that batteries be placed at strategic positions protecting the entries at each end of the harbour, to make it as impregnable 'as Gibraltar is'. Yet as the hot month of May was setting in, his pressing concern was the health of military personnel at work on the island.

> England has been proverbial in all her settlements for a total disregard of health—she sends out her bravest, and best soldiers—she raises ramparts around them without regard to money, more than if it had been of no worth; but she forgets that by placing these brave men in the neighbourhood of some marsh, or in the focus of some burning glass, she brings above their heads the pestilence which no ramparts can protect against and no courage stand.[100]

Most of the native Chinese, he observed, lived on the 'continental side', on the Kowloon Peninsula, while those that lived on the island were almost all on the southern side. This was no coincidence. The position of the new colony town was all wrong, it sat in the lee of prevailing summer winds. As Epsilon explained, 'anyone accustomed to pass the hot months of July, August, and September, must have noticed that the breeze coming from the sea, and giving life to all nature, struck in the bight before described, and on the land behind it, in the hottest days as early as 10 to 11 o'clock—whereas on the site of the proposed city, it was 3, 4 and 5 o'clock before a breath of wind was available.'[101] His next pronouncement would be prophetic. 'No doubt h.m.'s [Her Majesty's] plenipotentiary's medical advisers have looked at the site, and considered it healthy—that is, it may be very healthy from January till April, yet may be very unhealthy from May till December—let them try both seasons before they tie down unfortunate men, to die under their verdict.'[102] Epsilon encouraged and justified that the British seize land in Kowloon as 'strictly an act of self-preservation', as a long-term possession until such time as prospects on the island could improve. But it was not to be. Elliot ignored such qualms and proceeded with the land sale as planned.

Other, weightier viewpoints built upon Epsilon's. Commander Belcher, the noted surveyor of the coastline and waters around Hong Kong, had written a government memo months into possession of the colony cautioning the selection of a spot along the island as the capital merely because it was the first site chosen by the military for their encampment. Clearly frustrated, he felt his views ought to be leaked to the press. These were printed in the *Canton Register* in early 1842. The site had to offer 'as much space as is at present available and which can be extended hereafter with the least expense, delay, and trouble as well as the best suited for a comfortable mart'.[103] The next consideration was that of choosing the healthiest and most beautiful position. He determined that this was the area directly facing the Kowloon Peninsula, in other words, the area along the Wong Nai Chung Valley. Here, he felt sure, was 'the best site for an English town'. He gave numerous details of the advantages of such a site. He agreed with others as to seizing the Kowloon Peninsula, if only as a refuge point. Having the city placed opposite thereby afforded a direct route of retreat by citizens to this 'neutral ground' and an effective shelter from northerly winds.

Defence of Hong Kong would be relatively easy. Batteries could be built upon granite outcrops to command the entrance to the bay and the peninsula, and the city could easily be extended into the water by scraping down the low hills behind. Reclamation would become a signature method of land acquisition for the colony. If Kowloon fell to enemy forces, its peninsula could be protected by 'the large fort on Hongkong'. By cutting down the hills behind and filling the bay in front, 'you gain the largest level space for the site of a town that can be found along the whole range of the northern shore of the island of Hongkong'. Belcher also argued that it made much more sense to then extend the city eastwards rather than westwards with 'stone sea walls . . . which when filled in would afford an excellent wharfage', an increased depth of water allowing the deeper-draught ships to dock. As the principal Hakka stone quarries of the island lay nearby, 'the material for these works, of the finest granite, being close at hand, the expenses of their erection would be trifling'.[104]

Concerning health, Belcher observed that 'when it had been calm at the old or "western anchorage", a moderate breeze prevails in this strait, probably arising from an induced current caused by the rarefaction of the air when the sun has influence along the extent of the valley towards Titam Bay'. Settlers could construct 'excellent gardens' out of materials taken from the hillsides, the hills would then become surrounded by private residences, and wide streets could be formed that would remain cooler than most places as they would not see the sun until past the eleventh hour in the morning. Belcher concluded, 'it would indeed materially tend to the comfort, cleanliness, and salubrity of the town, if advantage were taken of the present abundant supply of water; which, divided into branches, should be separately available for consumption, supply of shipping well into the bay, and cleansing the town.'[105] As we will later see, this grand though eminently sensible idea in rerouting water was to belatedly jolt the government into action, yet with dire consequences.

'The Brick Fever Rages'

In spite of Belcher's misgivings, Elliot's land auction took place paying scant regard for any alternate proposals to relocate the town's centre. The lots appeared to have been hastily chosen by military surveyors based upon the simple pragmatic of accessibility to the new coastal road and finding the most level ground upon which to survey. This haste was surprising as there had evidently been enough time given for Parsee investors to travel from Bombay to Macau in order to participate.

Elliot's much-vaunted sale was first published as a peculiar 'Public Notice and Declaration' template dated 1 May 1841. The notice printed in the local press described 'the principles and conditions, upon which allotments of land will be made, pending her majesty's further pleasure', but left blank both the number and size of the lots to be put up, as well as the date of the sale.[106] However, the terms of sale was made clear: each allotment was to be sold 'upon the principles and practices of British law upon the tenure of quit-rent to the crown'. Unfortunately, the paragraph which was to follow would have repercussions in future relations between the government and the original purchasers, for Elliot offered a tempting carrot:

> But it is engaged, upon the part of her majesty's government, that persons taking land upon these terms shall have the privilege of purchasing in freehold (if that tenure shall hereafter be offered by her majesty's government), or of continuing to hold upon the original quit-rent if that condition be better liked.[107]

Quit rent, a method often adopted in British colonies at the time, was effectively a form of freehold purchase plus land grant payment set at an annual rate giving the payee the same rights and enjoyments of use as a full purchase in fee simple. The public notice's final version was published in the press on 7 June, in which '100 lots of land having water frontage . . . as also 100 town or suburban lots' would be offered at the annual rate of quit rent for auction at 10 am on Saturday, 12 June.[108] However, as there was 'no plan of the allotments' on view at Macau or conditions of sale, prospective bidders were obliged to go directly to Hong Kong Island where 'the dimensions of the respective lots will be specified and defined on the spot by the Commanding Officer of Engineers to whom parties are referred for further particulars'.[109] Elliot, having washed his hands of the business, the bidders or their designated agents were obliged to make their way directly to the island, alongside which they lived on boats. The situation then took a turn for the worse. Sickness had been spreading among the army and navy. Consumed by other pressing matters 'it was found that no preparations whatever for the sale on Saturday had been made, the Engineer officers stating as a reason . . . the non-receipt of orders to that effect'.[110]

Johnston, the deputy superintendent, then arrived and fifty lots were hastily surveyed though only thirty-four were auctioned off on the following Monday (14 June), the others held in reserve. It netted the considerable sum of £3,272 in annual quit rents. Bidders had arrived expecting the auctioning of two hundred plots and instead had to make do with just thirty-four—seventeen per cent, or about one sixth, of the expected amount.[111] It was hardly surprising then that bidding was fierce. Hong Kong's consequent reputation as a colony infamous for its exorbitant land prices was born of an artificial and accidental climate of competition brought about by an absurd lack of communication. Governor Pottinger would use this unfair precedent to his own advantage in the setting of land rents for his January 1844 auction. Another consequence was that the ill-considered auction established a pattern that prevented the subsequent development of a tight and orderly urban layout for the town.[112]

The first lot is recorded to have gone for £20 to a Mr. Robert Webster, though others fetched as much as £230 (Jardine Matheson) and £250 (P. F. Robertson). Jardine Matheson purchased three adjacent marine lots below Cantonment Hill for a combined sum of £565—the land on which they had already constructed their illegal godown. Despite demand for this very desirable location, gentlemanly feeling tinged with a fear of antagonizing the great trading house prevailed among the bidders. Jardine Matheson found 'at once bidding for the land it had occupied the full price to which similar lots had been run up, not a single bidding was made against it'.[113] However, it was the site purchased in the name of Captain Morgan for £205, known as East Point, which would become Jardine Matheson's principal residence and legacy.

The 'marine lots', as they became known, each possessed about one hundred feet of water frontage with varying degrees of depth of between one hundred to two hundred feet in length, extending across the beach by about three miles from West Point to East Point, and in varying degrees of density. The term 'beach' is somewhat misleading since, particularly along the west side, the cliffs plummeted down headlong for many tens of feet before meeting the sea. The higher, southward 'town lots' were more unevenly distributed and staked out as they undulated with the land contours.[114] Buyers were obliged to offer £500 as surety on the promise that within six months they would have erected property to a value of at least $1,000 on their respective sites. Some were unable to meet this pledge, either due to a lack of funds or an inability to hire a contractor and builders, as it had become 'extremely difficult to obtain workmen at any rate'.[115] These were eventually obliged to forfeit the plot and deed. The situation was critical at first, as 'but with a solitary exception, the works there cannot proceed for a want of workmen'. The Chinese authorities had issued strict prohibitions forbidding 'all mechanics to go to Hongkong, and erect buildings there for the English. Police runners have within the last few days been to all the master carpenters and master builders and bricklayers here, ordering them, on pain of death, not to go to Hongkong'.[116] Fortunately, the circumstances eased, and Chinese building labourers ignoring the threats scrambled across, in the process causing an expansion in the local population.

Johnston soon found a way to bolster the meagre June auction. He informally offered a third type of plot for sale to the public later that year. These became known as 'suburban lots', and were selected on various inland positions such as hillocks and within valleys. Generally less accessible than the town lots, they occupied what was believed to be good, healthy positions, 'and these, we imagine, extend over the whole island; their value is much less, and will of course be governed by circumstance'.[117] The bitter irony for purchasers was that, far from being healthy spots, several would become the first sites afflicted by malaria in 1843. Suburban lots became the 'canaries in the mine', alerting the city to an eventual onslaught of this brutal epidemic. Their diverse locations posed a riddle for medics trying to understand this pathology of terrain.

In his 1975 essay 'The Foundation of Hong Kong', Dafydd M. E. Evans argues that the government made two significant mistakes in its first land sale that would hinder future planning. The first regarded the initial size of the lots on offer. One hundred feet in width was large and could be broken down into smaller plots more suited to single residential or business units to be sold or built upon when needed. The second mistake, compounding the first, was that there were no safeguards placed in the lease agreements that prevented 'haphazard multi-unit development'. This imprudence led to a lack of visual homogeneity across the town, both in terms of building massing, relationships to neighbours, and styles of architecture. The obvious benefit to a developer was that this system was incredibly responsive to market sentiment as buildings could be erected as and when needed in the locations best suited. As Evans writes, 'developers built what they could, where they could, to suit the state of the market at any particular time; however it was not until comprehensive development began in later years of areas principally for Chinese occupation, that this homogeneity was approached.'[118] Crown leaseholders would sell off parcels of land. And with new multiple owners and not the original crown lessees attributable to non-performance of the covenants any semblance of regulatory control evaporated, such that by the late 1840s the government had all but effectively given up. It was not until 1856, when the first building ordinance was issued, that the government was able to regain some control over its urban planning. With control of the Crown licences 'irretrievably lost', the Hong Kong government missed a golden opportunity to craft the city's plan. After all, it was not long before that private enterprise allied with planning control in London had created Regent's Park's terraces under the architect John Nash and the elegant grid of housing blocks in Pimlico by the master builder Thomas Cubitt.[119] However, all of this seemed irrelevant for Hong Kong at the time. From the perspective of most original 1841 purchasers, the uncertainties of the colony's future prevented levels of speculative subdivision one would see a few years later. The political, economic, and, not least, health uncertainties of the island would first have to be resolved.

After Elliot's land auction, Johnston believed it was his duty to fill in some of the missing pieces and disburse land to other individuals and groups to encourage the embryonic components of a town to grow as quickly as possible. 'Town Lots', those properties 'contiguous to the road on the other side of the water', were the most peculiar and disordered, relying upon the nature of the terrain to maximise their curtilage and induce their morphology, 'their number and depth along the road varies according to the nature of the ground, which sometimes rises abruptly, not affording building rooms, whilst at other places, buildings may be erected a considerable distance in land'.[120]

Johnston allocated just two zones for Chinese settlers. These would be called the Upper Bazaar and the Lower Bazaar (**fig. 2.17**). The Upper Bazaar ran up the hillside as two parallel roads of 118 brick houses from the Queen's Road to the lower flanks of the prison (approximately along the line of the modern Graham Street). It was designated as a residential and shopping emporium for locals, with long narrow plots measuring about fifteen feet wide by thirty-five feet deep, sufficient for a shophouse.[121] The Lower Bazaar was a stretch of land at the current furthest extents of the Queen's Road to the west (up to the current line of Bonham Strand), its plots snaking along the shoreline. The advantages of sea access for the Lower Bazaar made it most desirable for small-scale Chinese importers—its more relaxed plot divisions exceeding the former with 150 plots of around twenty feet wide by forty feet deep but of a similar proportion to the Upper Bazaar, a plot ratio of 1:2.[122] Demand for these among the Chinese was understandably high. The annual ground rent for the former was set 'at the same rate per square foot as Town Lots', totalling £0. 18s. 3d. While those for the latter, with their desirable water frontages, was set much higher at the rate of £1. 2s. 6d., or the equivalent of $5.[123] Johnston's yardstick was simple, the prices realised in the June land auction would form the rates for all future sales whereby 'those apportioned since the public sale, are to pay quitrent in proportion to the prices realised at that sale'.[124] This simple mechanism would be adopted by Governor Pottinger, helping to calibrate the subsequent auction of January 1844.

Henry Pottinger's maiden stay on the island lasted for two days and a night in mid-August 1841. The future first governor of Hong Kong spent it in a tent on the beach. From here, as plenipotentiary and envoy of British trade interests in China, through which he was also the administrator of Hong Kong, he instructed Johnston to desist from further land sales, but Johnston disagreed and the envoy's instruction went unheeded.

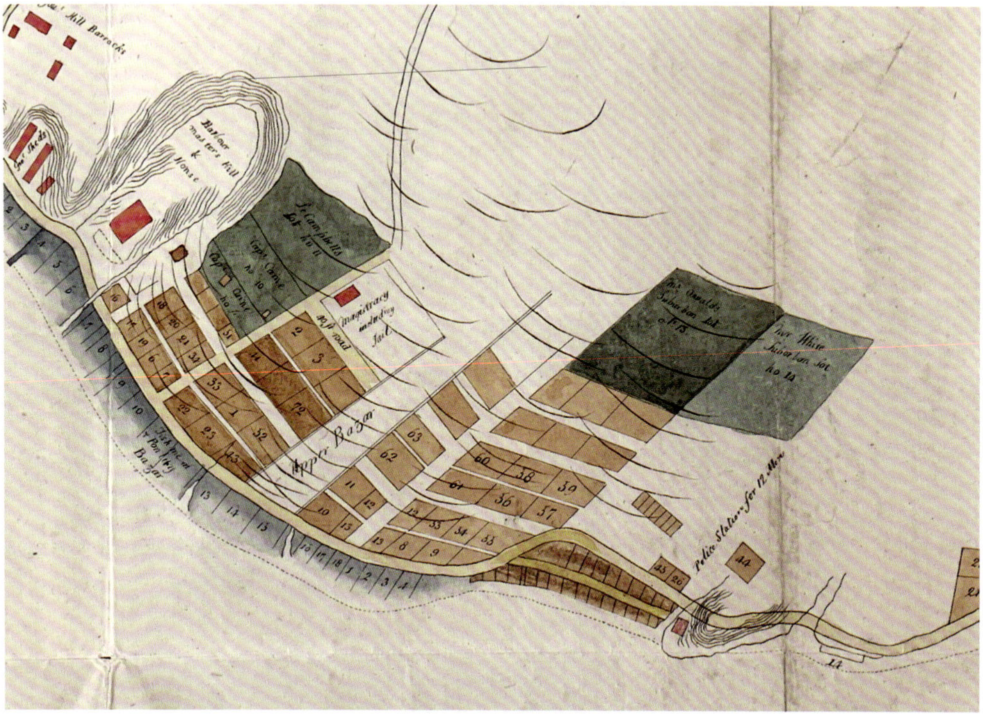

Fig. 2.17. Anon. (attrib. to Lt. E. W. Sargent), Upper and Lower Bazaars (brown) with Marine Lots (light blue) on 'Pottinger's Map' (detail), 1842. Ink and watercolour. © The National Archives, Kew (FO 925/2427).

Pottinger, soon abroad on trade matters, maintained his opposition to Johnston, writing repeatedly and increasingly emphatically before the start of his much longer sojourn on the island from February 1842, when he finally forced his deputy superintendent to cease all land disbursements.[125] The governor was adamant about freezing land sales until the British government had secured a binding treaty with Imperial China, thereby determining the future viability of Hong Kong as a British possession. Nevertheless, Johnston persuaded him to press on with road construction and to provide adequate supportive infrastructure such as ditches, bridges, and basic drainage in anticipation of a positive response from London.

The continuation of civil-works construction under Pottinger signalled optimism for the merchant community leading to a premature boom in capital-expenditure investment on the island. Another positive signal aimed at boosting investor confidence was that Pottinger quickly appointed a land officer to oversee and coordinate all the disparate

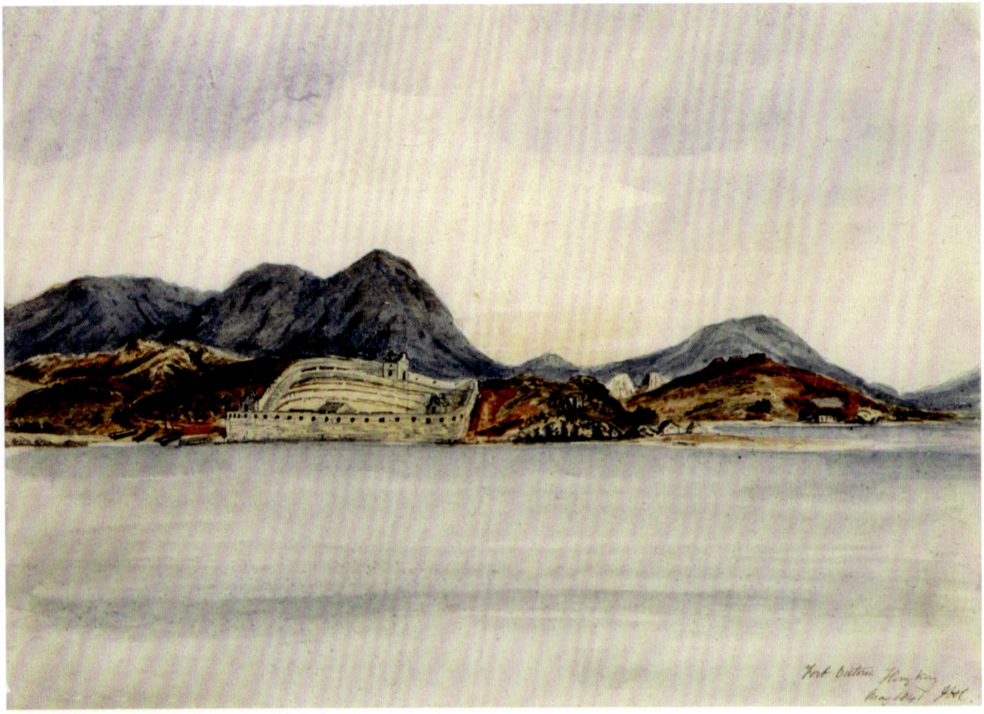

Fig. 2.18. J. H. Collins, 'Fort Victoria', Kowloon, 1841. Watercolour.
© Hong Kong Museum of Art Collection (AH1976.0020).

construction activities taking place, something that even the able Johnston was finding hard to manage. This would be a civil appointment, prior to which the colony had only a military overseer. Captain Cotton had been responsible for the construction of the first temporary barracks and the demolition of the Chinese forts opposite the island on the Kowloon peninsula of 'Cheem-sa-choey' (Tsim Sha Tsui).[126] Mockingly dubbed 'Victoria' and 'Albert', the valuable bricks from these two disabled forts were hungrily salvaged by looters and absorbed as spolia into the construction works of various buildings on the island (**fig. 2.18**).[127] Captain George F. Mylius, pay master to the 26th Regiment, was appointed to this civil post as land officer on 8 August 1841 and was given the assistance of one Lieutenant E. W. Sargent of the 18th Royal Irish. Sargent was a 'practical surveyor' to whom the first map of the north shore of the island—'Pottinger's Map'—is credited.[128] This was timely, as rumours had been spreading that Pottinger's reason for halting land grants was due to a plan he had been devising for the future layout of the town. Though there was no plan, public expectations allowed political manoeuvrability for Mylius enabling him to set about giving the town some coherence and orderliness under the pretext of minimising health risks 'as otherwise the town might be so irregularly built, as materially to affect the convenience and even health of the inhabitants'.[129]

Unfortunately, Mylius's post was proving burdensome to him. In addition to having to perform duties as the ordnance store keeper and as part-time post master, he had to take on much of the administration in running the rudimentary land office. His first bookkeeper, a young clerk by the name of Stanfield, committed suicide 'in a fit of *delirium tremens*' by shooting himself in the gut.[130] Following the tragedy, the office's financial accounts got muddled and Mylius mislaid several hundred pounds that he had borrowed from the military purse to purchase civilian construction contracts. Ultimately, he managed to clear up the mess before Pottinger left on a second trip to the north of China. The embarrassing experience, though, caused him to resign his post and return to his regiment.[131] Despite this, the captain had proved himself a well-respected and honest official, so much so that when a 'Committee for Lands and Roads' was appointed by Pottinger on 29 March 1842 with Mylius's name conspicuously absent from it, there was a great deal of public agitation. 'The only man whose acquaintance with the subject whose opinions and impartial judgement in these matters, would have commanded the respect and confidence of all, has been, strange to say, and we conceive unjustly excluded,' complained the *Canton Press*.[132] This was a legitimate concern as no member of the committee had prior experience in land leasing, surveying, or building. The members consisted of Major Malcolm (secretary of legation), Captain Meik (49th Regiment), Mr. Woosnam (surgeon and Pottinger's private secretary) and Mr. Pasco (2nd master of *HMS Blenheim*).

Since construction began on the private allotments, there had been complaints of encroachments onto government land, illegal shoreline reclamation by marine lot owners, and road construction refuse being dumped onto private property. These and other such issues had given much grief to the beleaguered Land Office. The committee's duties required that they investigate all of these complaints but more specifically they were charged with determining once and for all the demarcation of land boundaries and the legality of all terms of sale; to 'definitively fix the direction, breadth &c. &c.' of the Queen's and other public roads; and the 'immediate removal of any encroachment that may be found to have been unauthorizedly made upon them, the expense of such removal being chargeable to the individuals to whom the locations in which they have been made belong'. The purchasing or renting of land from native Chinese together with 'the reclaiming of land beyond high water mark must be deemed an infringement on the Royalties of Her Majesty'.[133] Pottinger would revive this Committee once again in late 1843 in preparation for the early 1844 land sale. George Malcolm turned out to be 'the life and soul' of the Committee, and his boundless energy and dedication was said to 'tire out three or four horses a day in riding about from one place to another'.[134] As mentioned, it was to Malcolm that, during his tenure, we can credit the construction of a central market for the town with, for the first time, a fixed scale of prices adhered to by vendors. Malcolm also had the foresight to insist upon the main artery, the Queen's Road, to be sixty feet wide with all crossing streets to have widths of fifty feet, a decision (with regard to the crossing streets) unfortunately, though at the time understandably, reversed by his successor, the land officer and subsequent surveyor-general, Alexander T. Gordon.[135]

There was a spurt of construction towards the end of 1841 and into 1842. Government estimates of the total population at the start of 1842 appeared to stand at 15,000 settlers,[136] though this was later rounded down considerably by an actual census. The 'native' population was counted in mid-March 1842 at a rather precise 12,361, including 2,100 boat people, 1,366 labourers, 600 hawkers and 439 prostitutes.[137] Unfortunately, as the elites saw it, there was little or no meaningful commerce taking place. Alexander Matheson would grumble in March, 'Buildings are springing up rapidly at Hongkong; but as yet there is little or nothing doing there in the way of trade.'[138] There was, however, increased optimism in the spring of 1842 generated by 'pro-trade' Pottinger and his officials in assuring that Hong Kong was almost certain to become a crown colony. The pace of construction got so fierce that a downpour of heavy rain causing 'a temporary interruption' in April was in itself newsworthy.[139]

Daily existence in Hong Kong was punctuated by clamorous sounds of construction and the arguments of drunken sailors and soldiers. Amid the cacophony there grew, alongside shredded nerves, an increasingly bitter criticism of greed and individualism that drove the shaping of the new colonial community. The absence of government was matched by the voluble sounds of uncoordinated, unregulated self-interest as the city took shape. This stew of anxieties was vividly described by an anonymous contributor to the *Canton Register* that April.

> From the land where fair Houris exultingly swagger,
> Where drunken Jacks reel, and the "scarlet coats" stagger,

Where government "cabbages" all the best land,
And its attachés prop up a large huckster's stand,
Where drains are much wanted, but never are cut,
And the queen's road's disfigured by many a rut.
Where the voice of the growler is heard loud and long
At the hybrid committee, for right or for wrong,
Where contracts are made that are never completed,
Where villains are cherished and honest men cheated,
Where projects are made by the wild teeming brain,
Which lull like the breeze, and cease like the rain,
Where the peaks of the hills are concealed from the sight,
And the daylight resembles the darkness of night,
Where the brick fever rages triumphantly high,
And the clamour of coolies is bourne to the sky,
Where the value of land is increasing each day,
For which fools pay large sums, and still willing to pay,
Where opium is vended by sleek oily men,
And the dice rattles loud in the gambler's den.
Where the Jacks fight it out in the broad light of day,
Whilst the police stand close by, on her majesty's way;
At which land if the merchants would but settle down,
And, by that means, establish a flowering town,
A mart I am certain would quickly arise
For their longcloths, their woolens, and other supplies;
And the isle to importance would speedily spring,
As the gay bird to heaven doth merrily wing:—
In idle enjoyment, for worse or for better,
In rambling metre I send you a letter.[140]

The next month, Alexander Matheson would write to London excitedly observing the 'wonderful rapidity' of development in Hong Kong despite lack of confirmation as to land tenure and that 'Several large store Godowns and dwelling houses are already finished, & many more in progress—and there is an immense Chinese Bazaar of brick houses exceeding in extent that of Macao, already crowded with shops of every description.—The place is now quite healthy; and with its fine anchorage, excellent roads, and picturesque scenery, it has already thrown Macao into the shade. I hope we shall all be comfortably established there in a couple of months'.[141]

Matheson's hopes withered. He had requested to his Calcutta agent the services of a competent designer and superintendent for the construction of various company buildings at East Point. His agent, John Lyall, sent over a Mr. F. Langer who travelled across with his family. Arriving in early August 1842, Langer touted himself in the *Canton Press* as a 'master builder lately arrived from Calcutta and about establishing himself in his business at Hongkong'. He asked for the opportunity 'of taking charge of the superintendence of such buildings as are now erecting, or furnishing plans and superintending the building of others to be erected there'.[142] Langer initially supervised the construction of the company's offices—an impressive three-story brick structure behind the godowns at East Point. These offices were easily the tallest buildings on the island. Unfortunately, the architect did not survive for long in the Hong Kong climate dying just over two months later in late October of, it was believed, a 'raging fever brought on by over exertion and undue exposure to the sun, and in the death of so able a master builder Hongkong has lost much'.[143] Matheson immediately wrote back to Lyall. 'I regret to inform you that we have this morning received intimation of the death of Mr. Langer yesterday at Hongkong. He had been ill for about ten days with fever contracted by imprudent exposure to the sun. He promised being very useful; & could not fail in time to have realized a handsome competency—as it is, I fear he will leave his family very destitute.'[144] But his own pocket was troubling Matheson more. 'I do not recommend you sending on another architect. In fact, I doubt if I shall venture ever again to trouble you with a private commission. You shew so total a disregard to my wishes & positive instructions I never contemplated, & certainly never would have authorized the advance of our money to Mr. Langer.'[145]

Another unfortunate was J. R. Burd (or Bird), a self-styled 'shipwright and engineer' as he described himself in the *Canton Register*.[146] He moonlighted in this job while serving as clerk of works for the Public Works Department.[147] He also supplied timbers and woods of various sorts. But he proved to be unreliable and increasingly fell into debt. By early 1843, Matheson sourly noted that 'Burd is at Hongkong. I have not seen him for some time & I know that he has not a dollar at present to pay anyone—his sandalwoods and other rubbish from Bally [Bali], being quite unsaleable.'[148] The victims of these early years in the rush to build Hong Kong, and there were many, lost either their lives or their livelihoods.

The Sickness Begins

For the next few years following the possession of Hong Kong Island, the presence of military installations, particularly the building of barracks, led to heated debates among the colonists. Their existence stirred emotions. At first these were makeshift constructions. The army had been burdened by renting costly transport ships, and this significant expenditure led to delays in building substantial troop accommodation on the island. By the close of 1841, freight expenses for 'three ships in conveyance of troops direct to Hong Kong' alone cost the Treasury a massive £20,772.[149] This reliance on rented vessels for long periods was a hallmark of the China Expedition during the First Opium War of 1839–1842, where attack positions and encampments had to be constantly reassessed. Buildings on land, therefore, had to be rapidly constructed and cost-effective. But these short-term measures in housing troops would be blamed for the high mortality rates that these soldiers suffered while living in them. The ultimate solution for Hong Kong's military would be to build more substantial barracks and ancillary facilities, a process really beginning in 1844. Yet this approach, in turn, appeared to confirm to civilians the long-term motives of the military on the island—to create a martial enclave. Conversely, it signalled a disinterestedness in Britain for Hong Kong to become a commercial entrepôt.

At the very start, before even the flag was hoisted at Possession Point, the wealthy merchant community had complained that Elliot's treaty had left an astonishing loophole for the Imperial tax collector. China, it appeared, was entitled to collect the same duties from merchants on the island as at Whampoa, which 'will reduce the British settlement of Hongkong to nothing more than a military station'.[150] The phrase 'military station' would echo through the minds of private investors for the next couple of years as a check on their enthusiasms. There were in fact legitimate grounds for this concern. Writing to 'the Plenipotentiaries on the Coast of China' in a letter dated 10 May 1841, the Governor-General of India, the Earl of Auckland—who as the main supplier of men and matériel effectively held civilian command over British forces in China—spoke in stark terms that Hong Kong ought to be considered chiefly as a depot for troops and a store for provisions for the forces stationed at the archipelago of Chusan. 'Sufficient provisions must be taken from Macao and Hong-Kong to supply the troops on the island [of Chusan] throughout the winter, independently of local resources.'[151] This view aligned with that of the Foreign Secretary, the Earl of Aberdeen, from whom Pottinger received instructions in June 1842 'that this Island should be considered a mere military Position, and that all Buildings, &c, not required in that light, should be discontinued'.[152] Subsequently, a major type of building constructed on Hong Kong Island was storage facilities—both military and naval—placed in the care of an officer of the Commissariat.[153]

As the military continued to expand upon the island and the civilian government delayed making its presence felt, by mid-1842 rumours had spread that the civil government was pulling out. Worse, the rumours continued, the expected departure of most troops from their Hong Kong garrisons for the northern campaign would leave the island bare of security and an easy prey to attack and plunder. Alexander Matheson, who had initially relied upon a military presence as a means of ensuring the safety of his built investments and the calming of his investors, voiced these fears to John Abel Smith, his parliamentary confidant in London that June.

> The apprehension of Hongkong being made a military station, without any civil Gov.[t] is daily causing more and more uneasiness among the British Community, and not without reason. In spite of the Plenipotentiary's Proclamation promising protection to the British Merchants and traders at Amoy & Chusan, which are military stations, the commander of the forces has thought it proper to withdraw all the troops, leaving in each place a miserable garrison of about 200 men. Should Hongkong therefore come under his rule we have no guarantee that he would not act similarly in regard to it—in which case there is no saying what the Chinese might not be tempted to try. With a garrison of 200 or 300 men, it certainly would not be prudent to have property stored on shore at Hongkong.[154]

Following a large troop depletion that very month, settler concerns were compounded by a sudden affliction among a large portion of the military left behind. It was thought to be malaria. The merchant community's fears of this disease and its sudden appearance was driven not just by risks to health and life, but also risks to their onshore investments by this significant loss of protection of the colony's outer defence and internal security. The fear, then, was complex, but the equation was simple. The longer it took to eradicate malaria, the longer it would cripple investor confidence.

It is highly likely that the illness suffered by troops in 1841, worse in 1842, and particularly across what became known as the 'Hongkong Fever' in 1843, was imported onto the island. After all, both larger outbreaks struck the encamped military the first and the hardest. Of course, the agricultural environment played a vital part, many of the rice-growing regions of southern China, including Hong Kong, formed ideal nurseries for mosquito larvae to develop within stagnant paddy. Yet many of the sick of 1841 and 1842 belonged to regiments that had suffered terribly from fever in the earlier China expeditions, such as those of the 26th Cameronian and their 1840 campaign to take the northerly, more temperate island of Chusan. These men were ideal carriers, of whom the local Hong Kong mosquito population fed off and became infected when the soldiers arrived in stages across 1841. This ensured a localised attack of the disease the following year—across the early summer of 1842. In turn, the returning sick 98th Regiment in October 1842 made further contributions to this vicious cycle.

At the close of the military campaign that would successfully culminate in the signing of the Treaty of Nanking (Nanjing) on 29 August 1842, troops from several divisions returned to their respective headquarters, many congregating at Hong Kong. Among these were the 26th Regiment, the largest contingent of European troops on the island, and the 39th Regiment of Madras Native Infantry (MNI).[155] From about the first week of July, sickness, which had been present but not prevalent, started to spread among those encamped. By October, this had grown to become a crisis that jeopardised the very security of the island. To allay the outbreak of fever, under instructions from Lord Auckland in September 1841, 7,500 batches of quinine and Dover's Powders (a preparation including opium powder and sulphate of potash to induce sweating) had been despatched from England under care of the medical storekeeper at Hong Kong for the China Expedition. But either these had failed to arrive or proved ineffective.[156]

Since June, the island had been left with a complement of about 1,400 troops. These consisted of the 18th, 26th, 49th and 55th Regiments, the Madras Artillery, the 39th MNI, the Ordnance Department, and the Sappers and Miners. The largest regiments encamped, the 26th Regiment and the 39th MNI, possessed about 480 and 640 personnel respectively. By July, twenty-seven per cent of the troops were in their sickbeds and four per cent were dead. At the close of August, the sick had declined to twenty-two per cent but with a further five per cent dead. At September's end, the sick had risen to twenty-nine per cent with another five per cent dead. Statistics show that since the spike in July 1842, there was a consistent percentage of sick and dead up to October.[157] These percentages were evenly spread across military divisions. Of this figure, it is likely that many of the same men remained sick, as the stable percentage of patients is highly suggestive of constant incumbents. Compare this to the European troops of the 98th Regiment and their four-month campaign by the Chu Kiang (Canton River), before moving up to Chusan, Nanking, and then back. In June, the monthly return of sick in hospital for the 98th Regiment showed only thirty-eight patients. This jumped in July to a staggering 241 with fifty-three deaths. In August, the figure doubled to 534 admitted, seventy dead. It then settled down to 285 admitted in September and 207 in October, with forty and fifty-five deaths respectively.[158] The main sicknesses were diarrhoea and intermittent fever. Dysentery was an ominous sign as it was associated with approaching death. The total number of European fighting men began at over 700 and collapsed to 375.

What can one surmise from these two sets of data? It suggests that though conditions were grim in Hong Kong it had not blown into an epidemic, as a much larger percentage of new sicknesses were being contracted on the campaign itself. In other words, it appears that the mission to wrest a treaty at Nanking in August 1842 inadvertently brought back with it the incubators of the more virulent 'Hongkong Fever' of 1843. Some later commentators such as the *Hongkong Register*, writing from the luxurious vantage of late 1845, shared this view as to the importation of the 1843 fever.

> Need we do more than merely allude to the miserable huts in which the military were crowded, in which no one would place a favourite dog, and that too after just arriving from the Yangtszekeang, where the seeds of disease had been planted in their constitutions.[159]

Nevertheless, Hong Kong for the troops in 1842 was dire enough. Sir Hugh Gough, lieutenant-general commanding the expeditionary land force, was appalled. He wrote to Sir Henry Pottinger, concluding 'I am persuaded that the north side of the island of Hong Kong will never be healthy during the hot and wet season (that is from about the middle of June to the middle of September) for Europeans'.[160] South-Asian and Southeast-Asian or 'native' troops had been as equally decimated in numbers as Europeans. Curiously though, against medical evidence, Gough baldly suggested that any necessary protection of the town could be undertaken by non-Europeans such as the Ceylon Rifles or the Malay infantry.[161] European soldiers, he decided, would be better off staying on the southern side of the island during these dangerous months 'being, altho within the tropics, open to the sea breeze, European troops are likely to enjoy health, and with proper precautions during the hottest weather may always take their share of duty.'[162]

Pottinger's reply, while stationed off Shanghai upon the steam frigate *Queen*, placed the first wedge between the civilian and military governments at Hong Kong. It also provides an illuminating discrepancy as to the perceived relationship between malaria and location. The consequences of this disagreement would unfold in land allocations over the following years. Gough believed that the source of the fever or 'ague' was location-specific, while Pottinger, himself an honorary major-general with twenty-seven years of continuous service in places such as Bombay and Afghanistan, held that it was endemic of tropical climates in general when complemented by a lack of sensible precautions.[163] Such debates about the distinctiveness of a locale upon the effects of a disease was a decades-old one between military medical practitioners in British India, so Pottinger's broad dismissal was unusual.[164]

> I am forced to record my total dissent as to the insalubrity of its climate, for although it may be visited with the diseases (chiefly ague and fever) incidental to all tropical regions during the months of Heat and Rain, yet experience has shown that with common prudence those diseases may be often avoided altogether and that they are seldom fatal even in those months; whilst throughout the remaining nine months of the year, nothing can be more delightful or salubrious than the climate.[165]

If Gough's thesis was commonly held, then why, Pottinger argued, were the merchants, the 'opulent British . . . flocking to the Island to reside' when they were comfortable enough ensconced in Macau? Troops, he claimed, were poorly managed while on duty on the island. He knew as a fact that they went about at all times 'without regard to heat, rain or cold. . . . Europeans in particular have been permitted to bathe for hours together under a Meridian sun'.[166] Their own commanders such as General Burrell sat, at enormous expense to the Treasury, on board transports cut off from their own officers and uninterested in the supervision of their men, the instilling of discipline, and the engendering of morale. In the meantime, soldiers imbibed the 'pernicious spirit of the country', *samshoo*, an intoxicating Chinese liquor, smuggled effortlessly onto the island. Gossip as to the causes of disease overran the newspapers too. By August, the *Canton Press* pronounced 'that either the climate or too liberal potations of Samshoo are causing the deaths of many soldiers of whom no less than 47 were buried last month'.[167] As the medical historian Mark Harrison notes, post-mortem diagnosis of chronic alcoholism among military troops became a classic cover for death by malaria, from which inflammation of the liver was a common symptom.[168]

The consequence of this was, at Gough's instigation, the setting up of a military court of inquiry the following month, in late November, 'for the purpose of inquiring into and reporting upon the causes which led to the sufferings and lapses in H.M. 98th Reg.t since its arrival in the Yangsekiang and in the Garrison of Hong Kong during the last hot season'.[169] The president of the court was Major-General Alexander Fraser, Lord Saltoun and included as its members a colonel from the Madras Artillery whose mess room the court occupied, two military surgeons, and a deputy judge advocate. The proceedings lasted for about one month. Throughout the trial, officers were asked to confirm or deny Pottinger's assertion that the men had exposed themselves to the sun and to excessive drinking. Each categorically denied knowledge of this. However, different viewpoints emerged from the proceeding as to what could have been the chief causes.

Lieutenant-Colonel Layton of the 39th MNI, arriving with the 39th Regiment on 22 June, described a grisly form of musical chairs performed between various military stations on the island as patients, for desperate want of space, were carried from their sick beds between encampments and transport ships.

> The sickness amongst the troops I consider to have prevailed to the same extent in each Corps and detachment, without regard to locality or other causes on this side of the Island. Those at Chuckchoo [Chek Chue] did not suffer so much. The Native troops suffered in the same proportion as the Europeans. Of three hundred of the 39th Regiment Native Infantry on shore at one time, a hundred and twenty were sick. Out of a Detachment of European Artillery stationed in Cantonment Hill Barracks, there were not sufficient men to fire the morning and evening gun.[170]

The sappers were just as afflicted, and this severely hampered the supervision of road construction. Layton, as part of an investigative committee, felt the most distressed by what he saw in the barracks at West Point, a standing camp situated on the far west of the new town. It is a military site long since forgotten save the trace of a name for the district below it, Sai Ying Pun ('West Military Camp').[171]

Soldiers at West Point had suffered repeated bouts of sickness since 1841 and would tragically experience much worse in 1843. Eitel described how in that first year they 'suffered most particularly' and consequently so too had the many Chinese encamped at the foot of the hill.[172] During the 1842 outbreak at West Point, buildings were overcrowded with the sick. All that could be done was to open the windows for better ventilation and cut away and drain nearby paddy.[173] After moving seventy men from the northwest to the southeast of the island and into the new barracks at Chek Chue while filling the adjacent naval stores at West Point with invalids, the admiral suddenly demanded his stores back. Fortunately, here at the beginning of August, the sickness seemed alleviated at Chek Chue sufficient that Layton, now commanding officer, found he could oblige. However, the same could not be said for the general state of health at stations along the north range of the island. Sickness prevailed within all the northern garrisons. The malady was not confined to a particular corps of the army. Rather it afflicted all ranks and both European and Asian troops. A further two hundred and fifty soldiers initially living on ships became sick after taking up their duties on the shore.[174] In Layton's own words, each barracks constructed 'became a hospital'. They could not keep up in the provision of these hastily constructed wards, and consequently, the accommodation proved 'defective' and overcrowded.[175] Furthermore, the sick lay unattended for most of the time, without any proper care—approximately six Chinese attendants to every one hundred men.

Seemingly unperturbed by the unfolding horror, the admiral instructed that the patients vacate one of the two hospital ships—the *Sulimany* and *Moira*—leaving the sick by the harbour, allowing the *Sulimany* its long overdue discharge from service. At the suggestion of the naval inspector of hospitals both vessels were vacated while the *Moira* was expanded by knocking down several internal partitions. This allowed the navy to accommodate an extra forty patients while freeing up medical staff to tend the shore-bound sick. Worse was to come. The *Moira* accidentally caught fire and patients were moved back onto the *Sulimany*. The *Sulimany* then leaked, and the sodden invalids were carried onto land with half their number squeezed into the barracks at West Point while the other half were carried about two miles across to the sickly barracks at Cantonment Hill or further east still to the small fort at Kellet's Island.[176] The management of the sick was turning into a fiasco.

Dr. Bell's own experience of West Point was one of bedlam. Having arrived on 30 October, late in the course of the sickness at Hong Kong, and accompanying the headquarters of the 26th Regiment, he proceeded to the barracks where he found

> the patients . . . in a state of extreme disability and many of them evidently rapidly sinking under their diseases. Their number amounted to one hundred and forty-four, besides several women and children, and they had not room in the wards even for the common hospital utensils, which were therefore placed outside in the open verandah.[177]

The arriving bulk of the 26th Regiment also experienced their fair share of sickness. The last regiment to depart Nanking, many were diagnosed as suffering from 'remittent' fever (a fever pattern in which the patient's temperature fluctuates daily) and 'intermittent' fever (a pattern of recurring fever episodes followed by normal temperature). It was a fateful revival of the symptoms European troops bore following their attack on Chusan's capital of Tinghae (Dinghai) in July 1840. Then, lack of native followers, duties under a burning sun, and poor provisions took their toll. In the case of the Chusan outbreak it was the climate that was chiefly blamed, believed to be an anathema to the 'European constitution', coupled with inadequate shelter. This had all happened in 1840. Now, arriving back at Hong Kong after departing in June 1842, where they had left their fit and healthy comrades, the regiment found 'a mass of emaciated, dying lads'.[178] They arrived not a moment too soon and immediately acted, providing followers, medical assistance, and their own transports as additional hospital ships. For many, however, it was too little, too late.

The court declared its findings on 9 December. The court asserted that climate *in combination* with crowded accommodation was the chief cause of the sickness. This intersection of climate and accommodation made it difficult to diagnose predominant factors. No specific location was held to blame. There was, they determined, as much sickness at West Point on the western edge of the town as there was sickness centrally and elsewhere in other barracks upon the northern shoreline. However, a general side of Hong Kong Island, its northern side, was blamed since most cases were recorded along this aspect of the island. The southern station at Chek Chue was deemed much healthier. The court believed that 'the sickness during the last hot season at Hong Kong is to be attributed to the effects of climate aggravated by the crowded state of the Troops at West Point. All the Medical Evidence state this to be their decided opinion.' Furthermore,

> On the question of locality, the Court is of opinion, that in the North or Town side of the Island, although the Europeans at West Point suffered most, still so much sickness prevailed amongst the Native Troops in the other barracks as to make it impossible to attach much importance to locality only—On the south side the station of Chuek Choo appears to have been decidedly more healthy.[179]

In conclusion, the court added that a lack of timely medical attention and treatment had been deficient. The charge by Pottinger of misconduct of the troops and poor management by their commanding officers was, unsurprisingly, dismissed.[180] In hindsight, the court made a glaring omission that would haunt debates on the future of the city of Hong Kong from 1843 and beyond. It offered no criticism or proposal as to what type of construction, in terms of form, space, and materials, might be considered sufficiently safe in protecting its military occupants. But this debate would follow, one in which the public works of the military and government would be held as debased against that of the palatial private works of merchant capital.

'The Rat Trap and the Bird Cage Orders'

As with the military, the civilian government was heavily blamed by settlers in setting a poor example for the population with its sub-standard building construction. Critics writing in the *Chinese Repository* in 1845 recalled that 'All the buildings early erected for government were every way very poor. The house of the magistrate is the only exception, and we are not sure that it was built by or for government'.[181] Captain William Caine, the chief magistrate, proved an easy target for this verbal assault. His residence gloried in its uniquely elevated position at the head of his compound and empire: a granite mansion atop a wooden palisade enclosure girdling a small prison complex, situated on a par with the government offices on the adjacent ridge and constructed well before them.[182] We see this dominance clearly in one of George Chinnery's few surviving images of Hong Kong during his six-month visit there in 1846 (**fig. 2.19**).

Captain Caine, the first officer to be appointed by Elliot in the administration of Hong Kong, had a head start over his colleagues and lost no time in asserting his pre-eminence. He was appointed under warrant as 'chief magistrate to the island of Hongkong' on 13 April 1841 though, surprisingly, this official notice took a few weeks to be published in the local press.[183] The Irish captain, a native of County Kildare, served in the Peninsular War against Napoleon in Spain, then spent a long period in India with his regiment, the 26th or 'Cameronian'. He was long acclimatized to the heat in which he developed his short temper, a love of rules, and a respect for rank, especially his own. He famously upbraided a visitor waiting at the veranda of his Hong Kong residence for not addressing him with the correct title. Caine maintained his 'old Calcutta style of living' by selling a bungalow he had built for himself to Dent & Co. as part of a private, uncatalogued purchase he had earlier made on the Queen's Road in front of Pedder's Hill.[184]

This house—described as 'a bungalow in a semi-Chinese style'—was the second brick building to be constructed by a colonist after Jardine Matheson's first godowns, and the first colonial house to be built.[185] It would eventually be absorbed into Dent & Co.'s magnificent garden of Green Bank and drawn by Edward Cree in 1845 (see **fig. 5.10**).

Consistent with his ease in adopting the local vernacular for a house style, Caine surrounded himself with local Chinese informants, and made dubious connections with some wealthy nouveau-riche immigrants such as the Tanka gambling boss Loo Aqui.[186] In the eyes of Chinese who first moved with the British to the Island, William Caine was the man in charge. When most of the British administration and the early European merchants were still living on boats offshore, Caine was busily involved in building the town both physically and socially. So, it was understandable that for any illiterate local living below, the symbolic authority of his dominant prison-magistracy compound inferred that as judge, juror, and jailer there was no other choice than to seek clemency or petition through his personage.

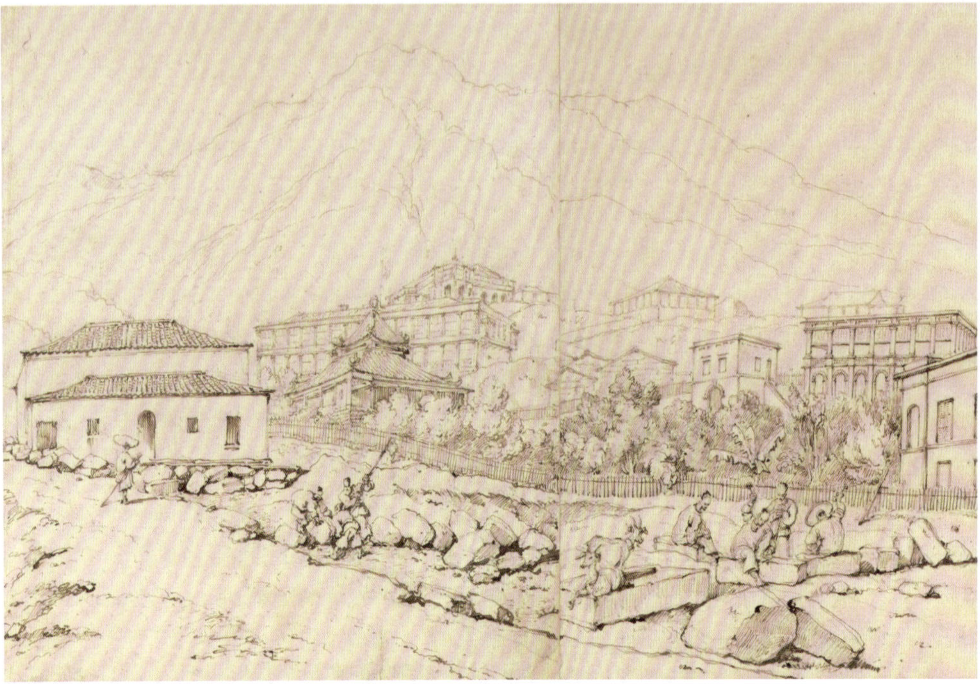

Fig. 2.19. G. Chinnery, 'Building on a Hillside in a Mountainous Village' (Caine's Chinese-style house with his magistracy and prison complex above), 1846. Graphite, pen, and brown ink.
© Yale Center for British Art (B1975.4.1064).

These unusual hybrid confections of Anglo-Chinese construction, such as Caine's, seemed to rise everywhere, providing useful political ammunition for Hong Kong's detractors. However, the conceptual bind these European critics found themselves in concerned the problem of how to apportion blame for the loss of semantic control over a western idiomatic style of architecture when, at the same time, westerners appropriated Chinese styles of architectural construction.[187] This blending served to confuse the lines of attack.

Some, blaming local labour, presumed that 'the bad taste displayed in the public as well as the private buildings' were due to the necessary haste in completing buildings in a climate where 'the want of professional architects allowed the Chinese bricklayers to display their art in the composite order, so as somewhat strangely to amalgamate their own predilections with the instructions given by their employers.'[188] *The Idler in Hong Kong* was one such anonymous and acerbic contributor to this debate. Spanning the course of three instalments in the *Canton Press* from mid-February to early March 1842, the *Idler* started by attacking the immorality of the settlement.

> If it be true, as I hold it that national character is evidenced by public buildings, I am puzzled to determine what is that of the Hongkongians, who have no forum, circus, agora, theatre and worse than all, no Temple of religious Worship. . . . If there be none of these, there *are* temples dedicated to the worship of Mercury, Morpheus and Venus; as is too obvious from their positions.[189]

Mercury was the god of wealth, commerce and, here, of thievery and gambling parlours. Morpheus, of sleep, here of narcotics and opium dens. Venus, of beauty, but also of sex and, here, of prostitution and brothels. In contrast, above the convenient temples of vice stood the inconvenient and remote servants of government. A building that had served as the rudimentary first Government House was now the Record Office and was 'so far removed that an *ardent* enquirer must, to arrive there, expose himself to risk of solar martyrdom'.[190] Caine's magistracy and prison, which included his own residence, also on a steep ascent above the town on the next ridge, pronounced itself so vividly in 'shades of Vitruvius, Palladio, and Wren, what can we say? How fitly express the utter disgust we feel at such monstrosities? . . . The magistracy—the mention of this mass of brick and stone, produces a feeling of nausea, so utterly revolting is it to every rule of good taste and fitness'. The Record Office, too, would not escape criticism. 'This edifice, moreover, boasts a pediment which is emblematically adorned, or rather hieroglyphically enriched; but the meaning thereof is wholly inexplicable to the builder and the Hongkong savans.'[191] He might just as well have been speaking of Alexander Johnston's own residence a little below it, where a later survey would record a confused side elevation of clearly local product, with the pediments over the upper windows a little too equilateral and the entire fenestration misaligned as the lower, upper, and even the parapet balustrade failed to follow the same unit of rhythm (**fig. 2.20**).[192]

This poor execution of a western classical façade signified more than just an unforgivable faux pas in taste. Coupled with the brothels and gambling dens below, it represented for certain critics a built manifestation of the lack of civility and care, indeed morality, of the governing elite. 'It is said', continued *Idler* in his verbal demolition of the Record Office, 'the Chinese artificer who executed it, was a wag, and that he has blazoned a sly hit at his obtuse and *barbaric* employers.'[193]

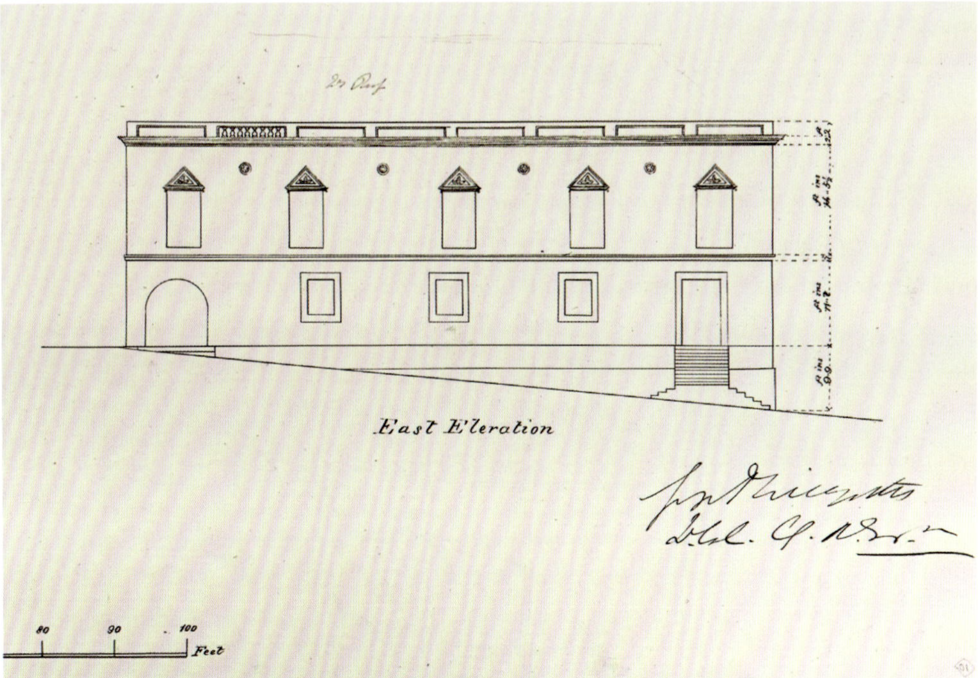

Fig. 2.20. Lt. Col. G. Phillpotts, Johnston's House, East Elevation, ca. 1842, in 'Phillpotts' Survey' (detail), 1847. Ink on paper. © The National Archives, Kew (MFQ 1/963).

In the line of fire, too, stood Jardine Matheson's first bungalow, constructed above their original godown, on Cantonment Hill. For *The Idler* this 'commanding site' stood 'disfigured by a hybrid erection, half New South Wales and half native production, and which is a foretaste of the architectural absurdities to be perpetrated on the Island'.[194] The bungalow, with its open Grecian veranda, built of course by Chinese, was dismissed in racist terms as 'a very feeble imitation of the rat trap and the bird cage orders'.[195] This, however, would not stop the future commander of British forces in China, Major-General Lord Saltoun, from happily moving in during the winter of 1842.

Only the Chinese shopkeepers of the Upper Bazaar, it seems, avoided the pitfalls of pretension and immorality. This was the first pair of streets in Hong Kong to be arranged perpendicular to the shoreline, climbing dramatically up the hillside. *Idler* praised the orderliness of this urbanism. The merchants having 'envinced in much good taste in their buildings, and if the plan in progress is carried out, the bazaar will soon surpass China Street in Canton; indeed, if the proposed width of the street is adhered to, with the sanitary regulations suggested: the China town at Hongkong will be among the most striking features of the new settlement'.[196]

There was, of course, pro-government propaganda to balance these attacks. In March 1842, the government gazette's license was granted to a new newspaper which soon moved its premises from Macau to Hong Kong—the first newspaper to do so. Entitled the *Friend of China*, it lost no time in distinguishing itself from its older rivals the *Canton Press* and the *Canton Register*, both pro-mercantilist broadsheets. In its second instalment, the *Friend* attacked the *Canton Press* as joined with a 'clique inimical to the interests of Hongkong'.[197] The *Press* was long noted for its vocal concerns about the unhealthiness of the settlement. This negative view was claimed by government factions to be a mark of anti-colonialism and a betrayal of Hong Kongers. The *Press*, infuriated, retorted:

> It is perfectly well known to every *impartial* person who has visited the island, that it is by no means the most desirable spot that could be chosen; the ground is nothing but a jumble of steep hills overtopping each other, and a very few valleys, with numerous ravines. The spot on which the town is building is sheltered from all southerly winds by the hills behind. . . . The heat in summer must be very great: and it will be a long while before any plantation near the town will give sufficient shade; for the island of Hongkong is now as bare of trees as Doctor Johnston represented Scotland to be.[198]

Having experienced a lack of cooling southerly breezes the previous summer, Hong Kong's settlers, most enduring their first winter, now complained of lying exposed to the piercingly cold northern winds, made worse by the sun setting behind the mountains before four o'clock.[199] In addition to the health risks, the very costs of building there—of levelling hills, diverting mountain streams, and the need to 'secure a foundation at great depth through quicksand'—were thought to be enormous.[200] Flawed though some of these perceptions were, especially about the sub-soil conditions of the island, within just the space of a year, Hong Kong's image darkened into a pestilential colony. Through the promulgation of such newspapers as the *Canton Press*, the island was gaining regional and international notoriety as an unhealthy and expensive concern for Britain. This tainted impression was to gain momentum over the next several years.

For those whose lives were intimately bound up in this adventure—including a melancholic writer to the *Canton Register* before his imminent departure—disease was an essential part of the settlement's charm.

> . . . Now night approaches, and the prong'd musquitoe,
> Flits round the candle as man follows fame;
> No rival insects in Madras or Quito
> Could use his powers with less fear of blame.[201]
> The rats gnaw hastily bamboos and planks,
> The house-top leaves are rustled with the wind,
> The frogs are croaking as by Indian tanks,—
> Oh, cruel fate—all this to leave behind!
>
> . . . Farewell, Hongkong—I never more shall plague you—
> No more shall tread your beach and grand parade,
> Except, perchance, some new and passing ague
> May lead back fancy to her China trade:
> And then in dreams, we three shall meet again,
> You, I, and old miasma—else, we sever,—
> But as I dread anticipating pain,
> Though pleasure follow—let us part for ever!
>
> —A Late Hong-Konian, 'At Sea', 14th March 1842.[202]

The writer records the regular nuisance of mosquitos in the first stanza but separates their actions from the colony's diseases in the second. So, it would remain—the cause disconnected from the effect—until the later rise and dominance of germ theory.

As we have seen, the fabrication of Hong Kong, and indeed it was a fabrication, involved the importation of almost all aspects of its cultural and physical life. A military presence was imported to provide protection and to assist in constructing the first toeholds upon the terrain. A Chinese labour force was imported to make the roads, level the ground, and reclaim the first strips of land. Surveyors were brought in to arrange the carving up of ill-considered plots for the purchase of commercial and private investors, by which a multitude of forms of construction were imported, from the makeshift mat-shed to the stately mansion. And with them came the shopkeepers, the gambling bosses, the publicans, and the prostitutes.

All these elements were predictable. What was not was the alchemy produced when the *imposed* intermixed with the *inherent*. Topography, orientation, climate, water, and vegetation were the raw elements of uncertainty. Ill-suited uniforms under a stifling heat, the fears of security balanced by hours of boredom trapped in small enclaves between the rocky fingers of mountains, and the subsequent habits and mood-swings of a fledgling community uncertain as to their roles and influences upon each other—these were the manufactured additions. However, there were other topographies, other terrains, such as those along the China coast, which exerted their influence upon Hong Kong's earliest development. Perhaps the most malignant and veiled influence was that of malaria. As will be shown, this accidental importation would, in the following year of 1843, help shape the perceptions and subsequent decisions of a variety of settler groups that would transform Hong Kong from a *collection* and into a *city*.

Notes

1 This, the most plausible of several theories, was first developed by Lo Hsiang-Lin, *1842 nian yi qian zhi Xianggang ji qi dui wai jiao tong* [*Hong Kong and Its External Communication before 1842*] (Hong Kong: Institute of Chinese Culture, 1959). See also Iu Kow-Choy, 'The Cultivation of the "Incense Tree" (Aquilaria Sinensis)', *Journal of the Hong Kong Branch of the Royal Asiatic Society* [hereafter *JHKBRAS*], vol. 23 (Hong Kong, 1983): 247–249.

2 Hal Empson, *Mapping Hong Kong: A Historical Atlas* (Hong Kong: Government Information Services, 1992), 22, 92. Dalrymple was aided in his discoveries by the earlier observations of Pedro Blanco made between 1759 and 1760.

3 There is speculation that the omission of this valuable information may have been deliberate.

4 Empson, *Mapping Hong Kong*, 23, 96.

5 Clarke Abel, *Narrative of a Journey in the Interior of China, and of a Voyage to and from that Country, in the Years 1816 and 1817* (London: Longman, Hurst, Rees, Orme, and Brown, 1818), 60.

6 Ibid., 60–63.

7 E. J. Eitel, *Europe in China: The History of Hong Kong from the Beginning to the Year 1882* (Hong Kong: Kelly and Walsh; London: Luzac & Co., 1895), 131.

8 Ibid., 132.

9 Ibid.

10 Ibid.

11 Ibid., 133.

12 Ibid., 168.

13 'Art. V. Notices of Hongkong: Situation, Shape and Extent of the Island . . .', *Chinese Repository*, vol. 14, no. 6 (June 1845): 293.

14 Ibid.

15 See the first iteration of Captain Sir Edward Belcher's 1841 map.

16 Ibid.

17 Eitel, *Europe in China*, 134. Dafydd Emrys Evans, however, thinks that this road was imagined by Eitel possibly as a means of justifying the local name given to the hamlet and the north shore: Dafydd M. E. Evans, 'The Foundation of Hong Kong: A Chapter of Accidents', in Marjorie Topley, ed., *Hong Kong: The Interaction of Traditions and Life in the Towns* (Hong Kong: Hong Kong Branch of the Royal Asiatic Society, 1975), 15.

18 D. McPherson, M.D., *Two Years in China: Narrative of the Chinese Expedition from its Formation in April, 1840, till April, 1842* (London: Saunders and Otley, 1842), 79–80; and as quoted in Evans, 'The Foundation of Hong Kong', 13.

19 *Canton Press*, 15 Jan. 1842.

20 Evans, 'The Foundation of Hong Kong', 18.

21 This can be seen when comparing similar advertisements posted by the American merchant C. V. Gillespie in the *Canton Press*, 17 July 1841 and 7 Aug. 1841.

22 *Canton Press*, 3 July 1841.

23 James Legge, 'The Colony of Hong Kong—From a Lecture by the Rev. James Legge, D.D., L.L.D., on Reminiscences of a Long Residence in the East, Delivered in the City Hall, November 5, 1872', *The China Review*, vol. 3 (1874): 164.

24 William Tarrant, *Hongkong Part 1: 1839 to 1844* (Canton: Friend of China, 1861), 33.

25 Eitel, *Europe in China*, 148. The earlier commencement of road construction can be verified through the watercolour studies of naval surgeon Edward Cree R.N. in Apr. 1841 (see below).

26 Tarrant, *Hongkong*, 33.

27 Ibid. This pass is now the eastern termination of Queen's Road East and not to be confused with the Wong Nai Chung Gap, above and south of the valley, which would be opened at about the same time.

28 Tarrant, *Hongkong*, 33.

29 *Canton Register*, 7 Dec. 1841.

30 Ibid.

31 *Canton Press*, 15 Jan. 1842.

32 *Canton Press*, 26 Feb. 1842.

33 National Maritime Museum, Greenwich, London [hereafter NMM], CRJ/5, 'Private Journal of E. H. Cree', 22, dated Wed., 28 Apr. 1841. See also Edward H. Cree, *Naval Surgeon: The Voyages of Dr.*

Edward H. Cree, Royal Navy as Related in His Private Journals, 1837–1856, ed. Michael Levien (New York: E. P. Dutton, 1981), 79.

34 CRJ/5, 21–22; *Voyages*, 78–79.

35 *Canton Press*, 15 Jan. 1842.

36 Cree, *The Voyages*, 79.

37 Frank Welsh, *A History of Hong Kong*, rev. ed. (London: Harper Collins, 1997), 134.

38 *Canton Register*, 11 May 1841.

39 Tarrant, *Hongkong*, 39. John Ouchterlony would go on to become the 'first historian' of Britain's war with China, with his jingoistic work *The Chinese War: An Account of All the Operations of the British Forces from the Commencement to the Treaty of Nanking* (London: Saunders and Otley, 1844).

40 Cambridge University Library, Jardine Matheson Archives [hereafter JMA]; C6/3, A. Matheson to J. Jejeebhoy, Bombay (Macau, 15 May 1843).

41 *Hongkong Register*, 1 Oct. 1844.

42 Gary Chi-Hung Luk, 'Occupied Space, Occupied Time: Food Hawking and the Central Market in Hong Kong's Victoria City During the Opium War', *Frontiers of History in China*, vol. 11, no. 3 (2016): 414.

43 Ibid., 416.

44 JMA; C5/6, J. Matheson to W. Jardine, London (Macau, 15 Jan. 1841).

45 JMA; C5/6, J. Matheson to J. Jejeebhoy, Bombay (Macau, 16 Jan. 1841). Matheson wrote this a day after his letter to Jardine.

46 Lindsay and May Ride, *An East India Company Cemetery: Protestant Burials in Macao* (Hong Kong: Hong Kong University Press, 1996), 4.

47 Tarrant, *Hongkong*, 11.

48 Ibid., 2.

49 JMA; C5/7, A. Matheson to J. Jejeebhoy, Bombay (Macau, 28 May 1841).

50 Tarrant, *Hongkong*, 14.

51 Ibid., 13.

52 JMA; C6/2, A. Matheson to J. Ouchterlony, Hong Kong (Macau, 26 Mar. 1842).

53 Tarrant, *Hongkong*, 14.

54 JMA; C5/7, J. Matheson to J. Jejeebhoy, Bombay (Macau, 19 June 1841).

55 JMA; C5/7, J. Matheson to W. Jardine, London (Macau, 23 Aug. 1841).

56 JMA; C5/7, J. Matheson to W. Jardine, London (Macau, 3 July 1841).

57 *Canton Press*, 23 Oct 1841, as translated from a Chinese public notice.

58 JMA; C5/7, J. Matheson to J. Jejeebhoy, Bombay (Macau, 7 Aug. 1841).

59 JMA; C5/7, J. Matheson to J. W. Henderson, Bombay (Macau, 19 June 1841).

60 JMA; C6/2, A. Matheson to J. Jejeebhoy, Bombay (Macau, 12 Jan. 1842).

61 Jonathan Andrew Farris, *Enclave to Urbanity: Canton, Foreigners, and Architecture from the Late Eighteenth to the Early Twentieth Centuries* (Hong Kong: Hong Kong University Press, 2016), note for plate 14.

62 *Canton Register*, 4 May 1841.

63 *Canton Register*, 31 Aug. 1841. Also noted by G. R. Sayer, *Hong Kong 1841–1862: Birth, Adolescence and Coming of Age* (London: Oxford University Press, 1937), 114.

64 Tarrant, *Hongkong*, 19.

65 Ibid., 41.

66 *Canton Press*, 17 July 1841.

67 *Canton Register*, 14 Sep. 1841. Advertisement dated 6 Sep. 1841.

68 *Canton Register*, 25 Jan. 1842. Advertisement dated 18 Jan. 1842.

69 *Canton Press*, 26 Feb. 1842.

70 *Canton Press*, 26 Mar. 1842. Advertisement dated 21 Mar. 1842.

71 *Canton Press*, 30 Apr. 1842. Advertisement dated 28 Apr. 1842.

72 *Canton Press*, 23 Aug. 1842. Advertisement dated 12 July 1842.

73 *Canton Press*, 16 July 1842. Advertisement dated 23 Feb. 1842, which reads 'GOODS and MERCHANDISE of all descriptions, received and carefully stored, in spacious, dry and secure Brick Gowdowns, at Hongkong . . . C. FEARON,—Macao'.

74 William C. Hunter, *The 'Fan Kwae' at Canton before Treaty Days 1825–1844* (Shanghai: Oriental Affairs, 1882), 12. For a recent and rich account of enclave life for western traders in Canton, see Farris, *Enclave to Urbanity*.

75 Shelia E. Hamilton, *Watching over Hong Kong: Private Policing 1841–1941* (Hong Kong: Hong Kong University Press, 2008), 33–35. As Hamilton describes, life as a member of Jardine's private 'East Point Police' was a very dangerous affair.

76 Carl T. Smith, *A Sense of History: Studies in the Social and Urban History of Hong Kong* (Hong Kong: Hong Kong Educational Publishing Co., 1995), 116–117.

77 Legge, 'The Colony of Hong Kong', 164.

78 *Canton Register*, 7 Dec. 1841.

79 Ibid.

80 There is confusion among historians as to whether this area should be correctly named 'Upper Bazaar' or 'Middle Bazaar'. Carl T. Smith preferred the latter based upon a categorisation by the Rev. Charles Gützlaff in his 1844 census (See Smith, *A Sense of History*, 41–47). 'Upper Bazaar' in his mind was an area of shacks, many illegally constructed, to the west above Lower Bazaar and approximately clustered around the sites of the Lower and Upper Lascar Rows (shown as Lot no. 70 on the Edwards–de Havilland Survey, 1843). However, considering most primary references such as government documents, surveys, and newsprint, use the former name 'Upper Bazaar', I prefer to adopt this.

81 *Canton Press*, 19 June 1841. The outlay was to be no less than a value of one thousand dollars.

82 *Canton Register*, 21 Dec. 1841, and (*Supplement to*) 11 Jan. 1842.

83 Christopher Cowell, 'Borrowed Verses: Code and Representation Within the First Travelogue of the City of Hong Kong, 1841–42', in Eleonora Sasso, ed., *Late Victorian Orientalism: Representations of the East in Nineteenth-Century Literature, Art and Culture from the Pre-Raphaelites to John La Farge* (London: Anthem Press, 2020), 133–162.

84 *Canton Register*, 21 Dec. 1841.

85 'The reports of most weight are that Howqua now says there is no chance of a peaceful settlement—that they are blocking up the river at Howqua's fort, halfway between Canton and Whampoa, that there is a large body of troops under mat sheds in front of the factories—all the above may be considered authentic.' JMA; C5/6, J. Matheson to James Adam Smith, Manila (Macau, 18 Feb. 1841).

86 'Art. VIII. Some Account of Her Majesty's Twenty-Sixth, or Cameronian Regiment, from Its Formation to the Present Time', *The Chinese Repository*, vol. 12, no. 3 (Mar. 1843): 160–161.

87 *Canton Press*, 15 Jan. 1842.

88 *Canton Register*, 21 Dec. 1841.

89 Hong Kong Public Records Office [hereafter HKPRO]; file: HKMS 140-1-1, 'Transcripts of Correspondence of Lieut. Thomas Bernard Collinson R.E.', Dec. 1838–29 Mar. 1846 [hereafter 'Transcripts'], Collinson to Mrs. Collinson, Boldon Rectory, Gateshead (Hong Kong, 23 Nov. 1845).

90 Ibid.

91 *Canton Register*, 11 Jan. 1842.

92 Ibid.

93 Ibid.

94 Ibid.

95 Ibid.

96 *Canton Register*, 11 May 1841.

97 Ibid.

98 Ibid.

99 *Canton Press*, 10 July 1841.

100 *Canton Register*, 11 May 1841.

101 Ibid.

102 Ibid.

103 *Canton Register*, 4 Jan. 1842.

104 Ibid.

105 Ibid.

106 *Canton Press*, 8 May 1841.

107 Ibid.

108 *Canton Press*, 12 June 1841.

109 Ibid.

110 *Canton Press*, 19 June 1841. The *Press* states 'thirty-two', but in fact thirty-four were knocked down the following Monday. The annual quit rent was likewise incorrectly stated as £3,116 instead of £3,272. 10s. See Sayer, *Hong Kong 1841–62*, 204–205.

111 To add to the confusion as to exact plot numbers sold, Ho Pui-Yin disagrees with this figure arguing that 'Pottinger's Map' (1842) together with the 1886–1887 report of the Hong Kong Land Commission demonstrated that 404 lots were auctioned: 39 Marine lots, 75 Town lots, 22 Suburban lots and 268 Bazaar lots. See Ho Pui-Yin, *Challenges for an Evolving City: 160 Years of Port and Land Development in Hong Kong* (Hong Kong: The Commercial Press, 2004), 26. This, however, does not tie with contemporary sources on the auction itself. It is much more likely that the 1842 map combines the first auction with subsequent land sales added to by Johnston, for which there is ample evidence of his activities; for instance, as encapsulated in the list of lots sold by the government from 1841 to 1843. See The National Archives, Kew [hereafter NA]; Colonial Office [hereafter CO] 129/2: 152–175.

112 Evans, 'The Foundation', 37.

113 *Canton Register*, 29 June 1841.

114 *Canton Press*, 26 Feb. 1842.

115 *Canton Press*, 26 June 1841.

116 *Canton Press*, 3 July 1841.

117 Ibid.

118 Dafydd M. E. Evans, 'The Foundations of Hong Kong: A Chapter of Accidents', in Marjorie Topley, ed., *Hong Kong: The Interaction of Traditions and Life in the Towns* (Hong Kong: Hong Kong Branch of the Royal Asiatic Society, 1975), 37.

119 Ibid.

120 *Canton Press*, 26 Feb. 1842.

121 Ibid. Or to be more precise, 14 feet by 36 feet, the size calculated for annual rents. See CO 129/2: 175. The number of houses is listed from this source.

122 Tarrant, *Hongkong*, 41. See also CO 129/2: 175.

123 CO 129/2: 175. However, the *Canton Press* confuses this with the annual rent for the Upper Bazaar. See *Canton Press*, 26 Feb. 1842.

124 *Canton Press*, 26 Feb. 1842.

125 Sayer, *Hong Kong 1841–1862*, 116, 118, 123. Pottinger's first stay on the island was from 21 to 22 Aug. 1841 returning to Hong Kong on 1 Feb. 1842.

126 CO 129/5: 143, 'Detailed Account Disbursements of the Land Department from June 1841 to January 1844—Military and Naval'.

127 Tarrant, *Hongkong*, 29.

128 Ibid.; *Canton Register*, 5 Oct. 1841. The 1842 map (NA; FO 925/2427) would become known as 'Pottinger's Map'. See Empson, *Mapping Hong Kong*, 160–161.

129 *Canton Press*, 19 Feb. 1842.

130 *Canton Press*, 12 Feb. 1842; Tarrant, *Hongkong*, 33.

131 Tarrant, *Hongkong*, 33.

132 *Canton Press*, 16 Apr. 1842.

133 *Canton Press*, 26 Mar. 1842.

134 Tarrant, *Hongkong*, 34.

135 *Friend of China*, 1 June 1844; Evans, 'The Foundation', 29. Evans does not distinguish between Malcolm's proposed widths of the main and cross arteries.

136 *Canton Press*, 12 Feb. 1842.

137 *Friend of China*, 24 Mar. 1842.

138 JMA; C6/2, A. Matheson to R. W. Crawford, Bombay (Macau, 2 Mar. 1842).

139 *Canton Press*, 30 Apr. 1842.

140 *Canton Register*, 10 May 1842 (The verse is dated 27 Apr. 1842).

141 JMA; C6/2, A. Matheson to Thomas Charles Smith, London (Macau, 10 May 1842).

142 *Canton Press*, 20 Aug. 1842 (Langer's advertisement is dated at Macau, 11 Aug. 1842).

143 *Canton Register*, 22 Nov. 1842.

144 JMA; C6/3, A. Matheson to John Lyall, Calcutta (Macau, 31 Oct. 1842).

145 Ibid.

146 *Canton Register*, 22 Feb. 1842.

147 Eitel, *Europe in China*, 177.

148 JMA; C6/3, A. Matheson to John Purvis, Singapore (Macau, 14 Jan. 1843).

149 CO 129/1: 267, Estimate of Expenses—1842 China Expedition, Treasury Chambers, 16 June 1842.

150 *Canton Press*, 23 Jan. 1841.

151 CO 129/1: 248a.

152 CO 129/2: 79.

153 CO 129/1: 257–258.

154 JMA; C6/2, A. Matheson to John Abel Smith, London (Macau, 3 June 1842).

155 CO 129/1: 163. As reported by Captain Eades (39th MNI) the Station Staff Officer for Hong Kong from 1 Aug. to 27 Oct. 1842 to the Court of Inquiry.

156 CO 129/1: 258.
157 CO 129/1: 153a–154a.
158 CO 129/1: 144–146a.
159 CO 129/13: 352, Davis to Stanley, 16 Dec. 1845, enclosing a copy of a recent article from the *Hongkong Register.*
160 CO 129/1: 118a, Gough to Pottinger, 7 Oct. 1842.
161 'Native' was the contemporary British military category for troops originating from their Asian colonies. For Hong Kong these generally referred to soldiers from India, Ceylon (Sri Lanka), and Malaya.
162 Ibid.
163 For information as to Pottinger's previous experience, see G. B. Endacott, *A Biographical Sketch-Book of Early Hong Kong* (Singapore: Eastern Universities Press, 1962), 14.
164 For instance, see Mark Harrison, 'Disease and Medicine in the Armies of British India, 1750–1830: The Treatment of Fevers and the Emergence of Tropical Therapeutics', in Geoffrey L. Hudson, ed., *British Military and Naval Medicine, 1600–1830*, Clio Medica, vol. 81 (Amsterdam, New York: Rodopi, 2007), 94.
165 CO 129/1: 120, Pottinger to Gough, 10 Oct. 1842.
166 Ibid., 120a.
167 *Canton Press*, 20 Aug. 1842.
168 Harrison, 'Disease and Medicine in the Armies of British India, 1750–1830', 94.
169 CO 129/1: 147, 'Proceedings of the Court of Inquiry', 29 Nov. 1842.
170 Ibid., 148.
171 The origin of the name remains contentious. See Alfred Y. K. Lau, 'An Outline of the Urban Development of Sai Ying Pun in the Nineteenth Century', *JHKBRAS*, vol. 35 (Hong Kong, 1995): 59–73.
172 Eitel, *Europe in China*, 175. The West Point buildings of 1843 before their demolition must have been substantial in that, as Eitel described in the 1890s, 'the cantonment lines can still be traced'.
173 CO 129/1: 147a, 'Proceedings'.
174 Ibid., 148a.
175 Ibid., 149.
176 Ibid., 149–150.
177 Ibid., 164.
178 'Art. VIII. Some Account of Her Majesty's Twenty-Sixth', 160–161, 166.
179 CO 129/1: 166, 'Proceedings'.
180 Ibid., 166–167a.
181 'Art. V. Notices of Hongkong', 291–298.
182 This initial palisade is noticeable both on the first plate of Ouchterlony, *The Chinese War*; and on a very early trade painting of the island probably dated 1842 (see fig. 3.9) entitled 'Hong Kong from Kowloon'.
183 *Canton Register*, 4 May 1841.
184 Tarrant, *Hongkong*, 44. The plot was one of Johnston's disbursements.
185 Tarrant, *Hongkong*, 14; Sayer, *Hong Kong 1841–1862*, 117–118.
186 Also spelt as Lu Aqui or Lo Aqui.
187 An added implication was that such dubious interblending was a symptom of the worst mercantile traits carried from Canton to Hong Kong. As Edward Denison and Guang Yu Ren note: 'By the 19th century, most of the factories [in Canton] were of a style that acquired the epithet "compradoric", an essentially derogatory term applied to the style that evolved from the merchants' best efforts at design, but was

evidently devoid of the architect's hand.' See Edward Denison and Guang Yu Ren, *Modernism in China: Architectural Visions and Revolutions* (Chichester, West Sussex: John Wiley & Sons, 2008), 36.

188 *Canton Press*, 19 Feb. 1842.

189 Ibid.

190 Ibid.

191 Ibid.

192 NA; MFQ 1/963 (War Office [hereafter WO] 44/593), Survey by Lieut. Colonel Phillpotts, entitled: *Plans &c. of a House, the property of A. R. Johnston Esq., proposed to be purchased by the Ordnance*, 29 Nov. 1847.

193 *Canton Press*, 19 Feb. 1842.

194 The identification of *Idler*'s target is corroborated by Colin N. Crisswell, *The Taipans: Hong Kong's Merchant Princes* (Hong Kong: Oxford University Press, 1981), 61.

195 *Canton Press*, 19 Feb. 1842.

196 Ibid.

197 As reprinted in the *Canton Press*, 26 Mar. 1842.

198 Ibid.

199 *Canton Press*, 26 Feb. 1842.

200 *Canton Press*, 26 Mar. 1842.

201 This is a curious line. It suggests that there was a possible awareness that the mosquito contributed to illness, despite the prevalence of miasma theory in explaining the causes of malaria. Yet this line also absolves the island insect.

202 *Canton Register*, 26 Apr. 1842.

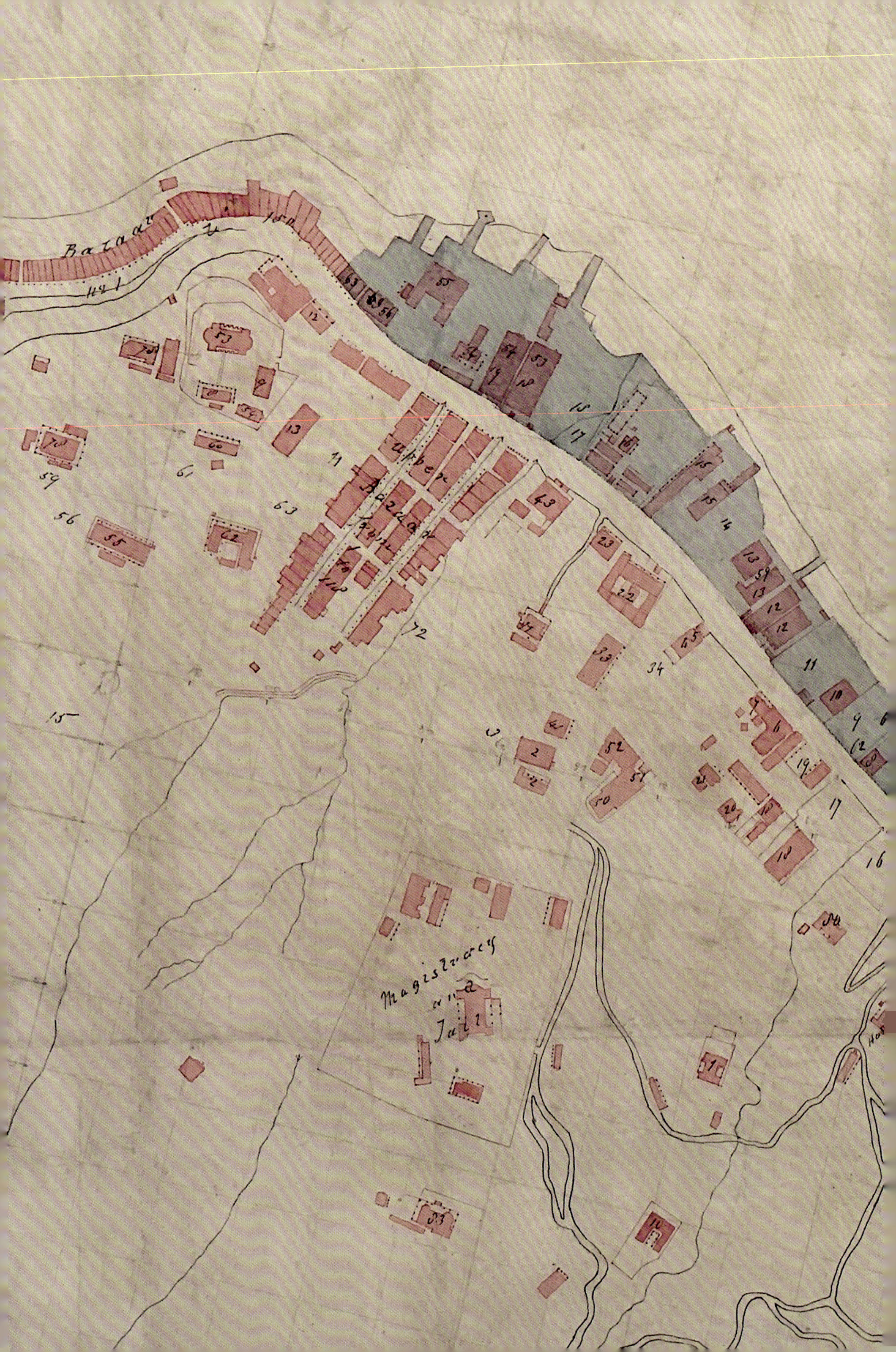
Bazaar
Upper Bazaar
Magistracy and Jail

CHAPTER 3

A Town Redrawn, 1843–1844

> Although I was charmed with the general appearance of the place, and the energy that was manifest in laying out the ground and pushing on building, I found many of the residents oppressed with gloom because of its unhealthiness. 1843 was, no doubt, a very sickly year, more so, perhaps, than any one has been since.
>
> —Reverend James Legg's lecture at City Hall, Hong Kong, 1872.[1]

The first milestone in Hong Kong's urban history marked a tragic pause in the growth of the young settlement. It fell during the tempestuous year of 1843 when malaria became an epidemic. This chapter explores this rupture, just over a year in the life of the new city colony named 'Victoria', from the early months of 1843 to the spring of 1844. Though a short period, it was of such significance for Hong Kong's early development that a degree of attention is needed.

As often the way with critical events in history, 1843 was both a year of celebration and a year of crisis, the two phases following in rapid succession. The first half was shaped by eager anticipation among both British and Chinese settlers for news of a ratified treaty with China, agreed in Nanking (Nanjing), which was duly exchanged in June. The second half was racked by a pestilence so severe that the very future of the colony seemed to be at stake. This time, it earned itself the sobriquet the 'Hongkong Fever' and dragged off with it about twenty-four per cent of the military garrison (generally British and South Asian personnel) and ten per cent of the European civilian population.[2] No firm data exists on Chinese civilians, but fragmentary evidence suggests comparable casualties. Yet both events conjoined into a single programmatic impulse. For, through them, the temporariness of Hong Kong, both physically and mentally, was swept away and in its place, for the first time, arose a coherent civic plan, a civic voice, and the confident alignment of an architectural and municipal grammar upon the island's peculiar topography.

From 'Old Warriors' to 'Queen's People'

The boom in construction during the latter half of 1842 alarmed Sir Henry Pottinger. It was a speculative rush caused by anticipation that London would soon accept the terms of a formal treaty with China. The more solidified the city of Victoria became, the harder it would be for him to untangle legitimate claims from illegitimate and assert whatever land-leasing policy the British government sought fit to impose upon the new crown colony. Alexander Johnston, his deputy superintendent, was continuing to disburse land quietly. So, following the initial signing of the Nanking Treaty in August 1842, Pottinger, its chief negotiator and co-signee, despatched a letter to Johnston in Hong Kong on 7th September.

> The confirmation of the cession of the Island of Hongkong to H.M. The Queen of England by the Emperor of China will no doubt have the effect of adding greatly to the value of land of all kinds on the Island and will make Individuals more desirous than even formerly, of obtaining grants on any terms. . . . I accordingly beg you will be so good as to decline to listen to any applications for allotments except those that are especially provided for in my instructions to you.[3]

Among his exemptions were the further construction of barracks, hospitals, and storehouses to meet the returning troops' needs from the China campaign, many sickly. However, all other applications were to be declined until Pottinger received instructions from Whitehall.

1843 began with keen anticipation from those fortunate enough to acquire a toehold on the island. Unfortunately, this air of optimism dissipated as the year went by. On 18 March, Lieutenant-Colonel George Malcolm, a man the entire colony had been waiting for, returned. As secretary of legation to Her Majesty's Special Mission in China, Malcolm had rushed to England carrying his precious cargo. He now returned on board H.M. Steamer *Vixen* clutching the ratified Treaty of Nanking signed by Queen Victoria.[4] The settler community was euphoric. Pottinger, at last, knew that the British Government intended to retain Hong Kong. In a letter dated 4 January, the foreign secretary, the Earl of Aberdeen, informed him that 'you will assume the Government of the Island of Hong Kong, then become a Possession of the British Crown, and you will make such Proclamation'.[5] Moreover, the Crown was so adamant in its claim that Aberdeen made it clear to Pottinger that Britain would defend its new possession even if Emperor Daoguang reneged in co-ratifying the treaty.[6] The Foreign Office's primary concern now was the defence of the island and the troops' health. The latter issue had rung alarm bells across Whitehall for the last two years and proved a severe embarrassment to the foreign secretary. 'You will be careful', he continued, 'to select positions for the Barracks which are most likely to be healthy, and you will not allow any building to be raised by private persons which can at all impede the circulation of air in the neighbourhood of the Barracks, or interfere with the free movement of troops if their services should be required.'[7] Aberdeen believed that a carefully planned layout of the city would significantly contribute towards maintaining a healthy settlement, crucial during this early and vulnerable stage. He warned that great care was to be taken in demarcating lots to private interests, as ample space had to be provided for streets, ensuring good ventilation. This measure would prevent 'the evil consequences which might ensue from too crowded an occupation'.[8]

As it happened, the Emperor this time did not decline ratification. Still, a delay occurred in the exchange of ratified treaties due to the untimely death of Imperial Commissioner Yilibu (named 'Elepoo' by the British), as well as some ongoing negotiations related to revising the trade tariff.[9] Yilibu's successor was the Chinese negotiator of the Nanking Treaty, Pottinger's counterpart, Special Commissioner Qiying (spelt by the British as 'Keying'). His imperial promotion was declared at the beginning of May, and by 4 June he arrived at Canton (Guangzhou) with his entourage. Qiying, the new imperial commissioner, was conveyed from Canton on H.M. Steamer *Akbar*, one of the largest and fastest steamers yet built, and evidently chosen to impress.[10] In the midst of 'much sickness prevailing at Hongkong on shore and afloat', he arrived in Victoria Harbour on 23 June, setting foot for possibly the first time in his life upon, what was technically now, foreign soil.[11] He descended upon a temporary jetty constructed for his arrival and was greeted by cheering crowds among whom gathered the disembarked passengers of four Chinese war junks, his mandarins and servants who had arrived a few days before him.[12] The jetty was not the only thing builders had hastily constructed. The first government house on Government Hill, a single-storey bungalow, had been quickly erected in preparation for his visit, as was Qiying's accommodation somewhat below it, 'a neat new building rented for them specially by Sir Henry'.[13] The exchanges of the ratified treaties took place on 26 June 1843, exactly two years and five months after Commander Belcher had first hoisted the Union flag at Possession Point (**fig. 3.1**).

At that moment, Sir Henry Pottinger became the first 'Governor and Commander in Chief' of Hong Kong, and the young city was now officially entitled to the name 'Victoria'.[14] Exchanges of hospitality also occurred during Qiying's short stay. Pottinger held a large dinner party in his honour. The Chinese aristocrat returned the favour by 'singing several Tartar songs, one of which he was heard to say was taught him by the

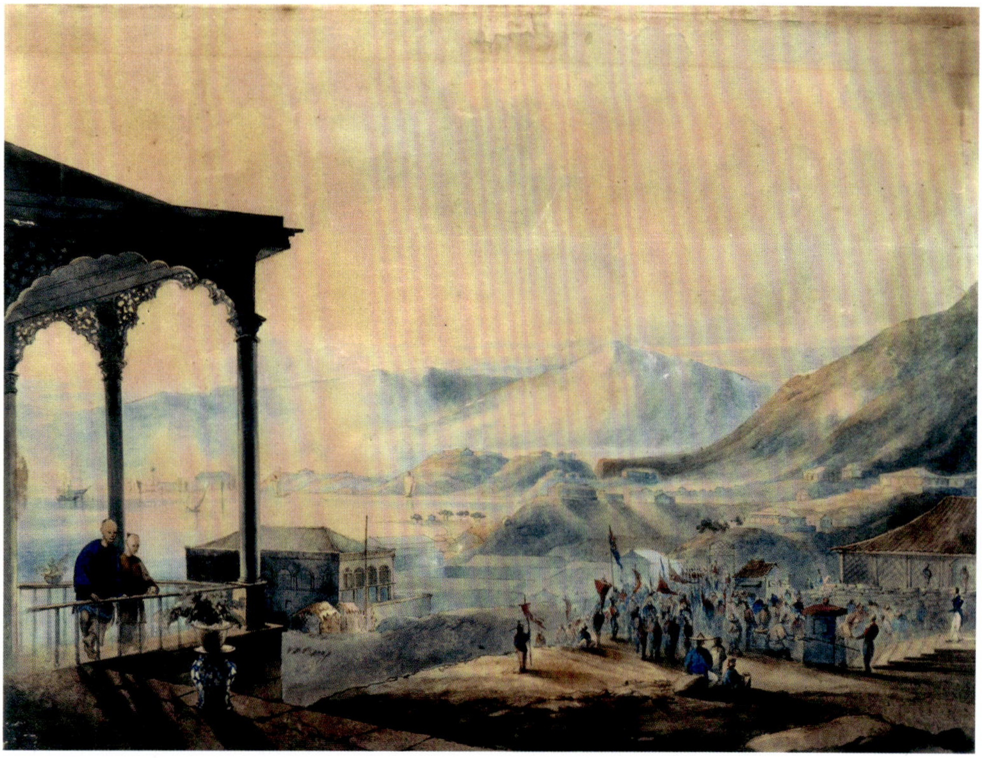

Fig. 3.1. Anon., Qiying Is Met by Pottinger at Government House, 26 June 1843. Watercolour. © Hong Kong Museum of Art Collection (AH1971.0001).

present Emperor's father'.[15] Finally, before he departed, Qiying was treated to a tour by boat around the island, and officiated in a remarkable opening ceremony—a short trip by Phaeton carriage through the newly constructed passage, 'The Gap'. It was a feat of engineering, despite its modest distance, that, for the first time, irrevocably linked the Wong Nai Chung Valley to the rest of the city by road and thereby, at a stroke, opened the city to the existing passes extending to the south side of the island.[16]

Now that the British government had decided to retain Hong Kong, the first thing that had to be solved by the London administration regarded streamlining various paths of communication and chains of authority for the future governor. Pottinger, before the treaty, had been plenipotentiary and superintendent of trade, receiving instructions from both the Colonial Office and Foreign Office (Lord Stanley and the Earl of Aberdeen respectively) and military instructions from the governor-general of India, the Earl of Auckland. Since Pottinger was to become governor of a crown colony, James Stephen, permanent under-secretary to the colonial secretary, wrote to his counterpart Henry Unwin Addington at the Foreign Office now urging the necessity of a single line of communication, preferably through his office, the Colonial Office. He offered to be a conduit, where necessary, to all the relevant parties.[17] In addition, this letter for the first time laid ground rules for the granting of land, and would be cited as guidance by other divisions within the London government such as the Colonial Land and Emigration Office, a consultative body advising upon policies of migration and land grants across the Empire.[18] These guidelines recommended that Pottinger first, 'abstain from alienating any of the Land in the Island, either in perpetuity or for any term, of greater length than may be necessary to induce & enable the Tenants to erect substantial buildings'.[19] This was especially true for land that might be in the most critical positions around the town, thereby restricting its future growth, or would likely be needed for 'military defences, . . . public works of utility, or ornament or public recreation'.[20]

James Stephen proposed that since Hong Kong would become a 'free port', it was essential to identify the principal means of generating local government revenue. In his opinion, this meant taxation of land 'as one of the chief means of maintaining the local Establishment'.[21] He even confessed a belief that the crown land of Hong Kong would soon fetch as high a price as that along London's Regent Street.[22] Finally, before any future land sales under these principles could be initiated, it was essential to establish the legal foundations of current land ownership. This measure was a particularly delicate concern for Stephen, as he wryly observed, 'It is a very perilous thing to enter into any engagement, express or implied, with mercantile people, without first weighing most maturely the terms of it'.[23] Stephen, therefore, sought an agreement with Stanley that a land census could be conducted, that 'an enquiry should be instituted by some competent and impartial authority in the equitable claims of all holders of Land to a confirmation, either permanent or temporary of their titles . . . with a just regard to the interests of society at large'.[24] This shrewd request would find incarnation that year in the form of Pottinger's independent Land Grants Committee. The committee would conduct a comprehensive review of land conveyancing, classification, and also determine paths of future growth. Such patterns, combined with the worst outbreak of fever yet encountered, would determine areas of population intensity and zones for urban development for at least the next decade.

Under pressure from the Foreign Office and with agreement from the Treasury, Stanley despatched a Royal Engineer to Hong Kong that spring to oversee and coordinate all the military works.[25] While the Foreign Office was determined to construct suitable barracks as fast as possible, it was in the Treasury's interest to ensure that this was done efficiently and economically (though a soldier's life would remain more costly than the price of dressed granite). The man sent was to profoundly affect the progress and design of both military construction and almost every element of the public works in Hong Kong for the next four years. Major Edward Aldrich R.E. sailed from Southampton on the wooden paddle steamer *Great Liverpool*, making Alexandria in eighteen days. He then travelled by various steam packets and horse omnibus to Cairo and the Suez. On his eventual arrival in Hong Kong on 10 June 1843, Aldrich wrote to the inspector-general of fortifications (IGF), Lieutenant-General Sir Frederick Mulcaster, conveying his initial views of the island. The major could see Hong Kong's potential. The city's rudimentary layout was clear enough, with its 'factories' (storehouses) and dwellings. But it needed order and discipline, something to be imposed amid a climate of disease and criminality.[26] Since such order was lacking, Aldrich was just the sort of man who was willing to impose it.

Meanwhile, Lieutenant John Ouchterlony, Hong Kong's chief military engineer, arrived back to the colony just in time for a nasty surprise. Landing from Manila with a large consignment of timbers for the public works, including around Cantonment Hill and in Chek Chue, he suddenly found himself out of a job.[27] Aldrich had immediately taken command, assuming the title of 'Commanding Royal and Superintending

Engineer'.[28] This was the first significant transfer of power in Hong Kong from the experienced Indian officers and troops, the veterans of the China Expedition, to the new forces sent directly from England, and it was a sign of the changing times. Two years later, Aldrich's understudy, the young Lieutenant Thomas Bernard Collinson, writing to his sister, would sadly reflect,

> The first generation of colonists from India have all left but one or two; many of them as I feel to my loss, dead: and their place has been supplied throughout all branches civil & military from England. The few old warriors look down upon the innovators & their improvements, like men who have been to Nankin; but the innovators themselves, dig drains, lay out streets & give names to places, establish London policemen from A to Z, keep lamp-lighters & lamps to light & won't look at the old warriors at all. This is the state of affairs in China—The English party in an agony to alter & amend everything & the Indian party vowing that everything was perfect before the 'Queen's people' as they call them, came.[29]

Under the Indian system, Ouchterlony had been supported by executive and assistant engineers, their salaries linked to their status and qualifications. A company of the Madras Sappers and Miners had, in turn, helped these officers.[30] As with the civil authorities, command lines had been muddied. Both London and Calcutta shared the power of instructions. But since military salaries were received in rupees from India, it was obvious which side possessed preeminent control. This arrangement was now reversed. The Madras Engineers were to be replaced by a detachment of the Royal Sappers and Miners, two civilian clerks of works, and three foremen of works to be directly commanded by the Board of Ordnance in London through the IGF, himself a member of the board.[31] Direct control from London upon approaches and expenditure of military works had tightened.

The arrival of new military personnel was not the only transfusion of blood from the British Isles. Since news of the treaty's signing, British newspapers were filled with events in China and the anticipated prosperity of the new colony it had acquired. Numbers of artisans, skilled labourers, mechanics, and junior clerks set off for Hong Kong, confident of finding lucrative work. Unwelcome job applications inundated Lord Stanley. These included a shoemaker from Edinburgh enquiring on the likelihood of 'mechanics' being needed, and a London-based draughtsman-cum-surveyor who had passed his 'examination at Woolwich "Academy"' and felt suited to join the Royal Engineers or Artillery at the new colony.[32] Needless to say, the applications of these individuals, in the main, were politely but firmly declined.

Following Britain's decision to keep Hong Kong, an accurate survey of the entire island was felt needed. It is unclear whether Thomas Bernard Collinson had been hand-picked or volunteered for this task. His brother Richard 'Dick' Collinson, a noted hydrographer, was already in China and had charted the soundings around Hong Kong Island with Commander Belcher in 1841.[33] But judging by the extraordinary draughtsmanship and attention to detail with which he prepared the 1845 'Ordnance Map of Hong Kong' and the accompanying 'Ten Outline Sketches' of the island, Bernard was already marked as a rising talent. Barely in his twenties, he had recently worked in Kilkenny on the 'Survey of Ireland' project, employing the latest techniques in recording height by using the contour line.[34] 'They have just sent me more Patts to drill into contourers,' he wrote to his father.[35] The young Royal Engineer was also exacting in his demands for quality equipment. Before he departed from Woolwich to Hong Kong he wrote on 3 April 1843 to Brigadier Major Matson at the IGF's department. 'I beg to recommend that the Telescope be 30 inches in length, and the instrument generally of the best construction Mr. Simms can make. I have also to request that the instrument may not be packed up until I have had an opportunity of seeing it.'[36]

Collinson departed Woolwich on 24 May 1843 and it took him five months to arrive in Hong Kong. Accompanying him were one sergeant and thirty-two soldiers of the Royal Sappers and Miners; the clerks and foremen of works, together with their families who would follow in the next departure.[37] This was another sign of the changing times—the paid passage of accompanying families—where civilian officers' wives and children attached to the military now ventured out for Hong Kong. Up to this point, Hong Kong, for Europeans, had been an almost exclusively male world. European women had been in scarce supply. The only women in large number had accompanied the South Asian soldiers of the Madras Native Infantry forces—a distinct concession. Lieutenant Collinson would also convey the tragic news of one particular woman, the death of Major Aldrich's wife. She was to have departed with the young lieutenant on the same vessel.[38] Perhaps this event and the subsequent lack of feminine temperateness explains Aldrich's increasingly hardened behaviour towards his subordinates and colleagues over the coming years. Reading through his letters, one wonders if Collinson, the unfortunate messenger, felt this the keenest.

Nevertheless, it was thanks to Aldrich that an accelerated building programme could soon begin, the Royal Engineers providing the benchmark for others to imitate in terms of design, procurement, and execution methods. As one military historian would proudly note, 'In the early days, a Sapper had no better than an even chance of surviving for three years against the ravages of ill health. That first little band of Engineers mapped the Island, built barracks and hospitals, tackled the drainage and provided drinkable water, so that, in a few years, the death-rate had been halved.'[39]

The 'Hongkong Fever'

Aldrich's arrival was timely for the military and their renewed desire for a substantial cantonment (a permanent encampment). On 3 May 1843, Sir Henry Pottinger rode to West Point—an area which today sits at the western edge of Sai Ying Pun—and spent the evening walking around the site surrounding the, by now, extensive military barracks. These ranged in three tiers upon the hillside above and to the south of the Queen's Road, beside which the road bent around and terminated.[40] 'All the indentation of the hill' recounted James Legge upon his first arrival that same month, '. . . was occupied with tents and huts peopled by the 55th Regiment'.[41] These barracks had been constructed on the orders of Lieutenant-General Sir Hugh Gough, probably in late 1841, and under the supervision of Captain Mylius. They cost just over $1,800, less than one fifth of the cost of the more substantial barracks constructed by Mylius at Chek Chue.[42] West Point had expanded under Major-General Alexander Fraser, Lord Saltoun's present term of office.[43] Pottinger, though, was more concerned that Saltoun was turning his attentions to the centre of the town, and developing an interest in commandeering the entire site of the Ordnance District (now known as Admiralty). This district comprised a strip of land at the base of Cantonment Hill, a zone at the heart of the city of Victoria and adjoining Government Hill. Saltoun wanted it as a secure military base, thereby jeopardising the urban continuity of the length of the city. Pottinger's hope that evening was that he could offer a suitable adjacent piece of ground at West Point to convince the major-general to continue to consolidate his base there. The following day, he wrote with some eagerness to Saltoun:

I had last evening an opportunity of examining the ground immediately around 'West

> Point Barracks', and, that, I am of opinion that a line drawn at right angles from the 'Queen's Road' up to the base of the mountains . . . and thence along the face of the Hills until it meets the Queen's Road beyond the bend that it must take above Navy Bay, will include an ample space for every purpose either for Buildings or Drill Parades.
>
> I have accordingly told the Land Officer to allot the ground in question for the Cantonment at West Point Barracks and to mark it off by Pillars, or Piles of Stones, in concert with the Acting Assistant Quarter Master General.[44]

He attached to the back of the letter a crude, unmeasured sketch of the marked-off area (**fig. 3.2**), adding:

> The whole of this ground will require a considerable outlay in clearing and levelling it, but when that is done, I look on it that there will not be finer or more healthy locations in the Island.[45]

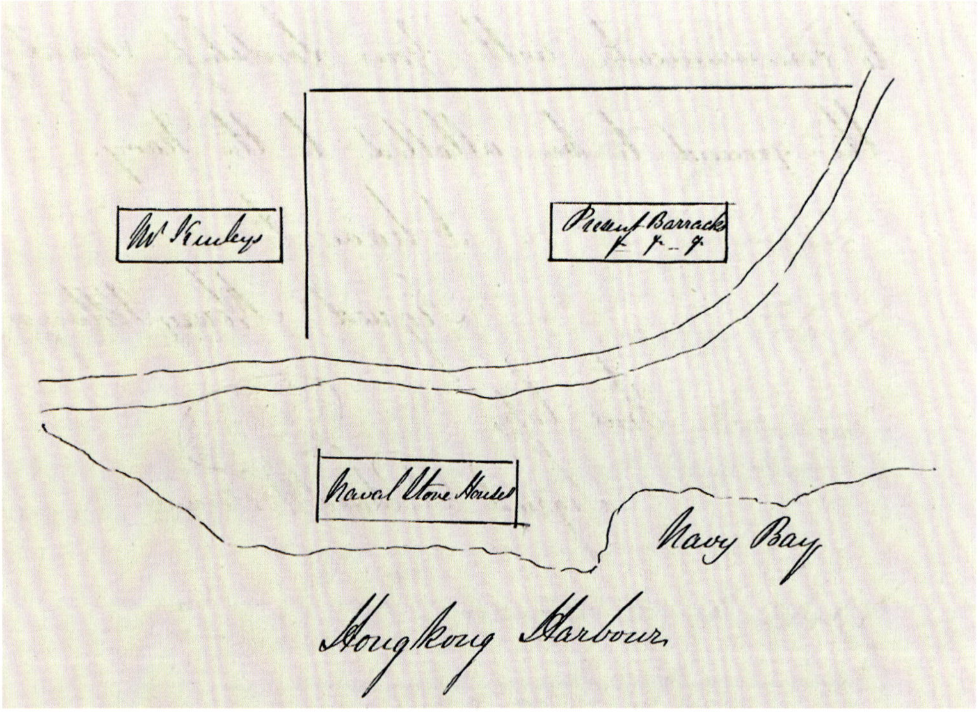

Fig. 3.2. H. Pottinger, Sketch Proposal for Extending the West Point Barracks, 4 May 1843. Ink on paper. © The National Archives, Kew (ADM 1/5530).

Saltoun was not the only interested party shifting his gaze eastwards to the colony's centre. Vice-Admiral Sir William Parker, too, desired his navy stores relocated in their entirety from Navy Bay, the small cove below West Point, to an area within the Ordnance District bordering the military, and where currently his 'Middle Stores' were positioned. The site, he wrote to Saltoun, was 'unquestionably infinitely superior in every point to any situation that has been hitherto suggested, inasmuch as it is in one of the best positions for security to shipping in this fine harbour; and where ships of the line may ride in safety at their Anchors'.[46] Parker also justified his selection by noting that the stores usually contained highly combustible materials, and could be better protected in the centre. And though he conceded, in terms of defence, that stretch of the shore was reasonably far from Kowloon's opposite coast, it was still within range of gunshot. No thought seemed to have crossed his mind about the risks posed to the heavily populated city by these centrally placed explosives. Aldrich doubtless had a hand in all this, quietly advising Parker while he accompanied him on the *Proserpine* steamer on 4 July.[47] It suited Aldrich's architectural ambitions to combine the military with the navy. It also suited Saltoun and Parker to consort to consolidate their hold on that central location, and events would soon transpire to achieve this.

In January 1843, the total number of rank-and-file soldiers across the Island of Hong Kong was 1,200 European and 550 Native troops (meaning native Indian, Ceylon and Malay). West Point that year was occupied by the Left Wing of the 55th Regiment of Foot and commanded by Major D. L. Fawcett. This force was the largest contingent on the island, an entirely European body of 500 men.[48] Sickness among the regiment had begun in the early part of May, much as it had done the year previously at West Point, with an increase in patients suffering from fever. But it was not until the end of May that cases of 'severe Remittent and continuous Fever began to prevail'.[49] From 20 May until 15 July, by which time Major-General Saltoun was forced to instigate a medical investigation, 408 patients were admitted, of which 294 were cases of fever. This was from an average strength of troops at the barracks of only 250 men. Thirty-nine men died during this period, twenty-five from fever. Out of a total of nine officers, all but two fell sick, while two subsequently died.[50]

There are few existing plans of the West Point Barracks; the most noteworthy is a small layout terminating the left-hand-side of the Edwards–de Havilland Survey, also known as 'Gordon's Map' (**fig. 3.3**). This survey of the north shore was made during the summer and autumn months of 1843. And so it records the last manifestation of the barracks at the point of abandonment and closure.

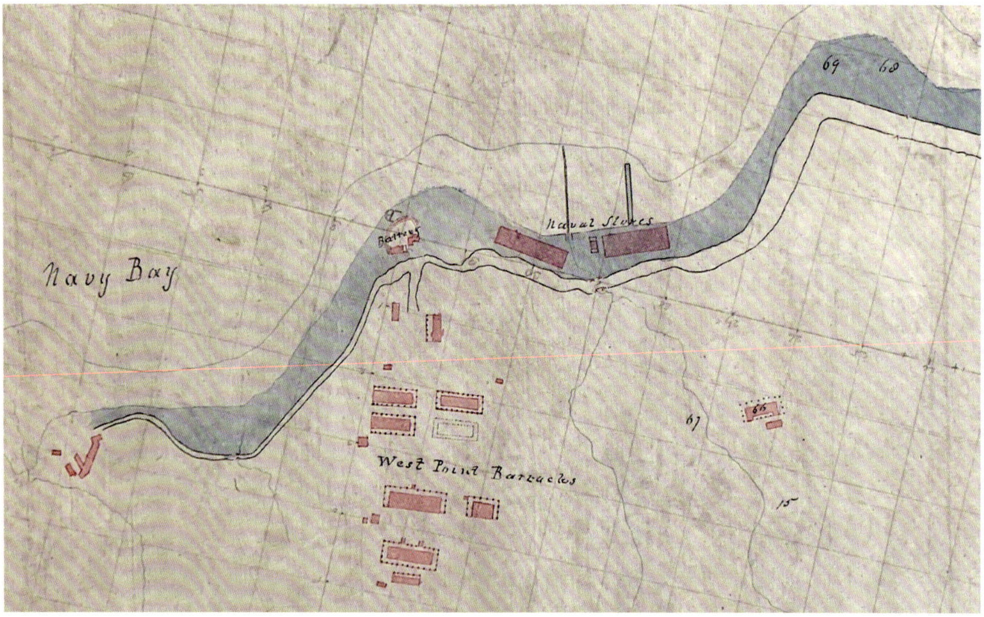

Fig. 3.3. Capts. C. Edwards and T. de Havilland, West Point Barracks (detail), 1843. Ink and watercolour. © The National Archives, Kew (MPG 1/156).

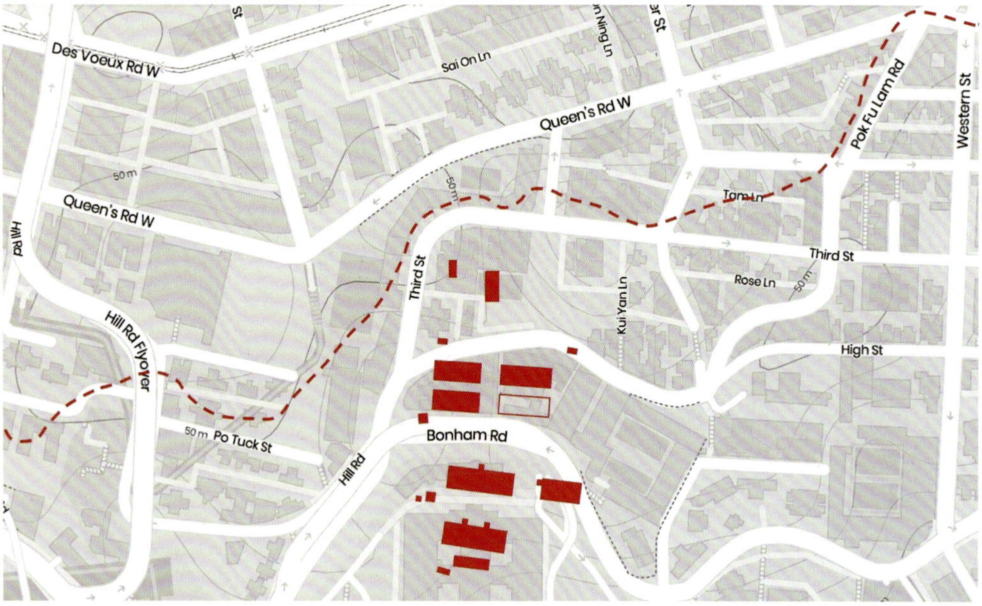

Fig. 3.4. C. Cowell, West Point Barracks (1842–1844) Overlaid on a Modern Ordnance Survey. © Author (base: Mapcarta.com).

Mylius had set the barracks in three clusters corresponding to three levels, quite likely on the terraces of abandoned paddy known to surround the area.[51] It is also probable that the military rudimentarily cut-and-filled upon these to achieve broader levels, accentuating already inherent land features. Road formations rarely change. Over time they become encased within bounded land ownership across wider networks, like insects in amber. This is true of the trace of roads created from the lost terraces at West Point. By overlaying a modern ordnance survey map it is easy to determine that these terraces now correspond with the areas contained between Third Street and Pok Fu Lam Road, Pok Fu Lam Road and Bonham Road, and at the uppermost level between Bonham Road and the Main Building of The University of Hong Kong, with what appears to be the upper latrines sited within the northwest courtyard of the Main Building, an area in which the Department of History recently sat. Unbeknown to its planners, the Main Building, completed in 1912, has been unwittingly placed at the locus of the outbreak of the 1843 fever (**fig. 3.4**).

All the barrack buildings at West Point had enclosing verandas. The upper two clusters stood raised from the ground, with steps leading up to a deck. The uppermost, the 'South Soldier's Barrack' with, what seemed, a rear latrine, was the earliest building group on the site.[52] The central cluster, the 'East and West Officer's Quarters', had verandas on three sides, the southern face buried into the hillside. The lowest cluster, the 'East and West Soldier's Lower Barracks', a set of three, have beside them on the plan the dotted outline of a fourth, quite probably recently removed—a possible location of sickness.[53]

Equally obscure are records of materials used for the various structures. In July 1843, a Chinese contractor, Amoon, won the tender to provide sundry repairs to the buildings. However, this sum also included work for the 41st Madras Native Infantry (MNI) Ordnance Barracks and Hospital. From this, it seems challenging to untangle and determine what material the West Point barracks consisted of. However, it was likely that the MNI were housed in mat barracks, as was the norm. Also, by far the highest costs were for carpenters and day wages for bricklayers, together with the purchasing of panes of glass. The materials at West Point were thought fit for reuse when it was finally demolished and sold by part at auction in 1844.[54] Therefore, the barracks themselves (apart from the additional 'tents' recounted by Legge) were not mat-sheds (they had panes of glass). More likely, they were of timber and brick, timber framing on brick bases—a similar

suggestion was that one *naik* (an Indian corporal) and three sepoys from the 41st MNI be employed to keep watch, and be granted a monthly allowance of four dollars for lamps.[66] A week later, and somewhat unexpectedly, the families of the 55th Regiment arrived from Calcutta. Many then heard of their husbands and fathers sick or dying, and themselves now bereft of accommodation.[67] Out of compassion, Pottinger felt compelled to sanction the hiring of houses and to build temporary accommodation. He thereby initiated what would become a lasting habit over the following years—the billeting of soldiers into private residences across the city, while the various barracks construction programmes got underway. Also, with new troops soon expected from England, Pottinger now realised the urgency of constructing barracks across the island, such as the ones planned to replace or augment the barracks 'at Chuk Choo and Saiwan, and any other point where they ought to be established'. However, he could not bring himself to suggest 'Cantonment Hill' at Victoria's core.[68] The struggle for the heart of the city was intensifying.

By August, the fever had become widespread, though most of the cases clustered at Victoria's western and eastern ends.[69] Its broad canvass of attack earned itself the name 'Hongkong Fever'. We have only a limited account of its effects upon the Chinese population, though, according to Johnston, they appear to have suffered as much under the new epidemic as their European counterparts.[70] The colonists had attempted to protect themselves with vaccinations since the first stages of occupation. The Chinese inhabitants, according to Johnston, had 'no remedies of their own except counter-irritation, produced by pinching and rubbing with the fingers and with copper cash'.[71] Those that were able fled the island, with some Europeans reverting to their earlier lives aboard ships. Many others returned to their old retreats in Macau. By 12 August, the Macau-based *Canton Press* reported:

> We regret to learn that much sickness prevails at Hongkong; invalids arrive here daily for cure and the Hongkong fever is of a very malignant description, and brought on probably not so much by the unhealthiness of the climate there as by too much exposure to the sun, which cannot always be avoided.[72]

The newspaper was obliquely criticising Pottinger's April instructions to investigate and halt much private construction work, solar exposure implying a lack of built and planted shade and, in turn, an unfavourable comparison to Macau.

On the night of 24 August, the East India Company's steamer *Proserpine* weighed anchor alongside the Praya of Macau. A feverish John Robert Morrison, son of the famous missionary Robert Morrison and the young Hong Kong government's chief Chinese interpreter and colonial secretary, was stretchered out. Accompanying him was his friend, Pottinger's private secretary, the surgeon Richard Woosnam.[73] It seemed at first that he would recover, but he relapsed, and nothing Woosnam or the colonial surgeon, Dr. Anderson, could do could save him. Morrison died five days later, on the morning of 29 August at a few minutes past seven o'clock. He was just twenty-nine years old. The newspapers were informed that 'the fever which terminated his life, and which must be called the Hongkong fever, combines we are told in its symptoms, the appearance of the jungle fever of India and of the yellow fever of the West Indies, and has hitherto in too many instances defied medical art'.[74] That evening his remains were conveyed to the Protestant Cemetery in Macau, with the entire foreign community there in attendance. The garden was among several 'foreign cemeteries' that dotted the trade routes into Canton (**fig. 3.5**).

Morrison's body was laid to rest at the south-eastern corner of the small cemetery beside his famous missionary father, due to whom there had been such high expectations placed upon the son. Morrison's brother followed the hearse, supported by Pottinger, Johnston, and Captain Balfour, the new consul for Shanghai. Amid the sombre mood, Sir Henry Pottinger announced that day in the press his 'feelings of the deepest and most unfeigned sorrow. . . . Mr. Morrison was so well known and so truly beloved, esteemed,

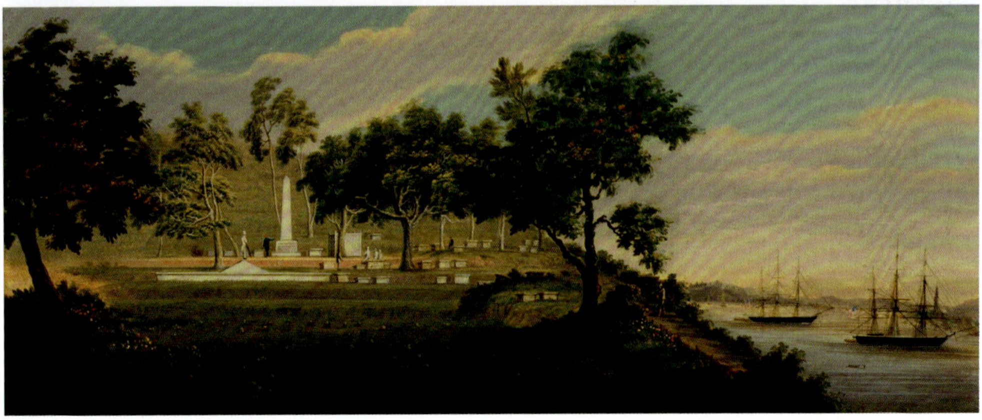

Fig. 3.5. Sunqua, 'View of Dane's Island Foreign Cemetery, Whampoa', ca. 1840. Oil on canvas. © Peabody Essex Museum, Salem (M20543).

and respected by all who had the happiness of his acquaintance and friendship'. The notice ended with the words: 'In a public point of view Sir Henry Pottinger considers the death of Mr. Morrison to be an irreparable national calamity.'[75] In private, he promised Lord Stanley that 'Her Majesty's Government will unfeignedly lament the untimely death of a faithful, devoted, and invaluable servant whose loss it is impossible to replace'.[76] These words proved more prescient than Pottinger realised. The subsequent signing of the Supplementary Treaty with China (the 'Treaty of the Bogue') would reveal gross incompetence on the part of the British in incorrectly translating at least two of the articles contained, and which would cast a permanent stain on Pottinger's administration, hindering Hong Kong's development and expansion.

Morrison's death may have led, inadvertently, to another who was dear to the governor. On 1 September, Major Eldred Pottinger of the Bombay Artillery, on his recent arrival to Hong Kong, was made an extra aide-de-camp on his uncle's personal staff.[77] His first official duty in October was to be the bearer of despatches to London, including the imperial ratification of the Supplementary Treaty, the same document that, had Morrison been alive, could have been translated swiftly and accurately. A place was accordingly reserved for him aboard H.M. Steamer *Spiteful*.[78] *Spiteful*'s departure was fatefully delayed until mid-November due to difficulties in agreeing on the final form of the Treaty, by which time Eldred, 'so well known by his heroic defence of Herat against the Persians', had died of fever. He passed away in the afternoon of 15 November, the very day *Spiteful* was finally able to depart Hong Kong for Bombay.[79] His uncle was in Macau, but unfortunately Henry Pottinger left that evening just before word would have reached him of his nephew's demise.[80]

The Valley Experiment

Along the city's eastern side, malaria wreaked havoc upon another vision of future development and cut down more lives. Jardine Matheson & Co., the largest and most influential of the Canton trading houses, had invested immediately and heavily in Hong Kong. Before the fever, they had been looked upon as a test case for the more timid merchants still to leave Macau or those that had recently joined the island's mercantile fold. Over the past two years, they had poured most of their capital into their enclave at

East Point, marking the most easterly end of the city of Victoria. Their asset comprised a distinctive spur of rock to the immediate west of the original Causeway Bay that jutted north-eastward into the harbour, with two sizable hillocks to the rear.[81] Both hillocks have since been flattened. The seaward or northern hill is now the area encompassing the Lee Gardens, and the landward or southern, then known as the 'Black Mount', is now Caroline Hill. All were collectively known as 'East Point'.

First, Jardine Matheson constructed a set of godowns (warehouses) upon the spur, then a three-storey office building behind, against which they built their hilltop residence upon the seaward hill (**fig. 3.6**). One of the distinctions of this arrangement was that the functions of the buildings remained discreet and separated, enjoying the newfound advantages of space, unlike the hybrid forms of cramped office–dwelling–storage that company officials were used to when living in Canton. Their two-story bungalow, dubbed East Point One, combined a Roman-arched rusticated base with a lighter Grecian upper-floor veranda of Ionic columns. A similar style would be adopted by Major Aldrich for his Officers' Quarters two years later below Cantonment Hill, East Point One possibly influencing that important architectural work later to be renamed Murray House. It was all a far cry from the 'rat trap and birdcage orders' of their first residence criticised by that uncharitable essayist back in 1842. On their more distant hill, the Black Mount, they built a sizeable bungalow, and within the dip were a set of stables.[82] Yet, despite quickly building a wall around the small enclave and guarding it with armed sepoys, the 'Princely Hong' remained troubled. Jardine Matheson could not shake off old opium-war storage habits and nagging doubts about the safety of land, choosing instead to store most of the bullion and all of their opium off-shore within anchored vessels. However, of all the places that would prove a sanctuary of health, East Point would stand out most notably and in stark irony, perched as it was upon the very edge of one of the most horrific locations identified during the 1843 outbreak. This outcome was peculiar, considering East Point's proximity to sickness and its modest elevation. For instance, in October 1843, at the height of the Hongkong Fever, naval officer Lieutenant Humphrey John Julian painted a sullen view of East Point and Causeway Bay from behind on Caroline Hill, standing by the villa of a Mrs. Moyan. East Point's hillock is revealed as a relatively low protrusion. But, there is a noted distinction. In contrast with the stark landscape surrounding, Matheson had now girdled one side of his residence with an extensive array of imported trees running down towards the peninsula to protect against the winterly northeast winds (**fig. 3.7**).

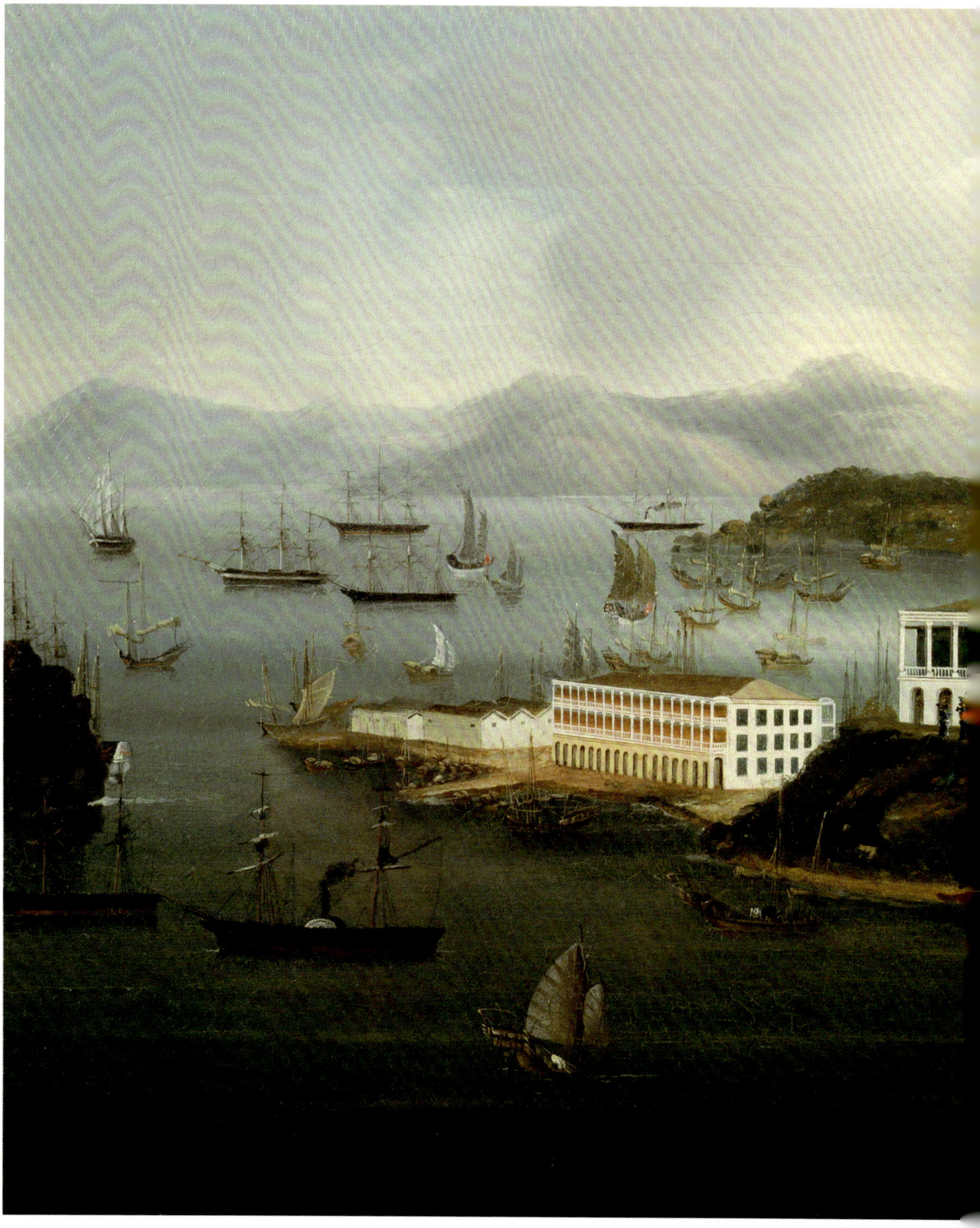

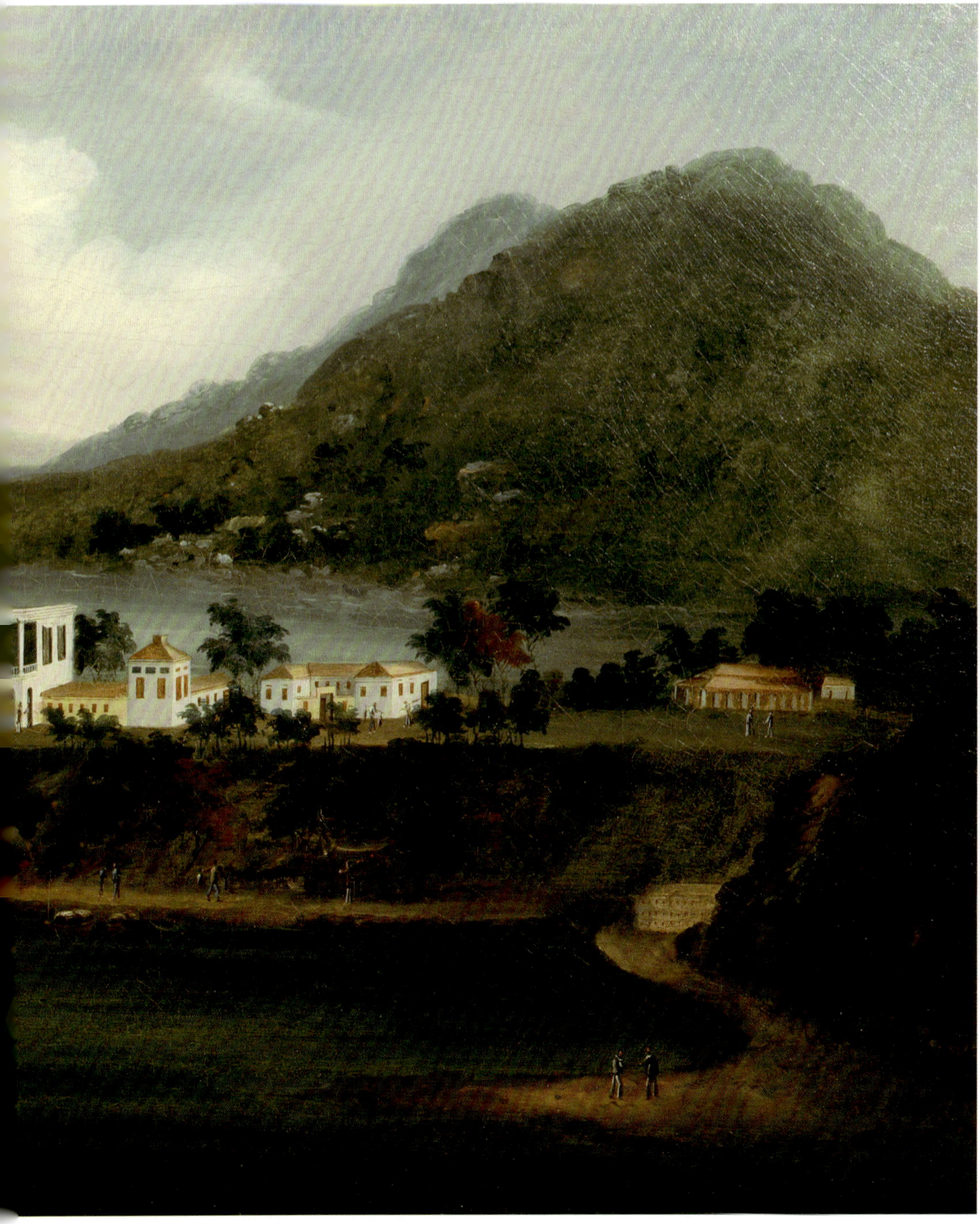

Fig. 3.6. Anon. (Chinese artist), Jardine Matheson's Residence, 'East Point One', ca. 1845. Oil on canvas. © Mr. Anthony Hardy, The Sze Yuan Tang Collection.

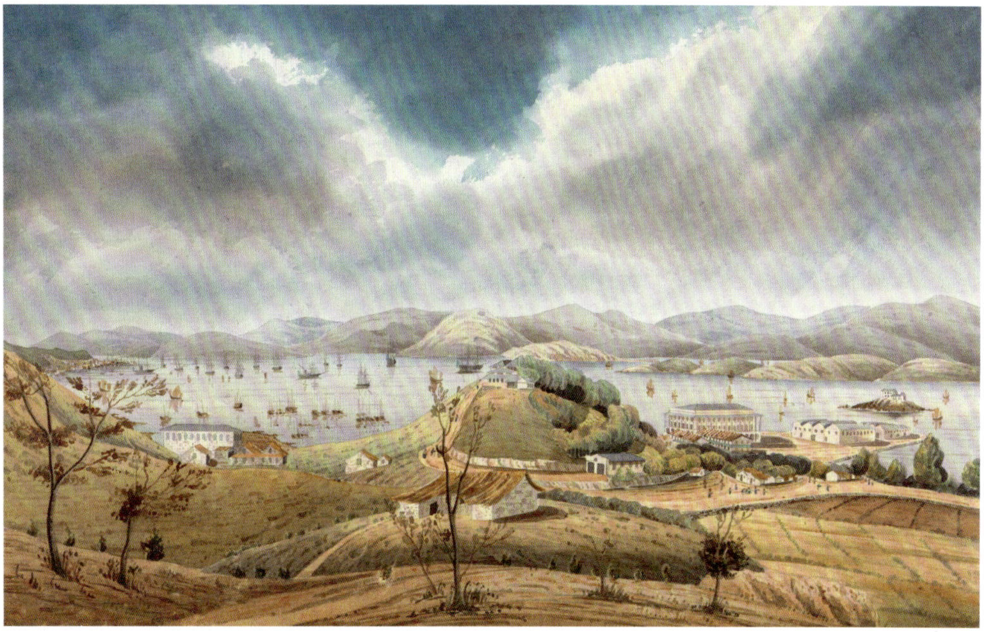

Fig. 3.7. Lt. H. J. Julian, 'Hong Kong Harbour', October 1843. Watercolour. © Yale Center for British Art (B1975.4.1305).

Alexander Matheson had felt obliged to relinquish some of his early purchases near Central, those below Cantonment Hill, for military use. East Point was at a considerable distance from this early clustering. Though it is unclear how much influence Matheson himself brought to bear, by early 1843, there were signs that Pottinger had begun taking Captain Belcher's initial thoughts much more seriously. The captain had, it may be recalled, urged the local government months into possession of Hong Kong Island to relocate the town eastwards into the Wong Nai Chung Valley (Happy Valley), that substantial flat area next to East Point. The valley lay as an abandoned network of paddy fields and streams within the largest area of naturally level ground to be had on the north side of the island. Belcher's 1841 report had spelled out the advantages in choosing the valley as the capital of Victoria, and a belief in this action may well have convinced Matheson to purchase this piece of land in the first place. Perhaps Matheson would be forgiven for finally believing that the 'mountain' would move to his 'Mohammed'. Instead, within months of colonial settlement, the military had decided to use the valley grounds as a makeshift cemetery. For instance, the funerary procession of Commander James

Brodie of the Royal Navy took place with great solemnity in mid June of 1841, as recaptured from memory a month later by Edward Cree in the earliest surviving view we have of the valley (**fig. 3.8**). The mourners entered from one of the only positions available at the time, through the northern cleft along the coast entering southwards. Brodie had died delirious, with ague (likely malaria). Two days later, Cree would see his friend Adjutant Wilson buried in a nearby plot, having just died of remittent fever.[83]

Now, in 1843, Governor Pottinger, owing—in his mind—to a disastrously ill-thought-out release of plots across the first land sale, felt acutely motivated to reinvestigate the valley option. The marine lots sold in 1841 had taken a significant percentage of the valuable shoreline away from government control. Future reclamation in front of these influential owners might first involve a protracted court battle, as it was legally unclear if they had a right to enjoy unhindered access to the shore.[84] The valley provided sufficient ground for quick resettlement of the core administration, residences of various classes, growth in commercial activity, and future expansion.

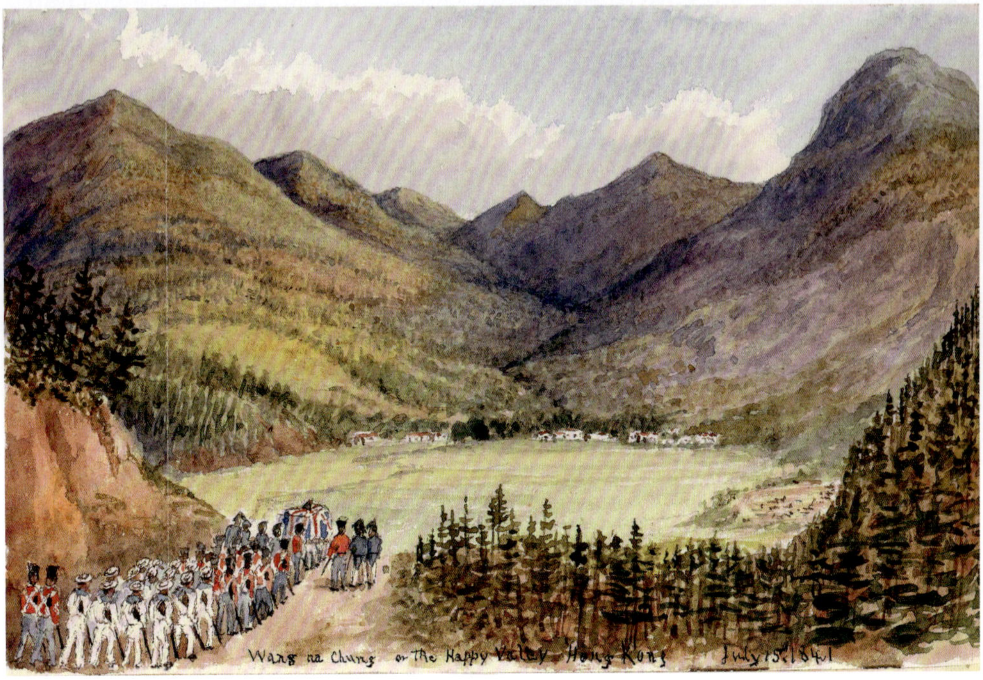

Fig. 3.8. Dr. E. Cree, 'Wang na Chung or The Happy Valley, Hong Kong, [drawn] July 15, 1841'. Watercolour. © National Maritime Museum, Greenwich, London (CRJ/5).

Pottinger, therefore, instructed his land officer and cousin, Alexander T. Gordon, to look into this. Indeed, Gordon, the moonlighting architect, had an additional interest in considering the area—it was adjacent to the land owned by his professional client, none other than Alexander Matheson. On 10 March 1843, Matheson wrote to him:

> We wish the building to be placed entirely in your hands. Appoint such superintendents as you may deem necessary, who are to be responsible to you, to whom of course, we shall look for having the work properly executed.
>
> We are not aware what your charge is, but shall of course be willing to pay the regular rate whatever it is. Our object is to have a solid & sightly building, & to have it furnished as speedily as possible.[85]

Gordon had taken over the job of overseeing the construction of the East Point offices from the late Mr. Langer, and due to the unfortunate collapse of one wing, completion was delayed until the following year.[86] It was not uncommon practice during the tenure of Pottinger for members of his administration to be engaged in private work. Indeed it was one of the only ways of keeping employees, as it was common to skim off the administrative talent to work for the top merchant houses in side-line ventures. This practice would be put to an end during the term of office of the next governor, John Davis, in 1844.

Meanwhile, on 6 July, Gordon submitted a report to the acting colonial secretary Lieutenant-Colonel Malcolm in which he recorded the 'present state of the roads and buildings in the Colony'.[87] Accompanying this report was his considered written plans for the means of rebuilding the city in the Wong Nai Chung Valley. He proposed a sea wall 'from a point at the foot of the Hill marked No. 84 on the survey, known as the "Morrison Education Society Hill" to one at that marked Suburban Lot No. 2, the property of Messrs. Jardine Matheson & Co.' (that being the hill upon which stood East Point One), in other words, a wall spanning across the mouth of the valley. He continued, 'Up the centre of the Valley, I would have a Canal, with gates to the Sea, sufficiently deep to admit of large junks (cargo boats) coming up.'[88]

Gordon's almost Venetian or Dutch scheme was well-thought-out and rich in merchant–civic qualities. Unfortunately, no drawn plan exists. He suggested that along the sea wall ought to be built a roadway supporting 'an extended range of warehouses'. The zone between this and the Queen's Road he proposed should 'allow only European Houses and Shops' and to the south of this a town for Chinese. Encircling all would be a 'road of sufficient width . . . at the foot of the surrounding hills; and all the streets to be parallel to the Sea Wall in the front, passing from a broad road on each side of the Canal into this circular road'.[89] The circular road would, in addition, unlock the entire perimeter edge of the valley, enticing the construction of villas around the foot of the hills.[90] Gordon, aware that the east–west direction of the primary streets he proposed might hinder the circulation of air, argued that this orientation was necessary to support the 'various small branches from the Canal' that would percolate into the Chinese town, allowing merchants to have cargoes delivered by junk to their shop fronts. 'I believe there is no reason to fear a want of good air,' he declared, offering that the generous width of these principal roads would mitigate any fears and that a north–south orientation could also be entertained for the European sector of the new town.[91] As a backdrop to all of this, Gordon proposed 'that the Queen's Road be continued entirely round the Island'. He saw this as entirely feasible though difficult in a few places. Yet its construction would benefit both the civilian population and the military, allowing for the swift movement of troops to any section. The whole of the Wong Nai Chung scheme, he suggested, be funded by a grant from the British government for the initial infrastructure of the sea wall and canal, with the lots let to tenants on the stipulation that they in turn build 'according to a given plan'. Alternatively, it may be paid for by letting the land in its existing state to a single 'company, which could probably be formed for the purpose' of constructing the entire project.[92] London's response would arrive the following January; however, malaria would make its decision known somewhat more rapidly.

At about this time, beginning in July, malaria struck along the island's east side.[93] The worst concentration of cases was in the same area Gordon proposed for the new city. William Tarrant, later anti-government editor of the *Friend of China*—then responsible for supervising the construction of roads in that district—recalled that 'indeed the intention of the earlier settlers appears to have been to make their chief quarters in that neighbourhood'. But of the rows of small houses initially constructed there, 'only a few . . . were ever occupied; their occupants dying of fever contracted within them'.[94] Mansions also appeared following the 1841 land sale. Mr. Mercer, Alexander Matheson's new agent, built his opposite to the new burial ground, but 'fever caught in it killed him; and down it came'.[95] By 1861, the published date of Tarrant's scathing history of Hong Kong, the only dwelling that remained standing was the bungalow of Mr. Stewart, an employee of Matheson, located at the head of the valley; 'Dr. Young's bungalow, just below it, being deserted immediately and carried away piecemeal'.[96] The valley experiment was a sorry affair. Groups of abandoned, unfinished houses littered the eastern side, including a deserted sanatorium belonging to Jardine Matheson at the summit.

From May until its eventual decline in November, the 'Hongkong Fever' would claim the lives of twenty-four per cent of the military personnel and a further ten per cent of European civilians. Accounts, though without statistics, also recorded devastation to the resident Chinese. Victims quickly filled the local Protestant and Catholic burial grounds to capacity. Both cemeteries, located in Ha Wan (Wan Chai) south of the Queen's Road, had now to be dug up. The bodies were reinterred at a much larger site on the western edges of the Wong Nai Chung Valley by the military makeshift cemetery (and where it remains), fittingly an area that now held as much terror for merchants as did West Point for the military.[97] The recommendation to relocate had been made by the Committee of Public Health and Cleanliness. Following the West Point outbreak, the governor had set up this body 'for the purpose of fixing a new site and for improving the method of conducting funerals'. As a consequence of their report a site was fixed upon 'East of Victoria . . . in a ravine on the right, after passing through the gap which is at the extreme end of the town. . . . A wall across the mouth of the ravine, with a gate in the centre, and a short road approaching it . . . considered as sufficient'.[98] Governor Davis would confirm this proposal to Stanley in late 1844, after another year of significant though not as severe mortality among the troops, noting that 'the burial ground originally allotted for the Protestant population was never extensive, while the great and unforeseen mortality among the troops has unhappily contributed to fill it very rapidly'.[99] This future necropolis, as was the tradition, would mark the shrunken limits of the post-fever city, at least for a short time, and provide an emotional cordon sanitaire for those living behind it.

A Link between Buildings and Miasma

1843 marked the outbreak of a third season of fever and an essential shift in hypothesis about its cause and remedy. Sir Hugh Gough's 1842 Court of Inquiry had concluded that climate, the crowding of barracks, and general locale—an inherent sickliness ascribed to the island's north side—had brought about the illnesses. There had been no mention as to the relative suitability of accommodation. Now, however, the medical profession, almost in unison, concluded that the cause was owing to the unsuitability of specific *modes* of construction. As the then pro-government newspaper, the *Friend of China*, reluctantly admitted in September 1843:

> We have not before dwelt on this subject, as we wished to allay all undue apprehension, but the removal of the Government to Macao, and the panic it produced if we may judge by the quick departure from our Island of almost all who could leave; compels us to advert to this painful subject and to say that the best medical Authorities uniformly ascribe the present sickness, not to any climatic or local influence of a deleterious character, but wholly to the absence of habitable houses and the suitable accommodations which are absolutely required for the healthy existence of Europeans in this climate and especially during this, the rainy season.[100]

The newspaper was taking a swipe at an unpopular government notification of 10 April, ironically, a notice that it had been the first to print since it also served as the official government gazette. If it were not clear enough, the *Friend* continued, 'But for the (we presume unavoidable) delay in the Land arrangements and the prohibition of building, we sincerely believe the fatal fever now raging, would not have been engendered.'[101] This was a daring attack on its proprietor and pinned accountability for the fever directly on Pottinger's administration.

The original notification alluded to was published in the *Friend* on 13 April, two months before the medical committee's fateful visit to West Point. It comprised of three orders. It first asked that all private holders of land provide immediate proof of possession to the Land Officer and that such '*terms* and *tenure* of holding all lands on the Island of Hongkong, were to depend solely on the pleasure, and commands, of Her Majesty's Government'.[102] This was not unexpected, despite later cries of foul play by landowners in January 1844, the second great land sale. There was a practical preparedness among existing purchasers that the quit rent ownership model promised under Elliot looked increasingly unlikely to be approved. What *was* a surprise to most of them were the following instructions concerning the forcible halting of construction, contradictory to previous pressure put upon them by the Land Office to ensure that each owner spend a minimum percentage of the plot purchase price in construction work. In other words, what seemed contradictory was that the halting of construction as now ordered would risk annulling the very stipulations of ownership that the government had initially imposed. The conditions upon which particular owners were required to halt such construction were more confusing. It was announced that the land officer, A. T. Gordon, had been instructed:

> . . . To prevent the commencement of any further buildings upon, or clearing away of, locations, until final arrangements can be made.
>
> . . . To put a stop to all Buildings that may be in progress on locations of whatever denomination, where the explanation, or proofs submitted, may appear to him to be at variance with his present instructions; and, also, in cases where the explanation and proofs now called for, may be delayed beyond a reasonable time.
>
> . . . The land officer has further been authorized and instructed, to summarily prevent, the progress of all buildings on locations which may, in his opinion, encroach on the present, or any future, line of roads or streets, and to oblige all persons to confine themselves to the exact dimension of the lots which were originally allotted to them.[103]

Believing, with this, to have fulfilled the instructions initially framed by James Stephen (and the Colonial Land and Emigration Office in London approvingly thought so), on 1 May, Pottinger wrote to Lord Aberdeen enclosing his notification to all inhabitants 'calling in all claims to land at Hong Kong and forbidding all further building or other operations on the same until such claims shall have been presented and substantiated'.[104]

This instruction was puzzling to landowners until they discovered that the original 1842 Land Committee had been so disorganised that it had kept no minutes of their actions and decisions. Consequently, Pottinger required a repeat performance of the entire process.[105] His government deferred working out who had legitimate rights of ownership. A new Land Grants Committee would painfully deliberate over this. In the meantime, purchasers found it hard to provide the precise boundaries of their property, let alone have the foresight to tell if it fell over the path of 'any future line of roads or streets'. Several parties were given notice by Gordon 'to remove the foundations of their house, just laid down at great expense, nearer to the water, although these foundations are within the boundary of their water frontage lot'.[106] The notice brought about an almost complete halt to construction. It was this cessation—'the absence of habitable houses'—coincident with the worst and most generalised attack of malaria since colonisation that joined to provide the community with a new and terrible thesis: that the fever was induced by the combined effects of form, construction quality, materials, and siting of built accommodation in Hong Kong.

At the nub of these factors was the state of health of the interiors of buildings. For those of a religious disposition, the selfish, interior-living habits of 'Hongkonians' had finally received their comeuppance. 'Our success in the late war has been remarkable.

What has been our public acknowledgements to Him that "fighteth for us"?' intoned one 'member of the Church of England' in the *Chinese Repository* of November 1843, smarting from delays in rebuilding the colonial (mat-shed) church.

> We have now a good number of public buildings in the island, and others are in progress: have we laid the foundations of a church? There is no lack of industry among us: have we remembered to give that industry its lawful repose on the first day of the week?
>
> . . . Our life here is emphatically in the midst of death; bear witness the records of our hospitals, of our military messes, of private families. Surely this is a time to make some unusual demonstration of our absolute submission to our Maker's will, and our utter dependence on his mercy; instead of seeking excuses for the evasion of his laws, and giving our sole attention to scientific speculation for our relief![107]

However, for most others, 'scientific speculation' was all that hope could cling to. Following the closure of West Point and the enormous panic that deaths across the city were beginning to produce, Pottinger was now finally persuaded that a plausible link existed between unsanitary locations and miasma. On 16 August 1843, he appointed two surgeons, Mr. Young and acting Colonial Surgeon C. A. Winchester, together with Clerk of the Police Court C. B. Hillier and Land Officer Gordon, to form a Committee of Public Health and Cleanliness. The committee would have the authority to investigate, formulate, and implement any rules thought necessary to impose upon the colony for improved cleanliness and, therefore, health.[108] In the end, no rules were implemented. But their findings would be enshrined in the cumbersome and encyclopaedic 'Preservation of Good Order and Cleanliness Ordinance' No. 5 of 20 March 1844.[109] The Committee did, however, recommend and undertake four projects at the cost of a mere one hundred and fifty dollars. These four items were the clearing and enlarging of drains at the west end of the city; the provision of a new drain along the Queen's Road; the raising of the road near the Lower Bazaar, which flooded during rainstorms; and the provision of a new watercourse along the Upper Bazaar.[110] Yet a concerted effort emerged to provide cohesive drainage and sewerage across the lengthening road network, and it would grow to become a key concern during Governor John Davis's administration. Till the end, Pottinger would maintain his belief in dismissing 'the theories that have been laid down either as to the peculiar advantages of one situation over another judging from past experience or as to the peculiar insalubrity of this Island over any other part of the Coast of China'.[111]

Davis, as will later be shown, maintained the opposite view, convinced by location-specific advantages. And this conviction reshaped the city. Still, the success of the sanitation and construction projects in Hong Kong from 1844 onwards would, in a way, not contradict either viewpoint. Location problems could be overcome and therefore discounted as inherent, irredeemable features.

In his 1845 Blue Book report as colonial surgeon, two years after the great fever outbreak, Dr. Francis Dill remarked upon the relative healthiness of the past year. The general state of health was one 'which is to be accounted for by the improved state of the Colony, improvements in drainage, in roads, and in dwellings more adapted to the Country'.[112] He was perhaps the most explicit about his beliefs as to the causes of the fever and its prevention in a paper read that same year before the China Medico-Chirurgical Society.

> In my opinion the chief exciting causes are, exposure to the rays of the sun, sleeping under the direct rays of the moon, and exposure to the night dews; the atmosphere is much more charged with miasmatic vapour at night than during the day, or rather the poison is concentrated along the surface of the earth. Badly constructed dwellings placed either in immediate contact with the damp earth or which is still worse, elevated a few feet, leaving a space without ventilation, which becomes the receptacle of foul and confined air, and farther the dwellings being occupied before they are perfectly dry, must appear one of the most prominent sources of fever.[113]

Dill, admittedly, was now writing in a time of respite and felt that the changes brought about by a revamped building programme had demonstrably reduced the incidence of fever.

Reverend James Legge agreed with Dill, feeling that it had been a combination of ground conditions and poor dwelling provision that were the cause of the fatalities. In the reminiscences of his time in Hong Kong, Legge recounted that 'there was no subsequent year of sickness and mortality so great as that of 1843', the year of his first arrival.

> The mortality was mainly owing to the want of accommodation for the multitudes who kept pressing into the new colony, and to the miasma set free from the ground which was everywhere being turned up. I remember visiting officers who were living in small huts reared on the hill behind the general's house. It was no wonder that one after another they were seized with fever, and either died, or were invalided home. Then the drains were for the time all open, and an atmosphere of disease, which only the strongest constitutions and prudent living were able to resist, might be said to envelope the inhabitants day and night.[114]

Legge believed that, apart from the effects of Pottinger's confusing notification to halt construction, inhabitants had accidentally increased their exposure to the disease by the poor quality of buildings already constructed. If the British government had been more confident and clear in its determination to retain Hong Kong in 1841, then 'the small and rude beginnings would not have been what they were in the middle of 1843, if they had not dated from before the treaty of Nanking'.[115]

Somewhat closer to these terrible events, Captain Arthur Cunynghame, the aide-de-camp to Major-General Lord Saltoun, returning to London in 1844, immediately published a memoir of his time in China. Entitled *An Aide-De-Camp's Recollections of Services in China*, Cunynghame's account of his short stay in the territory records some of the worst months of the fever besieging Hong Kong in 1843. For Cunynghame, the steep terrain leeward of prevailing winds posed a fundamental problem.

> The town itself is long and straggling, from the nature of the ground upon which it is built—a strip of land at the base of the hills; and from the circumstance of their rising so immediately behind it, screening it during the summer from the prevailing winds, the south-west, they cause it to be very hot, not allowing a breath of air to circulate freely through the streets.[116]

The gloomy mood affected some painters of the time, a few of whom would play upon the threats thought posed by the landscape, exaggerating in height and darkness the oppressiveness of the screening slopes and mountains upon which the city of Victoria seemed to perilously perch. In one vivid example—likely painted during the outbreak—even the tones and colours of the landscape have taken on a sickly hue of bile-ish greens, mouldy blues, and a jaundiced sky (**fig. 3.9**). Hindrance in the air movement suggested itself as a critical factor to several observers. The military began to share in this theory. One contract went out in late August 1843 for 'cutting down a tongue or wedge of Land to improve the ventilation of the lower rooms of the new Officers Quarters at Chek-Chu'.[117]

Furniture design was also affected by the desire for air circulation, with the Commissariat purchasing sixty cane-bottomed cots.[118] When air appeared to circulate freely, and other aspects of the landscape such as drainage and vegetation were considered favourable, other factors had to be found to account for the unhealthy nature of a location. The military suffered sporadically and extensively across many of their settlements, West Point being just the most notable at the start of the 1843 outbreak. However, these

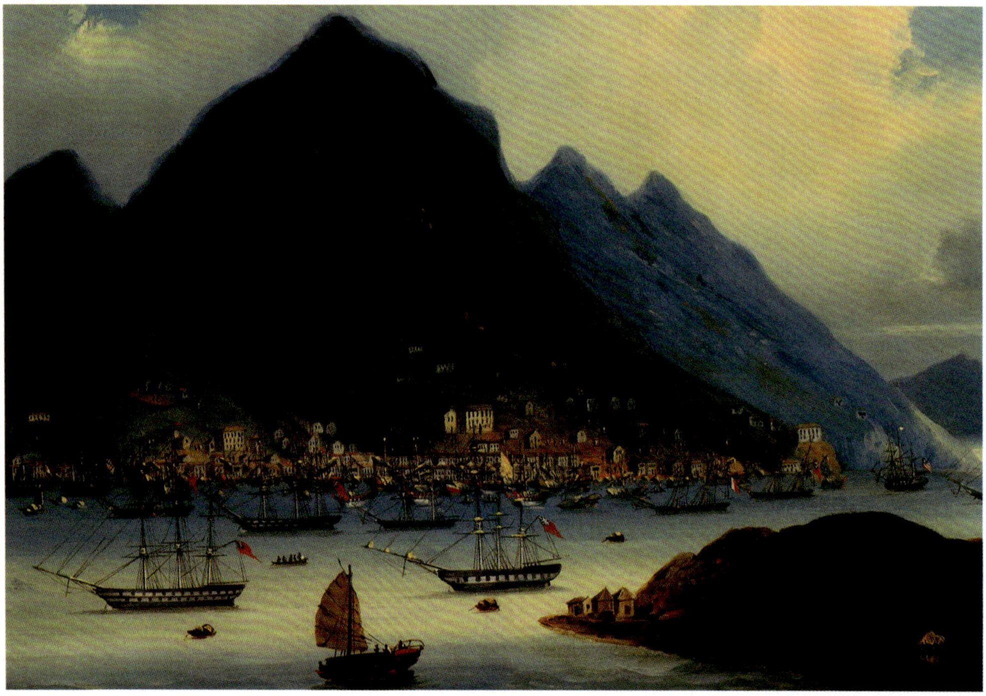

Fig. 3.9. Anon., 'Hong Kong from Kowloon', 1842–1843. Oil on canvas. © Castle Fine Arts, Inc.

settlements had been dispersed widely across various terrains and coastal orientations around the island. For instance, Cunynghame alluded to a similar incident occurring at the small barracks constructed in Sai Wan (now Chai Wan), located along the northeast, and described by him as 'by far the prettiest part of the island'. So he concluded that, as with other barrack locations, the only possible common denominator in the sickness among stationed troops was poor construction and cramped conditions. 'I am inclined to think,' he recalled, 'that it was there owing, as well as elsewhere, more to the want of good and sufficient accommodation than any other cause.'[119] A newer barracks designed to house about a hundred men was being built as he wrote. Doubtless, this would be robust and generous and, therefore, healthy. By 1844, across Hong Kong, a revised programme of substantial, spacious barrack construction was underway from what had previously been considered the more healthy location of Chek Chue in the south to Sai Wan in the north.

Nevertheless, a shrewd understanding of the attributes of a site was held by island elites as fundamental to health preservation. Cunynghame, in particular, lamented the situation around the Wong Nai Chung Valley. 'Many private dwellings have been commenced,' he wrote. 'Most have yet proved very unhealthy and in consequence have been little inhabited.'[120] Using it to test his theory of poor site selection, Cunynghame declared what he thought were the 'two causes' of disease. The first he attributed to lack of air movement caused by a secluded position and the restriction of sea breezes. Such movement he considered partially attributable to paddy cultivation. The second source was 'from the neighbouring hills being encumbered with shrubs and tangled woods, miasma from the paddy-fields and decayed vegetation being extremely prejudicial to health'.[121] Medical practitioners would argue out the details. Was it owing to 'exhalations from the deserted rice grounds' in Hong Kong as Dr. John Wilson, Medical Inspector of Naval Hospitals and Fleets, would later suggest in his published *Medical Notes on China* in 1846?[122] Or was it 'that the principal causes are the natural marshy swamps, the decaying brushwood, as well as the cultivated rice fields', as counter-proposed by Dr. Dill that same year?[123]

So, what precautions could be taken to improve the health of residents of the city? For the medical officers of Her Majesty's Naval Hospital, a newly-built edifice perched on the southern slopes above the Queen's Road and immediately east of Saltoun's Cantonment Hill residence, even its 'moderate elevation' seemed to have enhanced the chances of survival.[124] Subsequently, for an increasing number of experts from the new chattering class in Hong Kong, *height* was evidently *right*. The higher the elevation above sea level, the safer it seemed. As one article in the *Chinese Repository* wrote in August 1843, 'We learn that the hospital for seamen is now ready to receive patients. This institution is situated near the preceding, [the Medical Missionary Society Hospital] in an elevated and healthy position.'[125] Ever since European surgeons in India had persuasively argued of a link between higher altitude and recuperative health in the early 1820s, the British had sought to climb. But these hill stations sat upon mountain slopes thousands of feet above sea level. Here, in Hong Kong, such aspirations were miniaturised. In imitation of East Point One, soldiers and medics sought to slice the tips of hills, producing a series of elevated coastal plateaus for the building of barracks and hospitals. Edward Ashworth's remarkable view over the Seaman's Hospital from Morrison's Hill and towards the town, drawn around 1844, dramatically shows the effect of such surgical refashioning (**fig. 3.10**). The practice of this early habit would lead to the creation of the 'Mid-Levels' area above the Western (now Central) District shortly after.

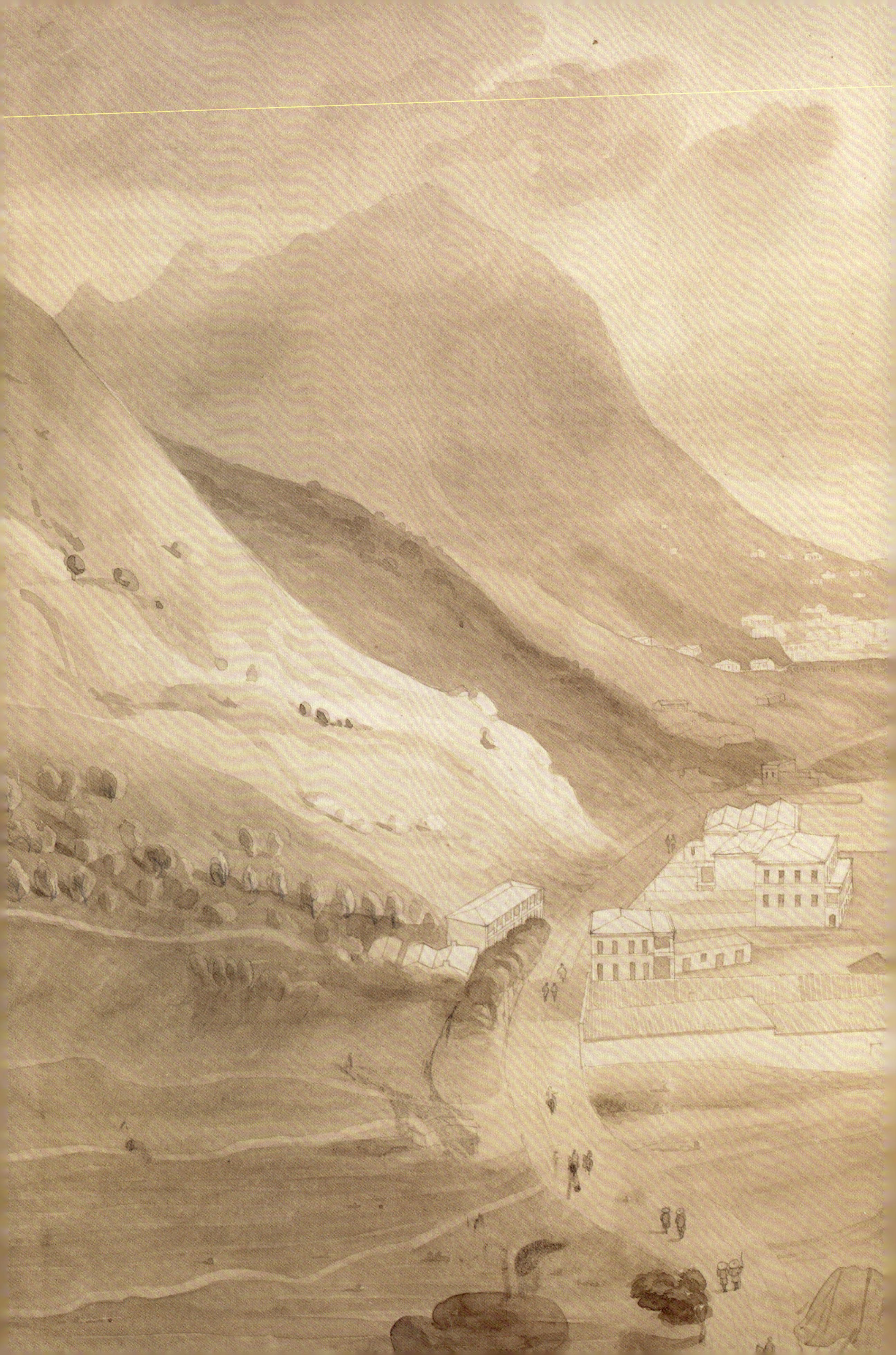

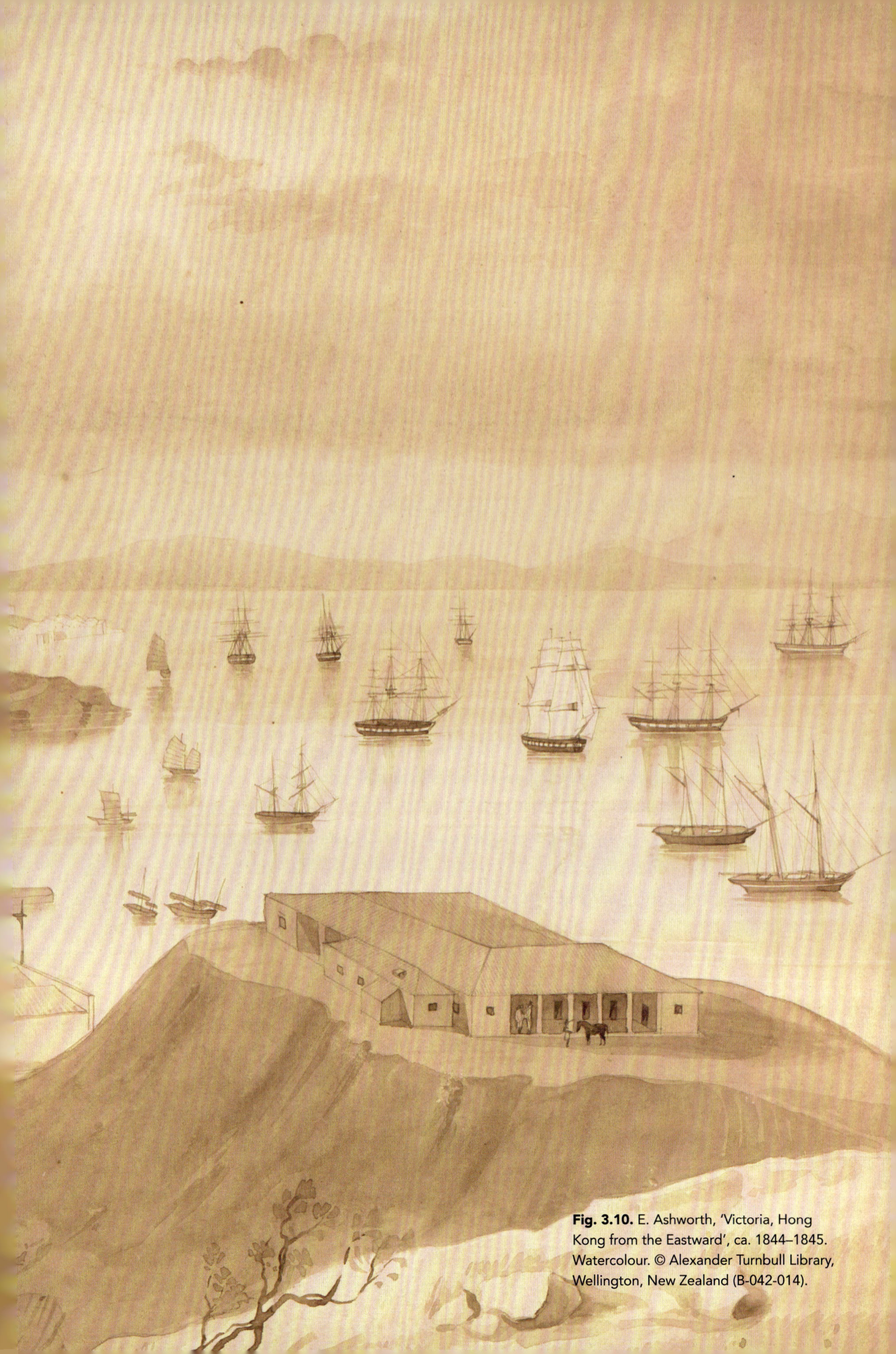

Fig. 3.10. E. Ashworth, 'Victoria, Hong Kong from the Eastward', ca. 1844–1845. Watercolour. © Alexander Turnbull Library, Wellington, New Zealand (B-042-014).

Of course, height alone was thought insufficient. The camp at West Point had sat elevated but in an unhealthy location. There seemed little point, therefore, in rebuilding upon the site. The barracks were soon demolished, their parts auctioned off to the highest bidder. Eight lots, one for each of the barracks, outbuildings, and guardhouse, were sold, and their pieces entirely removed by early March 1844.[126] By the time Collinson, Hong Kong Island's first surveyor, set his theodolite upon this stretch of land later that year, it was as if West Point had never existed except for the faint ghost of its lines, still visible into the 1890s.[127] The naval stores and the circular battery to the north along the shoreline near Navy Bay would remain, but a significant new highway, the Pok Fu Lam Road, would cut its way through the old barracks running neatly along Collinson's elegant contour lines to descend into an area named 'Aberdeen' (see **fig. 4.19**). This road was the third artery after the Wong Nai Chung Gap and Tai Tam Gap to connect the island from north to south.[128]

Before its destruction, however, West Point held a secret. As workers lifted the boards from the platforms in preparation for the barracks' removal, they discovered that 'the floors were totally rotten, and beneath them a quantity of water was lodged'.[129] This account was recalled in 1846, at the time, the healthiest year on record. West Point's lingering importance was that it would serve as the *anti-model* in almost all respects of how *not* to build in Hong Kong. It was the cause célèbre of Governor John Davis and his colonial surgeon, Dr. Dill (incidentally, both of whom were not yet present on the island in 1843). As Davis said to Gladstone, then British colonial secretary, the troops had once been 'lodged not in Barracks, but in ground floor hovels, the boards of which were in close contact with the wet earth below'. He implied by the reverse that now, following Major Aldrich's designs, they had been elevated upon solid, well-built masonry. 'I had not been a month on shore,' he continued, 'before I gave my assent to Major-General D'Aguilar erecting the new Barracks where they are now completed.'[130] In stark contrast, the West Point barracks 'were not only surrounded, but actually built upon a swamp'. Davis had learned from this and constructed a 'catch water drain'—also with the involvement of Superintending Royal Engineer Aldrich—running along the base of the hills above and across the extent of the town 'which formerly kept that part in a perfect swamp'.[131]

Gone too, for the military, were the casual positioning and orienting of buildings, particularly when their backs were to the southern slopes of hills. If only they had consulted the merchants. The 'old China hands' professed some early knowledge in this art of orientation, presumably, knowledge gleaned from their Chinese compradors. Alexander Matheson had, as far back as January 1842, advised a client intent on building in Hong Kong that

> As an old resident in China, I strongly recommend your having the entrance to the South West, and if possible no entrance to the North or N. East—as in winter it would be a thorough obstacle to keeping your house warm. I conclude you will like to have a surrounding verandah.[132]

Perhaps the titans of commerce indeed held the answer? In a few months, the *Friend of China*, formerly a loyal supporter of government policy, had switched its allegiance to the merchant class. It had some justification. The government had repeatedly skipped to Macau with most of the wealthier residents, some of whom were reluctant to return. Yet amid this exodus, at the two wealthiest companies' bases—Jardine Matheson & Co.'s East Point, the rocky promontory enclave, and Dent & Co.'s magnificent offices in Central—the worst period of Hong Kong's early history also saw the near completion of their grand projects of construction. These buildings must have been seen as beacons of hope as they took shape. For the *Friend of China*, the juxtaposition of trauma and triumph took shape in a single entry on 14 February 1844. The afflicted 55th Regiment had now received their orders for immediate embarkation for England. And lesser merchants remained cautiously penned in Macau. Yet 'the princely establishment built by Messrs. Jardine Matheson & Co. and also those by Messrs. Dent & Co. and other firms, are nearly completed. We anticipate at an early date, the removal from Macao to this Colony of every British House in China'.[133] It felt as if a nightmare had been quickly shrugged off.

Meanwhile, until the end of his term of office in March 1844, Governor Henry Pottinger had stubbornly maintained his beliefs against mounting opposition. 'He does not concur,' wrote his private secretary to Major-General D'Aguilar's assistant military secretary that month, 'in the theories that have been laid down either as to the peculiar advantages of one situation over another—judging from past experience—or as to the peculiar insalubrity of this Island over any other part of the Coast of China.'[134] He would soon be replaced by a governor who did.

Fire, Insurance, and Opportunity

As malaria ravaged the community, good-quality dwellings were increasingly believed to protect life. In this regard, property insurance played an essential role in crafting the built character of Hong Kong. It is not surprising that before 1843, most forms of insurance in the colony related to marine cover. In that year, however, the first forms of property insurance were offered, and these primarily protected against fire damage. One can trace both a cause and effect of this development.

Since construction began on the island in early 1841, it suffered many localised fire outbreaks. Some were accidental, some deliberate—either through arson or burglary. Many building materials did not help, often matting, leaves, bamboo, and timber. However, by 1843, a sufficient amount of building stock was amassed on the island of a solidly built, secure, and relatively non-flammable nature that could encourage an insurance company to view it more generally as a low-risk enterprise for investment. In turn, the introduction of insurance cover encouraged greater conformity in the methods and materials of construction and even in the relative positions and density of buildings (space permitting). As this insurance cover soon extended to the other treaty ports, Hong Kong found itself at the vanguard of safer approaches in construction related to fire risk, which could be replicated in other settlements, such as Shanghai. Disaster elsewhere also offered an unexpected opportunity. A catastrophic event at Canton in the winter of 1842 induced a favourable view of Hong Kong's new mode of building.

At about half-past four on the wintry afternoon of 7 December 1842, at the eastern face of the Canton Factories site, a mob of Chinese gathered around the Company's garden next to the river near the Creek, Dutch, and the New English (East India Company) Factories. We can see the layout of the grounds in one of the most accurately drawn depictions of the factories made between the fires of 1822 and 1842 (**fig. 3.11**).[135] Since that morning, this crowd had been growing following a local quarrel with several drunken Lascar sailors. The crisis, apparently, was fuelled by the sight of two women walking brazenly in the garden—something most unusual and irregular.[136] The Lascars fled to the Creek Factory and were pursued. A few of the crowd began pulling down the garden fencing. At about half-past six, dinner for the American merchants was interrupted by news that the American Consul had fled to seek the protection of Chinese Hong merchants. As one of the party who was present later recounted,

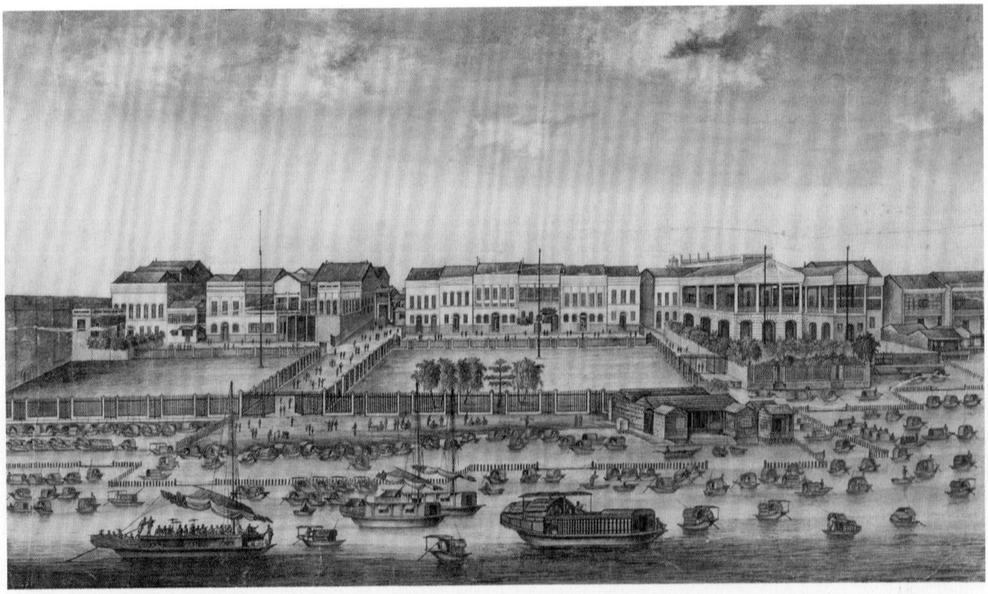

Fig. 3.11. Anon., View of the Factories from the Pearl River, ca. 1839–1840. Ink on paper. © Peabody Essex Museum, Salem (E81458).

> We thought the gentleman a little nervous and much excited, and rather laughed at his fears; but as the noise in the American square increased, we left the table, and from the verandah saw an immense mob in the square and about the factories. All seemed forcing their way to the English factory. We soon saw a light as if they had fired a building, and presently discovered it to be the English flag staff . . . then commenced the destruction of the company's factory, (a very extensive range of buildings, offices &c. &c. occupied by several different mercantile concerns).[137]

These factory buildings were indeed extensive, having evolved since the great fire of 1822 from the original Hong merchants' layouts from whom they were rented. Over the years, they grew into a veritable rabbit warren of spaces, punctuated by light wells, enclosed courtyards, and private and public rooms. There were even factories behind factories, access to which was sought via arched passages running through the front offices (**fig. 3.12**).[138] The lower floors were the most compartmentalised, consisting of godowns, store-rooms, counting rooms, the comprador's rooms, apartments for his assistants, servants and coolies, and the treasury—a massive granite strong-vault buried deep within and sealed by iron doors. This additional protection was considered essential after the expiration of the Company's tea monopoly and

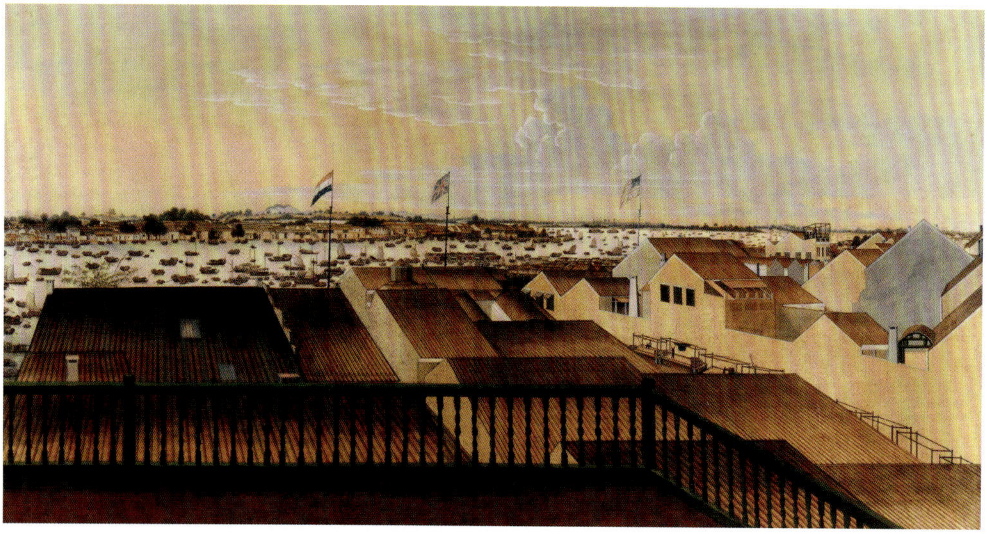

Fig. 3.12. Anon. (possibly Tonequa), Panoramic View of Canton Across the Rooftops of the Foreign Factories, ca. 1810. Gouache on canvas. © Hong Kong Museum of Art Collection (AH1989.0002).

banking system in 1834. The upper floors consisted of dining and sitting rooms, with bedrooms for the merchants at the uppermost.[139] It was a manufactured death trap.

The Lascars took refuge in the Creek Factory, pursued by a crowd of Chinese who directed their fury against the range of buildings between Hog Lane & the Creek, breaking the windows and battering the doors. The riot leaders broke into the Company Factory. They placed wood shavings against the pillars of the large hall for which, somewhat ironically, repairs were underway for the imminent reception of Sir Henry Pottinger. The tinder took, and the entire range of the factories soon lit up the night sky.[140] The mob then set fire to the rear factories bordering Hog Lane and Thirteen Factories Street, assisted by a light northerly wind that spread the flames across from the Company Factory. It was almost as bad as the great fire of 1822 (**fig. 3.13**). The Americans feared that the crowd would mistake them for British.

> One of our number was soon called a Hongmo (Englishman), when Fanqui (foreign devil) and Hongmo were repeated with such violence, and the rush so great, that we found it impossible to move farther, and retreated to our former quarters, where we had a full view of the spreading rage of the fire, expecting every moment it would pass Hog Lane to the American factories.[141]

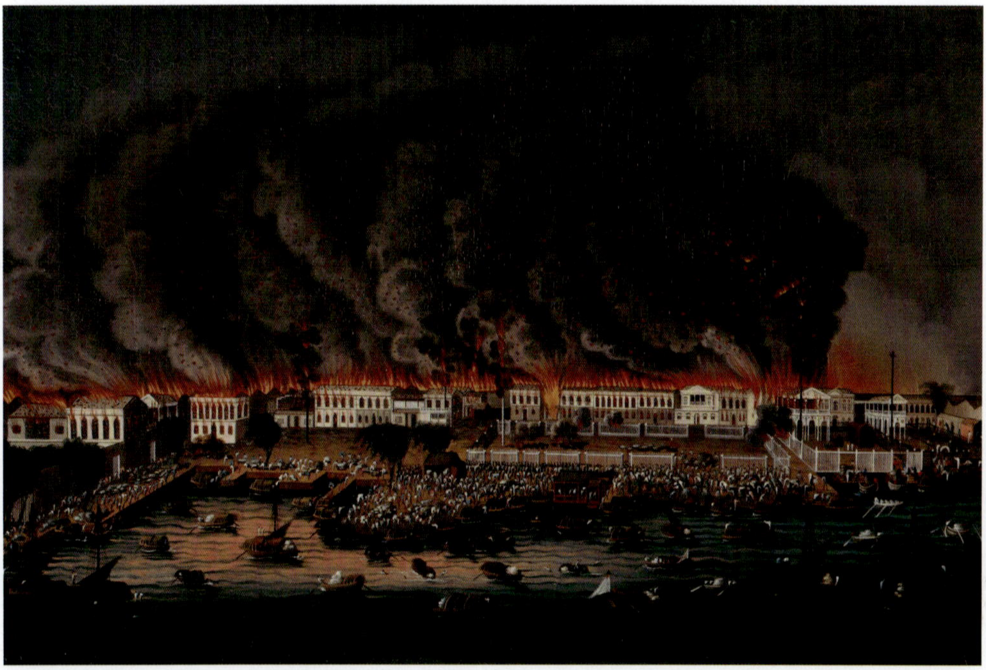

Fig. 3.13. Anon., Fire at the Canton Factories, 1822. Oil on canvas.
© Hong Kong Museum of Art Collection (AH1964.0211).

They were saved by the arrival of three American vessels, which rescued the remaining foreign residents who had been unable to flee sooner. The British sent no aid. The gap created by Hog Lane protected the American Factory and those around it from the conflagration, but the Dutch and Creek Factories next to the Company Factory shared in its fate and were destroyed (**fig. 3.14**). National indignation inevitably met self-interest. The Chinese protestors began looting all movable objects, though much of the treasure had been tipped down wells, ferreted away, or still contained in the relatively impregnable treasuries.

Alexander Matheson, sitting in Macau, was one of the first to be told of the catastrophic events. He wrote to his recently knighted business colleague Sir Jamsetjee Jejeebhoy that 'news reached us of a most serious riot at Canton which has terminated in the destruction by fire of the English, Dutch & Creek Factories with all the valuable property they contained, including a large amount of specie'. Though he assumed the incident was sparked by the quarrel with the Lascars who sought sanctuary within the Creek

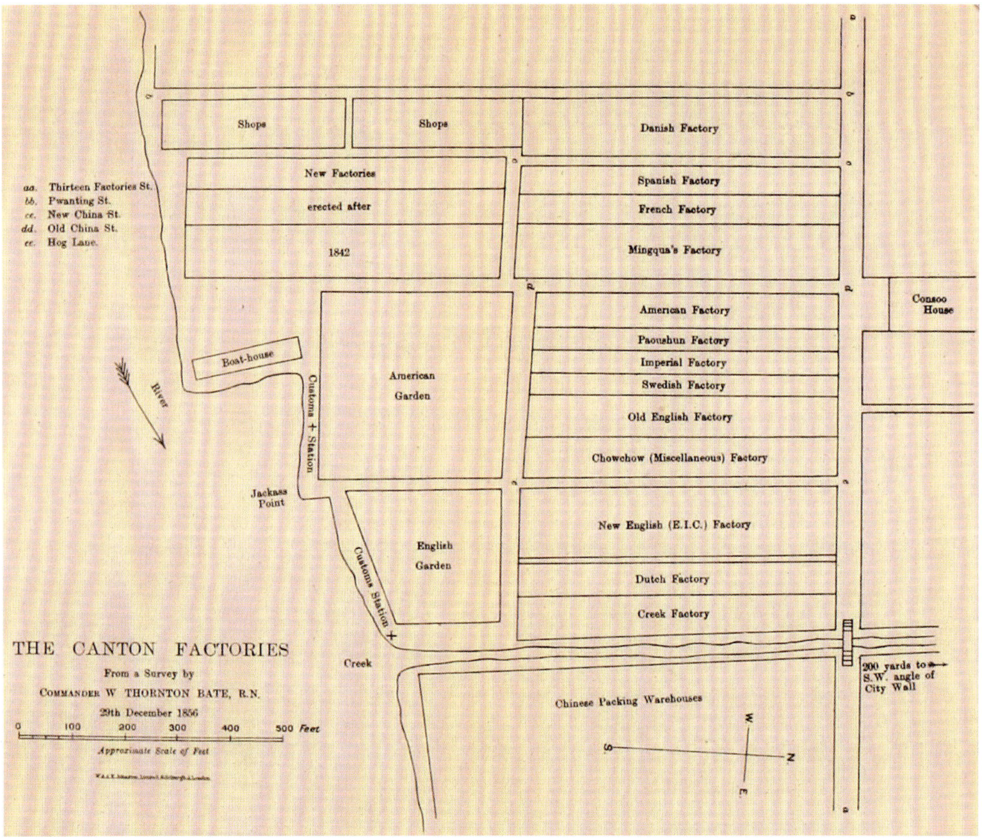

Fig. 3.14. T. Bate, 'The Canton Factories' Layout', 29 December 1856.
W. C. Hunter, *The 'Fan Kwae' at Canton*, London, 1882.

Factory and were followed by the mob, he declared, 'Our opinion is that the authorities, including Howqua, willingly allowed the mob to act for the purpose of intimidating the foreigners, & deterring them from bringing their families to Canton.'[142]

A British military steamer eventually arrived offering protection to the desolate site but was then promptly recalled. Pottinger sharply rebuked the drunkard Lascars, reserving particular ire for the merchants who had taken their wives to the factories before the Nanking Treaty had been ratified.[143] All of this settled the mind of Matheson. Hong Kong, for better or for worse, despite the island's health and land-ownership problems, seemed the only viable choice for his company's regional future. But how to turn such risk into profit? The Canton fire provided the answer, and the answer came swiftly. Two months later, he confided to his parliamentary relative at Westminster, John Abel Smith, that:

> At Hongkong alone can we have anything approaching to security of property, and we think that in a very few years the principle part of the foreign trade will be carried on there.
>
> I mentioned in a recent letter to my Uncle, the desirableness of establishing at Hongkong a branch of one of the London Fire Insurance offices. Such an agency would be a great convenience to us and we shall feel obliged if you will kindly procure such for us. All the new warehouses building at Hongkong are well built, the lower storey generally of granite, and the upper of brick. There are not better risks anywhere the buildings being most substantial, and nearly all of them close to the water's edge.[144]

The idea of acting as agents for an overseas fire insurance firm was further encouraged by a spate of insurance advertisements recorded in local Macau and Hong Kong newspapers from the close of 1842. These included the 'Phoenix Marine Insurance Company' and the 'Hindostan Insurance Society', both firms from Calcutta, offering general-risks policies for merchant vessels.[145]

While fire insurance was a new phenomenon, shipping insurance had been offered in Canton since 1805 by various groups of country traders. The first had been the 'Canton Insurance Company', alternately managed in five-year periods by Magniac-Jardine (the former incarnation of Jardine Matheson) and Dent & Co, but after 1835 remaining in Jardine's possession. Dent eventually formed a firm called the Union Insurance Company, moving its headquarters to Hong Kong in 1841.[146] However, with the late 1842 boom in speculative construction on Hong Kong Island, there was now a need for insurance specifically tailored to those with land-based property interests. In mid-July 1843, Jardine Matheson & Co. advertised themselves as agents to the 'Alliance Fire Assurance Company of London'. They accepted two classes of coverage.

> 1st.— On Buildings of Brick or Stone, covered with Tiles, Slates, Metal or other incombustible material, together with their contents, when such buildings are isolated from all other.
> Rate of Premium ¾ per Cent per Annum.
>
> 2nd.— On such Buildings and their contents when not isolated at the Rate of 1 per Cent per Annum.[147]

They also offered coverage for a fraction of the year with rates of three-quarters and one-third of the annual payment for six months and three months respectively, and with insurance caps of £10,000 for first-class and £8,000 for second-class risks.

During 1843 and well into 1844, bolder and better-organised night attacks targeted isolated European residences across Hong Kong's northern coastline. These were often conducted by Chinese ferried secretly across from the mainland peninsula. Among the signature attack methods was the smashing of windows with stones followed by lobbing in incendiaries, including fire pots.[148] Often, the assailants would flee at the sight of firearms, usually grabbing what they could. Yet the most significant loss to households could be scorched or burnt contents left in the aftermath. The new insurance plan allowed cover for both the fabric of the building and its contents as a single risk or separately if required. It also held out the promise of participation by policyholders in profits after five successive years without claims.

For several years, Jardine Matheson & Co. corresponded directly with the Alliance Fire Assurance Company's London secretary, Mr. A. Hamilton. As the years progressed and competition grew, Jardine Matheson reminded Hamilton of the balance between acquiring new clients and the relative climate of risk. The London-based Alliance always sought the more conservative path. By 1845, Hamilton, recognising the reality on the ground of a fully formed city, authorised the granting of policies to non-isolated buildings at the lower premium of three-quarters of a per cent.[149] Nevertheless, reassurances had to be provided that policies for properties contiguous with others were at secure distances from the next policyholder and therefore non-communicative or else covered under the same policy number.[150]

A complex network of insurance agents soon formed across Southeast Asia and China, with Hong Kong becoming a vital hub. Jardine Matheson's insurance business evolved, providing multiple agents and a portfolio of interested parties for other agents elsewhere for whom they could offer the services of their British or Indian partners. In May 1846, they procured a three-year contract as agents in China for the 'Bombay Insurance Society', recommending an acquaintance in Manila as an agent there.[151]

Also shared across the region were innovative, often indigenously inspired forms of construction, some of which would be rejected by insurers. One such was the introduction of the flat roof—some eighty years before it was to appear in the architecture of European Modernism. In India, native construction had employed flat roofs made of wood with an upper, compressed layer of dried leaves and earth.[152] Brevet Major H. J. Savage, the commanding Royal Engineer at Mauritius, a colony whose early growth coincided with that of Hong Kong, was contemplating the use of flat roofs for his barracks. He saw the form as conducive to health, in which 'removing the Walls, and substituting Flat Roofs, covered with Bitumen, in place of the present shingled ones, would, I am of opinion, be most desirable as it would very much contribute to the health and comfort of the Troops quartered in these Barracks'.[153] This was known as an *Argamasse Roof*, a term taken from the Portuguese for a type of cement made from crushed tiles and lime. It was described as 'simply a flat terrace with 6 to 8 inches of concrete on the beams and planking'.[154] The system would continue to find favour as an approach in that colony for several years.

Flat roofs were of dubious benefit in restricting the convection of air and the subsequent cooling of the lower portion of a room. However, it seems that its 'health and comfort' lay in its internal treatment, providing a finished, level ceiling. The exposed underside of the timbers of pitched roofs, on the other hand, was often infested with wood-destroying white ants (termites), the upper-side shingling at risk of decaying and subsequently admitting water penetration, generating damp air inside and potentially accelerating collapse.[155] In Hong Kong, as early as 1841, Lieutenant Ouchterlony was promoting the use of flat roofs for military and civil construction.[156] But with the shift from mat-sheds to easily-sought Chinese clay tiles, roof pitches remained necessary. Nevertheless, the advent of a standardised form of property fire insurance had the effect of stifling such experimentation across all the treaty ports, so that by 1851 Jardine Matheson would write to their insurance partners in London of construction in Shanghai:

> In reply to your communication of the 24th Dec. ulto. we beg to inform you that the Godowns at Shanghae belonging to Messrs. Sykes Schwabe & Co. are built with stone brick walls and tiled roof. A Mr. Dallas who has recently arrived here from Shanghae informs us that at one time it was in contemplation by Messrs. Sykes Schwabe & Co. to cover the roof of their Godowns with tarred felt, but so soon as they were aware that the Insurance Offices would not take the risk, they immediately gave up the idea and covered them with tiles on the English model.[157]

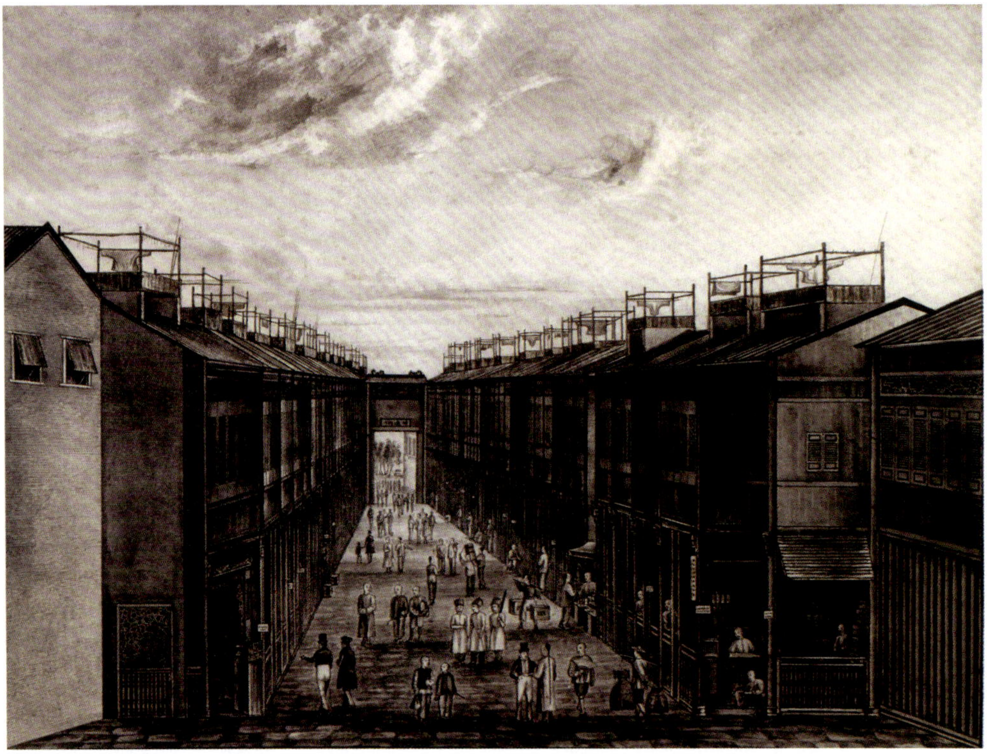

Fig. 3.15. Circle of Youqua (Chinese), Trading Houses on Old China Street, Canton, ca. 1839. Ink and grey wash on paper. © Hong Kong Museum of Art Collection (AH1994.0004).

Another significant opportunity arose from the fire at Canton, or rather a second fire, which was to benefit Hong Kong immeasurably. On Tuesday, 24 October 1843, one of the almost annual conflagrations that seemed to occur somewhere within the massive city broke out, though somewhat distant from the Factories, towards their northwest.

The close crowding of the Chinese buildings during the colder, drier season, coupled with the habit of keeping firewood in open rooftop stores, assisted the spread of the fire (**fig. 3.15**). By the next day, aided by an unfavourable southerly wind, it had spread across to the merchants' quarters, destroying the Danish and Spanish hongs and New China Street between, as well as a part of the French factory.[158]

The blaze effectively cleared the opposite end of the site, what little had remained after the recent arson. One month later, rumours spread in the press that the British authorities had agreed to rent from the Chinese Hong merchants the entire scorched site, including the British, Dutch, and Creek factories area, for a twenty-five-year lease and a ground rent of $6,000.[159] The rumour was soon confirmed. On 12 December 1843, Pottinger issued three government notifications in the Hong Kong press. Two announced the imminent Hong Kong land sale in mid-January and delivery of leases to owners of marine and town lots under the Land Grants Committee. At the same time, the third gave notice of the sub-leasing of land to merchants on the Canton Factories site, which the British had now acquired. Part of the site would be reserved for a new British consulate, and part was allocated for the construction of a small church. The significant point was that the government now demanded that warehouses would form only a minor portion of the land use. The rest would be houses 'according to a plan which will be furnished by government'.[160] In other words, the fire had produced, and made physically manifest, the inevitable division in trade functions between Canton and Hong Kong offered by the new treaty. Canton would now become the front office, Hong Kong the back storeroom. The Cohong system was abolished, minor merchants could now operate a 'just-in-time' policy in transferring goods across to Canton purchasers as and when needed, and therefore Hong Kong would prosper as a 'bonded warehouse' to Canton. Perhaps above all other factors, this new arrangement provided the economic lifeline for Hong Kong in its first faltering years following a miserable 1843 and helped to regenerate the city.

The Survey and the Land Committee

It was Lord Aberdeen who initially prodded for a complete survey of Hong Kong Island in a despatch sent to Sir Henry Pottinger during the new year of 1843.[161] The foreign secretary's instructions bore fruit two years later with the publication of a ground-breaking four-portion survey by Lieutenant Thomas Bernard Collinson of the complete island. Pottinger communicated his orders to Major-General Saltoun on 6 April, explaining that he had been instructed 'to have the Island of Hong Kong carefully surveyed and examined'. The survey would provide the British government with three vital pieces of information: an understanding of the general potential for colonisation across the island, help in identifying the most suitable sites for fortifications and barracks, and to illustrate potential pathways for future city expansion. Pottinger was acutely aware of a likely conflict between military and civil interests arising from the second and the third requirements. In the meantime, needing to conduct a general land survey, Pottinger decided to focus on the third requirement; to plan for the city's future growth. The new land committee was instructed to resolve both the terms of leasehold (as directed by the home government to be the accepted form of land release) and determine individual rights and fulfilments undertaken by current purchasers. Therefore, a careful plan of the town was needed to assist, a survey of the northern face of the island.[162] Pottinger made clear his priority to Saltoun.

> I am very anxious, however, to have the Northern face of the Colony, from "West Point" to the location to the Eastward belonging to Mr Burn, surveyed as soon as possible, that the Streets and Squares and the sites for Public Buildings may be laid down and fixed upon so as to enable me to grant land to the numerous applicants who have been long awaiting to obtain lots.[163]

Accordingly, Saltoun asked Captain Clement Edwards of the 18th Royal Irish, an Assistant Quartermaster, to undertake the survey. Two weeks later, on 23 April, he appointed Captain Thomas de Havilland of the 55th Regiment to join Edwards and help speed up the process. Saltoun requested that de Havilland be transferred from his current post as Military Magistrate at Chusan (Zhoushan) Island to the civil department of Hong Kong, where he would assist. In this endeavour, Edwards was aided by Lieutenant E. W. Sargent of the 18th.[164] They were to be overseen by Land Officer Gordon throughout. Their mission was 'minutely surveying, measuring, and laying down the lots of ground, that have been already sold, or granted on any terms, to individuals within the colony'.[165] These, though, would exclude the lots already earmarked for future military needs. De Havilland was freed from his earlier obligations to Aldrich, but Aldrich at first refused to release the survey books of the northern side of the island that had been undertaken sometime earlier, his proprietorial instincts getting the better of him.[166] The survey team would all be paid in rupees and consist of several European and Chinese overseers, eight coolies, provided with all of the surveying instruments available at the government's disposal, and the use of a house on Cantonment Hill, adjacent to Major-General Saltoun's, to act as their offices.[167]

By mid-May, a parallel survey project was underway, as Edwards was now also commissioned by the Admiralty to chart a portion of territory around Cantonment Hill and southwest in the bay of Shek Pai Wan. Here the Admiralty wished to expand its naval interests (**fig. 3.16**).[168] Both surveys—the civilian and naval—would serve opposing ends: one to present an increasingly conjoined, civic image of the city of Victoria; the other to to intervene and

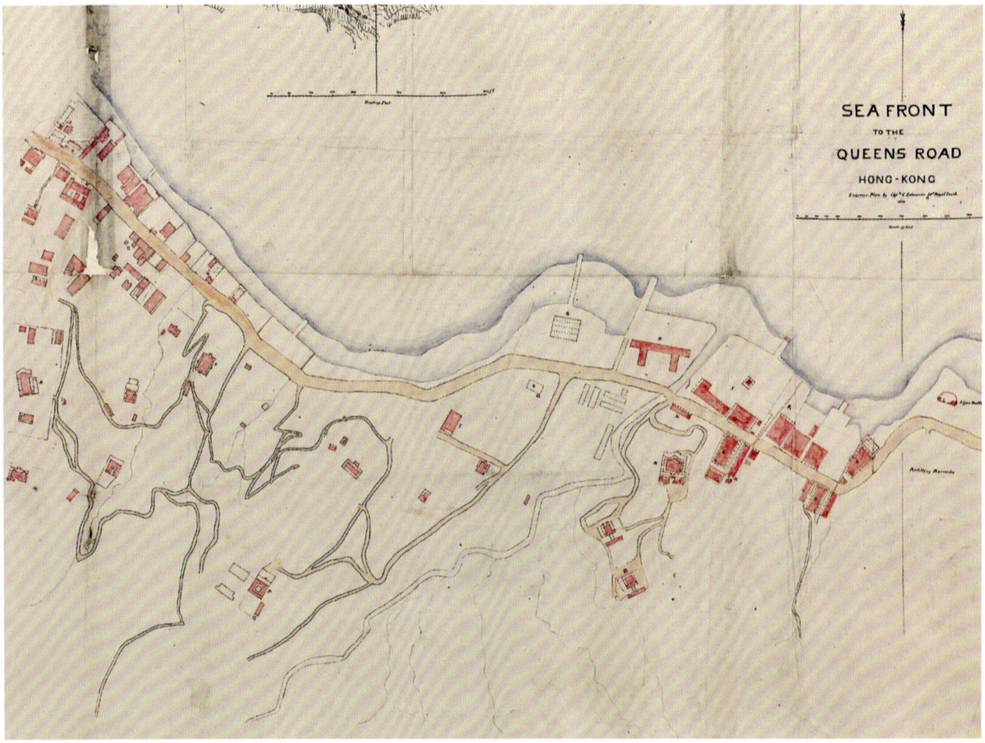

Fig. 3.16. Capt. C. Edwards, 'Sea Front to the Queen's Road, Hong Kong', Admiralty Survey (detail), 1843. Ink and watercolour. © The National Archives, Kew (MR 1/381).

disrupt for strategic military purposes and to find secure enclaves. It is ironic how the same survey team was commissioned to aid the realisation of these two conflicting endeavours, presenting an almost identical graphic format in their surveys of the northern shore.[169]

Since August, the first month to witness the widespread effects of the 'Hongkong Fever' across the colony, the Land Office had been thrown into a state of disarray, with most of its meagre staff lurching from sickness to respite. It took until mid-November for the department to resume an air of normalcy, though that was not before further tragedy placed the city survey in crisis. As the governor recorded to Stanley,

> The sickness which has unfortunately prevailed in this Colony during the last three months, and by which every creature belonging to the Land Officer's Department—including that officer himself—has been incapacitated for duty—and Captain de Havilland, I lament to add, died.[170]

De Havilland died on 5 September, having been in his post for just over five months.[171] His physical decline had been aggravated by overwork as Lieutenant Sargent had been relieved of his duties in early July due to his own ill health and sent to Chusan 'for the benefit of the change'.[172] A new, young professional surveyor, Charles St. George Cleverly, was appointed assistant surveyor as a replacement. In the years to come, he would eventually rise to the post of Surveyor-General. He received an annual salary of £500, half that of his superior A. T. Gordon, and set to work completing what would become the most detailed survey to date of the city of Victoria.[173]

The city survey was eventually delivered to Lord Stanley accompanied by a despatch dated Christmas Day 1843. Captain Brooke of the 55th Regiment, a survivor of West Point, conveyed it in person.[174] Pottinger described it as serving both as a survey of the city's existing layout and indicating the nature and location of future public works proposed by his cousin Gordon. Brooke would be on hand to offer Lord Stanley 'the fullest explanation as to the localities, &c.'[175] The Edwards–de Havilland Survey, now known as 'Gordon's Map', therefore served as protection against military encroachment upon Pottinger's broader urban scheme. A delicately demarcated continuous blue band, presumably denoting the tidal zone, had the added effect of visually uniting the city into a constant strip of marine frontage. What was also immediately apparent with this new plan was that, for the first time, it orientated the city due north. An earlier survey, 'Pottinger's Map' of 1842, had been orientated in reverse, that is, from the perspective of a boat dweller looking upon the island (see **figs. 2.7**, **2.9**, and **2.17**).[176] Here now was the first, most significant cartographic contribution from the perspective of the land dweller and a sign of commitment to remain by the new, post-treaty government of Pottinger. A light grid of squares overlays the entire map, and within this, buildings sit, inked in rose pink. The setting out of a cartesian grid across the whole surface of a survey map had been a method prescribed by Captain Dawson in his survey work in New Zealand before 1840.[177] Two or three copies of his report, previously disseminated to several colonies by London, had been sent to Hong Kong under recommendation from the Colonial Land and Emigration Office.[178] But Edwards and de Havilland adopted a far earlier technique in displaying the buildings themselves. The positions of street arcades, open verandas, and courtyard spaces were meticulously indicated against the walls and private volumes of buildings. It was a method that matched Edwards' Admiralty survey. The former, however, continued where the latter abruptly ended, demonstrating that now, between Pedder's Hill and reaching the end of Lower Bazaar, the elements of a built environment had knitted to such an extent that they began to display, for the first time, a genuine sense of urbanism.

The method used by Edwards and de Havilland followed Giambattista Nolli's famous plan of Rome published in 1748, where public space, arcades, and courtyards remained as negative space, a blank figure-ground, against the solidly hatched buildings that bound them (**figs. 3.17a** and **3.17b**). This Enlightenment method was to have a strong influence on future city cartography. In this respect, Pottinger's plan announced the emergence of Hong Kong as a new, classically civic city to the educated eye. And yet one must also remember that this plan was created during the sickest months on record—where shade, correct orientation, and good ventilation were now considered essential to survival. Under these circumstances, the Nolli plan for this new 'Rome' took on an added meaning, echoing the original sentiments of Lord Aberdeen—in the civilising effects of a well-planned city lay the hope for an end to the fever.

But the Edwards–de Havilland Survey had a much more immediate and mundane purpose. Almost like a visual Domesday Book, it meticulously recorded property ownership through a numbering system placed upon each building or vacant lot. This method allowed its use as a tool for Pottinger's new four-man-strong Land Grants Committee, of which Captain de Havilland was an initial member.[179] The other three members were the land officer, A. T. Gordon; the colonial treasurer and financial secretary, Charles Edward Stewart; and the legal advisor to the government, Richard Burgass. Quite literally, the map's development charted that of the committee itself as it went from property to property, painstakingly determining the legality of every entity. What is absent from the survey is as interesting and revealing as what is shown. The area above and around Lower Bazaar extending towards West Point was covered by 'numerous tenants of mat sheds', all occupied by Chinese. The committee recorded none of these illegal or semi-legal structures in their survey.[180]

The committee was established in late August 1843 with instructions 'to inquire into the equitable claims of all Holders of Land, to define the classes to which particular lots shall henceforward belong, as well as their future annual rent'.[181] They also had the unenviable task of determining whether each holder had complied with their covenants regarding land improvement, which doubtless infuriated those who had been obliged to cease construction earlier that year. Out of their deliberations emerged a set of proposals that would have far-reaching consequences in terms of future land auctions and the solidifying economic disposition of each section of the town. The latter was perhaps the most radical: linking the town and suburban lots to their specific circumstances. Apart from the expensive

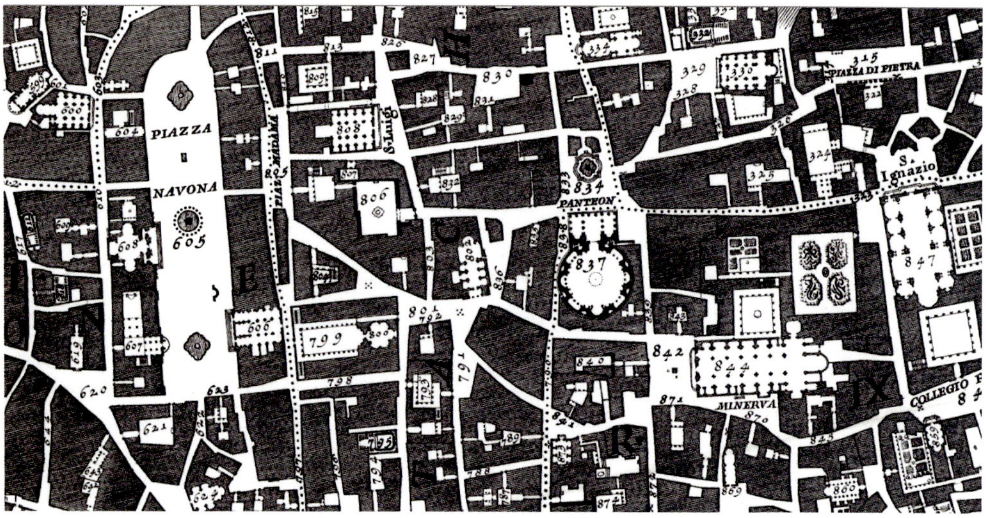

Fig. 3.17a. G. Nolli, *La Pianta Grande di Roma* (The Large Plan of Rome) (detail), 1748. Etching.

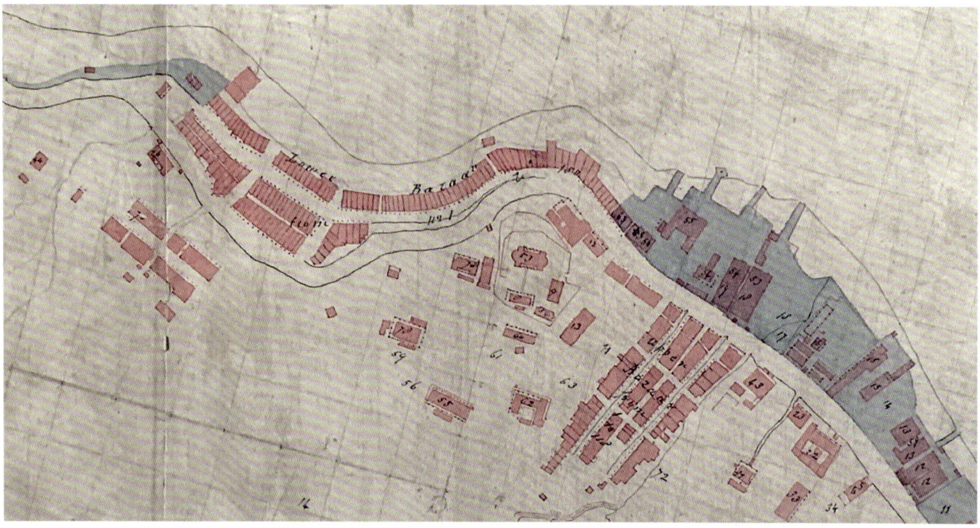

Fig. 3.17b. Capts. C. Edwards and T. de Havilland, Upper and Lower Bazaars (detail), 1843. Ink and watercolour. © The National Archives, Kew (MPG 1/156).

marine lots, these others were dispersed across a wide diversity of terrain. As a consequence, some were now perceived to be considerably undervalued while others were somewhat overvalued. Eighty-eight town lots had been granted to date with seventy-five paying an annual rent of £20 per 105 square feet, now thought to be a considerable bargain.[182] The committee proposed a classification system for these plots under thirteen classes in total, as 'from the very uneven nature of the ground in the Island, it could not be fairly assessed if divided into a smaller number'.[183] The experiences, still raw, of the Hongkong Fever must have inevitably contributed to the consideration of the criteria. Contributing factors were, among others, the height above sea level, the nature of the approach to each lot, and the potentiality of each site for improvement.[184] In addition, by the careful analysis of each case, the circumstances and behaviour of the individual owner, and the capital expended on improvement, the committee was able to build up a comprehensive economic zoning plan, thereby reinforcing the value of one section of the city against another. Apart from its distance from the centre, in essence, land closer to the southern edge of the Queen's Road and by which the ascent was negligible or gradual would be rated highly. Those properties which had a difficult approach and for which a larger expenditure had been made to remedy the inherent problems of the site would be placed in a lower class.[185] As an extension of this logic, it was clear that improving the city's infrastructure—its roads, sewers, and drains—could enhance the value of subsequent land released at auction.

Finally, the committee recommended that the length of a leasehold should be seventy-five years and that any new lots sold should be fixed at an upset price commensurable with those of corresponding lots. The classification system made it easier to evaluate lots by this new criteria rather than purely by location. This system determined the upset prices of all lots put up for auction at the new land sale of 22 January 1844. It would become the first tangible yardstick to measure the value of land and, by extension, build a consensual picture of value for each portion of the island, giving birth to the concept of 'districts'. It also reinforced the privileging perceptions of height, level, access, and connection.

A Battle for the Centre

'Connection' was also the key to another debate that was raging. A battle of two visions for the city's future spread across 1843. Malaria would not just form a backdrop to this

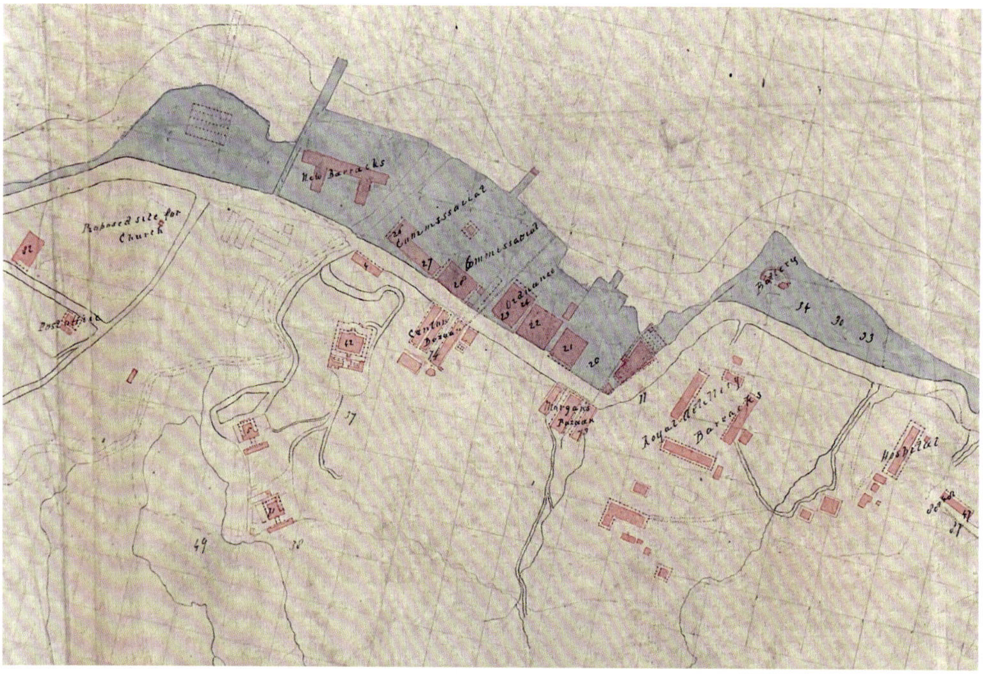

Fig. 3.18. Capts. C. Edwards and T. de Havilland, Ordnance District (detail), 1843. Ink and watercolour. © The National Archives, Kew, London (MPG 1/156).

struggle but would directly intervene in the decision-making. The combatants were Sir Henry Pottinger and Major-General Lord Saltoun. The prize—a thin strip of land below Cantonment Hill, which would ultimately form an area later known as Admiralty. On one side was the civilian government's civic concern for a unified shoreline where a mercantile community might lavish their considerable expenditure upon fine palaces and godowns, make good use of the waterfront, and visually start to tie the city together. On the other was an inward-looking, isolationist concern for the well-being and control of troops within a new, self-contained, fortified military cantonment, where all the necessities of provision and good governance were at Saltoun's disposal as he sat on the hill above as overlord.

This strip of coastal land had become known as the 'Ordnance District' (**fig. 3.18**). It comprised part of the earliest military settlement that had straddled the Albany Nullah at the beginning of 1841 and covered part of the foot of Government Hill. Lieutenant Ouchterlony had constructed temporary mat-sheds here for the arrival in September

1841 of the 98th Regiment, the Staffordshire, 'along the harbour shore just north of the Queen's Road and some around the land now occupied by Flagstaff House'.[186] It then became a depot for provisions for the China Expedition of 1842, and, on instructions from the governor-general of India, the Commissariat was established here together with ordnance stores. Yet, at the same time, a mixture of godowns, two market bazaars, the Canton and Morgan's Bazaars, and residential buildings dotted the area, and there was no apparent determination by Pottinger to remove them.[187] On the contrary, he considered it necessary that the shorefront area to the north of the Queen's Road was safeguarded from further military encroachment. For, by now, this meagre strip had become one of the most valuable patches remaining to lease from the Crown and would, to his mind, comprise an eminent centre-piece for the January 1844 land sale.

A remarkable view of the Ordnance District has recently come to light. This image corroborates the only other known view to exist, Murdoch Bruce's *Queen's Road Looking East from Canton Bazaar* (1846), and appears to be contemporaneous.[188] It was sketched by the architect Edward Ashworth in 1844 or 1845 before Aldrich dramatically reconfigured the district (**fig. 3.19**). Though Ashworth's study shows significantly more of the streetscape than Bruce's, both demonstrate each architect's desire to accurately depict the evolving city, despite their adoption of certain picturesque modes of representation. Aldrich's new arrangement established the basic layout of an area later to become Admiralty. Ashworth's view was taken beside the Albany Nullah and along the Queen's Road, looking southeast towards Ha Wan (the future Wan Chai). We see that the Canton Bazaar to the right (south) backs onto Cantonment Hill (now Hong Kong Park), and the Commissariat with its walled compound to the left (north) backs onto Victoria Harbour. According to the 1843 Edwards–de Haviland Survey, behind it, one can see the verandas of the two-storied properties of the minor hongs, Messrs. Gemmell & Co. and Fletcher & Co., both soon removed to turn the area into a military enclave. Up on the hill, straight ahead, are the square buildings of the Royal Artillery's powder magazines, with Mount Cameron to the right. Here, along the barren-looking Queen's Road, we see a remarkable intermingling of cultures: a variety of Chinese hawkers and workers mill about, with a South Asian sepoy or lascar in the foreground, and two Europeans, possibly seconded military, patrol as policemen to the far left. Taken at the height of the day, one gets a sense of how relentlessly exposed were the early settlers in Hong Kong to the raw light and heat of the sun.

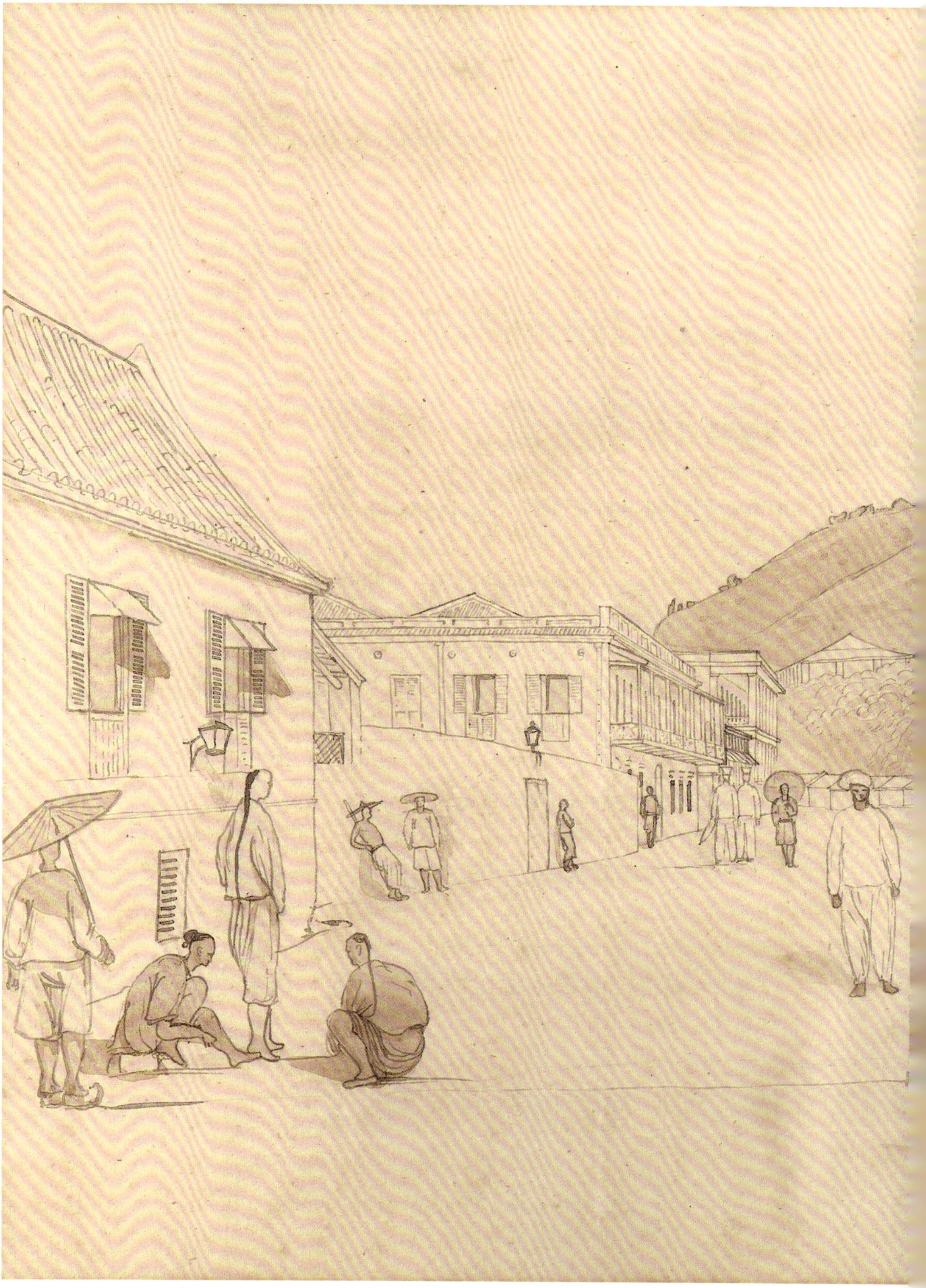

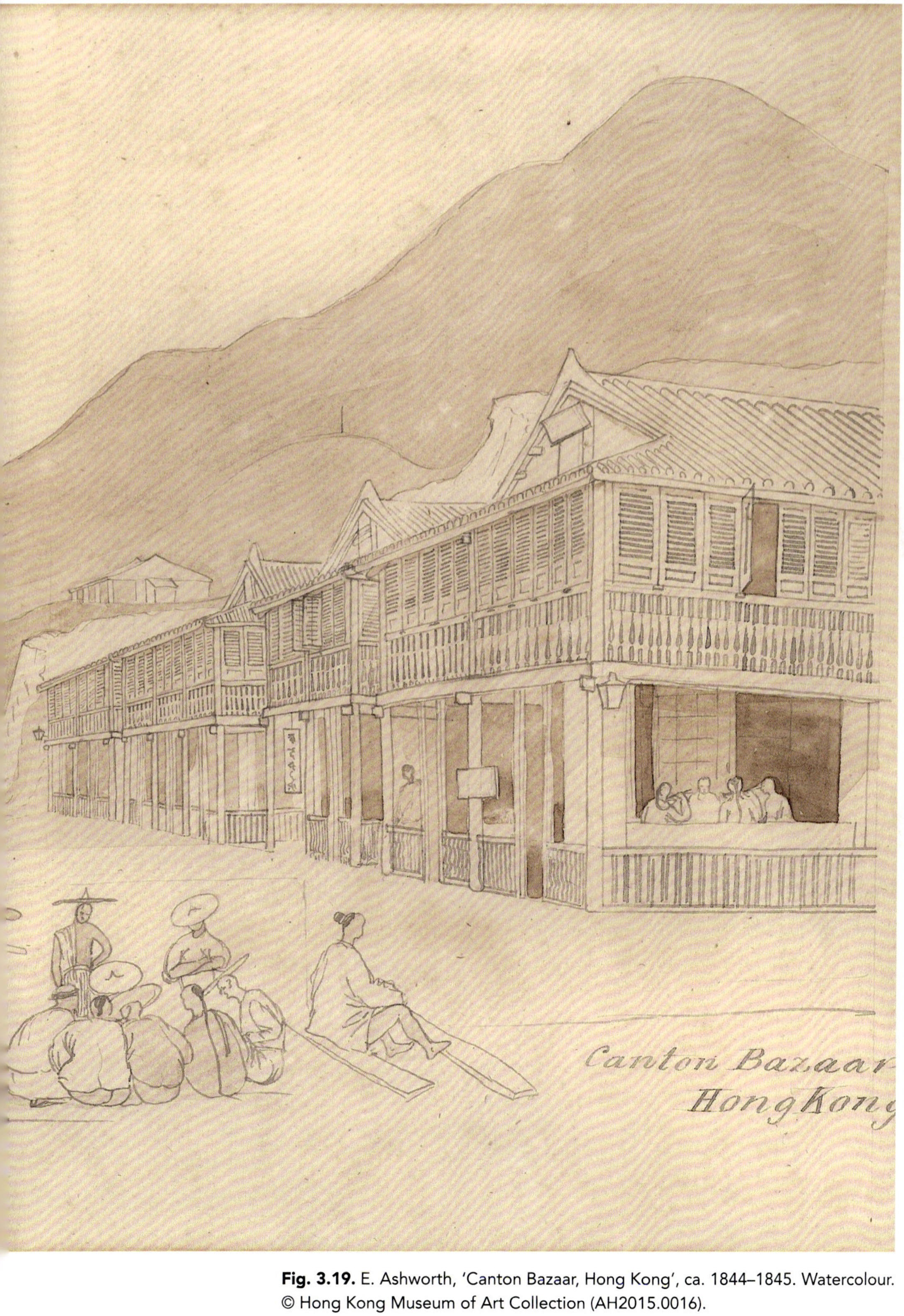

Fig. 3.19. E. Ashworth, 'Canton Bazaar, Hong Kong', ca. 1844–1845. Watercolour. © Hong Kong Museum of Art Collection (AH2015.0016).

Pottinger had always been sympathetic towards the need for barracks—he saw these as relatively mobile bits of kit, responsive to government needs for land and their reacquisition.[189] However, he had drawn the line at the intense fortification plans adopted by Aldrich under Saltoun. In late July 1843, as the stakes mounted, Pottinger, through his secretary Richard Woosnam, took the unusual action of publicising his disagreement in the local newspapers.

> A plan has been proposed by Major Aldrich of the Royal Engineers for laying out and fortifying the centre part of this city. . . . His Excellency the Governor further directs me to acquaint you that he has not himself, after full consideration, seen cause to recommend Major Aldrich's plan to the authorities at home.[190]

The army and navy had already planned to concentrate military forces within the central portion of the city before the outbreak of malaria at West Point. Now, with the ratified treaty and the prize of permanence assured, a tug of war between the civil government of Pottinger and the armed services for possession of this prime real estate seemed inevitable. However, as Pottinger, the ever-mobile Plenipotentiary was frequently absent from the island performing his diplomatic and trading duties, Hong Kong–based Saltoun as general commanding officer was able to steal the initiative.[191]

In mid-June, one month before the medical committee gathered at West Point, Saltoun directed Aldrich to 'examine this place [Hong Kong] with a view to the best defensive positions being selected'.[192] It was likely the first significant instruction given to Aldrich after he arrived in Hong Kong on 10 June. Saltoun also passed on proposals for a comprehensive cantonment plan that Ouchterlony had formulated while executive engineer.[193] This plan was known to Pottinger, as he had previously protested about its encroachment across the Albany Nullah onto Government Hill and north across the Queen's Road onto the valuable shorefront, causing him to reiterate in early May:

> I consider it will be a most excellent arrangement to assign to this Cantonment all the land lying between the Ravine that runs along the Eastern side of 'Government Hill' and the Ravine that divides 'Hospital Hill' from the location belonging to Messrs. Holliday Wise & Co., merely reserving a frontage towards the 'Queen's Road', of the depth of the ranges of shops know by the names of the 'Canton and Morgan's Bazaars'.[194]

He would allow 'four great roads' to penetrate the Canton and Morgan's bazaars and two other locations along the Queen's Road, provided the cantonment remained discreetly set back and screened by commerce on two sides of the principal artery of the city.[195]

By 28 June, Aldrich had produced a sixteen-page report: his *Memoranda with reference to Barrack and Hospital accommodation and with reference to internal Defence. . . .*[196] He blithely ignored all of Pottinger's concerns, even going one step further by suggesting that the entire area should be 'confined entirely to the Military Department. . . . The whole being thus under military surveillance, military discipline will be best preserved, the military duties carried on with fewer sentries, and the arrangement will most materially contribute to preserve order among the civil population'.[197] What seems surprising in this document is that, with cases of the 'Hongkong Fever' multiplying around him as he wrote, as well as intimating that he had served in the malarial West Indies, Aldrich appeared almost exclusively focused upon the compressive virtues of defensible space and surveillance rather than the expansive ones of ventilation and contagion prevention.[198] Surprisingly, considering the impact of disease as the major cause of mortality for troops in China, Saltoun neither instructed nor did Aldrich overtly contemplate a strategy for dealing with this at the same time. This absence may have been because Lord Aberdeen's recent January 1843 despatch from the Foreign Office had made it abundantly clear to consider ventilation and barrack positioning and need hardly have required re-mentioning. Moreover, in his subsequent designs of the Officers' Quarters (later named Murray House) and Headquarter House (later named Flagstaff House), ventilation, shade, and elevation were inimitable components of Aldrich's thinking (**fig. 3.20**). Regardless, the epidemic of the following months would consolidate Aldrich's proposal and undoubtedly add to his leverage in Whitehall. In Aldrich's reasoning, it was not just the strategic defence of a town that was required but the creation of a self-supporting military community within it. A military enclave would offer ease of access to goods, provide medical treatment offered by a 'general hospital', administrative offices, and even a military prison.

From the start, Aldrich focused on the Ordnance District, that valuable strip of land along the shore which so concerned the governor. Regardless of the civil government, he was determined to commandeer the site for a cantonment. In addition to defence, the army desperately needed barracks. Significant reinforcements of troops were on their way to the new crown colony, a detachment of the Royal Sappers and Miners and seven hundred soldiers supplementing the 98th Regiment, fresh from Britain.[199] Aldrich, therefore, integrated the defence and accommodation programmes to strengthen his hand. He requested the acquisition of existing adjacent buildings, both military and civilian, which sat vulnerably within the district, blocking his designs. Large-scale accommodation was of immediate need, so Aldrich demanded the use of the commissariat godowns and the quarters for native (South Asian) and Chinese commissariat officers as temporary barracks for the European troops. He also asked that ordnance stores be relocated to other sites freeing up building stock and land.[200] As a temporary measure for the officers, the major proposed 'immediately securing . . . the private Godowns on the East side of the new Building lately erected as an Ordnance Store . . . for the Mess House and for Officer Quarters'.[201] He would soon get permission to design an entire barracks system, its layout based upon Ouchterlony's earlier plans. However, as if belatedly recalling Saltoun's instructions, Aldrich then combined this with an encapsulating argument on defence terms.

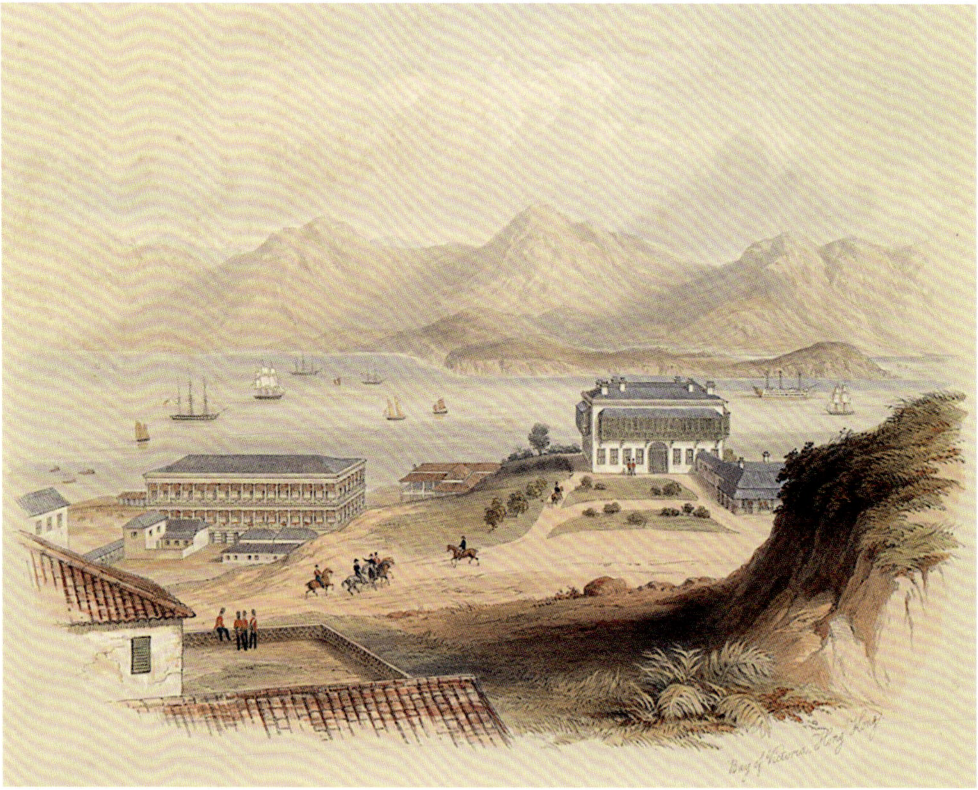

Fig. 3.20. Lt. G. M. Martin, Ventilation and Shading Devices Shown on the Officers' Quarters (left) and Headquarter House (right), Title Page to *Operations in the Canton River in April 1847*, London, 1848. Hand-coloured lithograph.

> I therefore consider the present cantonment the ground best selected to afford from its central position flanking fire from Batteries East and West for the protection of the Town on these sides and by inclosing the right and left of the position planting the gorge with prickly pears &c. giving to the whole the character of a permanent field position advantage of command.[202]

In concluding his memorandum, Aldrich seemed to reveal his actual anxiety, that military security lay in the prevention of attack *from within* Hong Kong Island.

> In a few words a defensive district including all necessary Commissariat and Ordnance supplies and water, and wholly confined in occupation to persons under the restraint of military Discipline constitutes that which I consider essentially necessary to possess in the occupation of any Colony and particularly so where the population of the Island is composed of aliens of every variety of religion, and it is truly fortunate that there is the means of this position being so arranged.[203]

Saltoun promptly forwarded the report to the governor on 29 June, and somewhat disingenuously distanced himself from Aldrich's zealous conclusions claiming that he had spent the intervening time between instruction and receipt in Macau.[204] He also partially absolved himself, admitting to Pottinger, 'this plan you will observe from the very absurd way in which locations have been given, interferes considerably with what has been considered private property.' Saltoun then pinned down Pottinger by offering him a fait accompli. The governor was 'to decide whether this or any other plan of fortifications drawn out by the officer duly authorised to do so and approved of by me as commanding the forces shall be caused into execution forthwith, or whether it is your pleasure we shall wait for the approval of the Master-General and Parliament'.[205]

Having had his conditions for site selection bluntly ignored, Pottinger must undoubtedly have felt the bind. Writing back to Saltoun on 4 July, he concluded that 'the fullest consideration upon it has led me to doubt whether it is that which is best calculated to afford general protection to this City as a future great emporium of commerce'. Pottinger explained that 'a part of my presumed arrangement was to have recovered a frontage along the whole extent of the Queen's Road on both sides for shops, warehouses, dwelling houses, &c. &c., and to have had other streets running off from it at right angles'.[206] This was a conclusion coincidentally reached by his cousin Gordon's 'present state of the roads and buildings in the Colony' report, which, as earlier mentioned, was submitted to Malcolm two days later.[207] All the governor could now do was again repeat his determined belief that the West Point area was the ideal position for a cantonment 'which I had sketched in my own mind for this side of the Island long before I heard that Major Aldrich had been ordered to China'.[208] He argued the logic for 'Fortifications to the West of the City (beyond the Naval Arsenal, Depot, &c.) to command the Western or Principal entrance to the Bay of Hong Kong.'[209] The fifty-foot-wide Queen's Road, Pottinger offered (echoing Gordon) would be extended, kept in good repair, and thereby able to afford rapid deployment of both troops and gun carriages to any point along the northern coast, 'and in such an extreme case, the public as well as private buildings would be, of course, appropriated for temporary Barracks, or Hospitals, or any other purpose to which they could be usefully applied'.[210] But it was July, and the micro-political world around him had shifted with the climate of sickness.

The governor sent his dispatch to London on 17 July in the hands of Lieutenant Colonel Malcolm. Attached to this compendium of documents was the correspondence between Pottinger, Saltoun, and Aldrich, and Gordon's 6 July report. Pottinger availed of the Gordon Report, comparing it favourably against Aldrich's proposal. He argued fiercely on economic grounds. 'Situated as I am it is my duty to say, that I think that carrying out those plans will interfere very much with the increase and prosperity of Hong Kong (Victoria) as an Emporium of Trade, which was, I believed, the sole, or, at least, the Chief, object in securing its cession.'[211]

Pottinger, as we now know, was unlucky. The untimely epidemic at West Point was followed by a whole-scale evacuation of the area seventeen days after Pottinger's reply to Saltoun and just four days after his report of the entire situation to Lord Stanley in Whitehall, including Aldrich's memoranda, his remonstrance, and all. Certainly, it scotched any idea of a cantonment in the vicinity of West Point and Navy Bay. Months passed as the Hong Kong administration waited for a decision to reach them from Whitehall. Nevertheless, whether or not the epidemic directly impinged upon London's decision, the removal of Pottinger's alternative left Aldrich's proposal to secure the area desired relatively unchallenged. The city would be bisected.

As it chanced, Lord Stanley did indeed fall behind his man. He wrote on 9 December, 'Her Majesty's Government agree with Sir Henry Pottinger that the prospects of Hong Kong as a mart and as a colony are not to be sacrificed to other purposes.'[212] It was, however, a pyrrhic victory. Where else now were the military to go? The Ordnance

District and the area above it would become a cantonment in all but name, though soon known as the Murray Barracks (within the larger Victoria Barracks complex) and Admiralty. Bit by bit, Aldrich and the army would add building elements into Pottinger's 'no-go' zone, with private property edged out.

The process began almost at once. Riding on the coattails of the recently constructed naval hospital nearby, Saltoun's replacement the new commander Major-General George Charles D'Aguilar instructed to build a military hospital. By this health pretext, he would gain possession of the valuable north side of the road along the shore. 'The site now proposed for the Military Hospital is not within the ground which was allotted for Cantonments,' piped Pottinger's private secretary helplessly. 'It is almost superfluous to add, that by far the most valuable part of the Crown Lands in this Colony are those which are washed by the Harbour and which are consequently—peculiarly adapted for mercantile purposes.'[213] He was powerless to prevent it. As the land around Cantonment Hill was progressively removed from civilian use, a predictable sequence of events unfolded.

First, it became clear that Central had to be consolidated, requiring expansion up the steep mountainside—the urban grain of the city realigning itself. The Chinese Upper Bazaar in Pottinger's and subsequently Davis's eyes emerged as an planning blunder, a blockage needing speedy removal.

Second, this need for the Europeans to climb was reinforced by a belief that higher-altitude dwellings would protect inhabitants from the fever. Despite his location-based scepticism as to malaria, the first governor had no doubt about this matter. In a letter to Saltoun in October 1843, Pottinger assured him that 'the experience of even the past season is strongly in favour of the superior eligibility of the tops of hills'.[214] Pottinger would use the January land sale of 1844, later reinforced by Davis, to push the resident Chinese out of Upper Bazaar and into an expanded lower area of Tai Ping Shan to the west. This brutal act was the first example of eminent domain, the expropriation of land for public purposes, in Hong Kong's history. Pottinger initiated an increasingly habitual instinct by the colonial government of compulsory purchase as a mechanism of urban control. Ironically, this would eventually include plague-ridden Tai Ping Shan itself under the resumption ordinance of 1894.[215] The removal allowed remedial re-configuring of the street system, which included additional streets such as the new Wellington Street. In conjunction with this re-formed street circulation, the government provided sales plots of a greater topographical spread than had previously been offered under auction.

Third, the Murray Barracks and Admiralty would inevitably cut off Central from the wealthy residential and commercial quayside of the Spring Gardens, located in present-day Wan Chai. Here is where the homes of the elite had been hastily captured in watercolour by George Chinnery and, later, more leisurely lithographed by the architect Murdoch Bruce. Its survival as a suburb relied upon a good connection to the commercial and civic centre. As neither Central nor the Wong Nai Chung Valley (its plans abandoned) afforded such hope, Spring Gardens itself would eventually be vacated by European traders and their families to become a significant Chinese part of the city. At the same time, Europeans would climb for the steeper reaches of Mid-Levels.

And so, like a plant abruptly pruned, the malarial outbreak of 1843 had the combined effect—both west and east—of cutting the city of Victoria back to its initial root, thereby influencing the tendril lines of subsequent growth for young Hong Kong. There would be further upheavals over the next few years, mainly of an economic and political nature, which would threaten the colony's development, including a climate of increasing disenfranchisement with Sir John Davis's administration, but nothing quite like the trauma of 1843. This period was both the nadir and the reforging of the city. The internal, segregated worlds of discreet interests—that 'Hongkonian' way of life—were gone. In their place was an increasing desire by the community for municipal governance. The variegated terrain of the city had seemed to present hidden dangers and benefits concerning health, and therefore it had to be understood and tamed. One example of this taming would occur through land surveying, whereby T. B. Collinson would introduce the added dimension of altitude through contour-lined maps. Also, *how* to build was now as important as *where* to build. Consequently, a healthy property intermingled with the badge of status. A shifting thesis for the causes of malaria would continue, however. As will be seen, the politicisation of health would evolve into a more sophisticated attack upon the very fundamentals of the colony itself. The future of Hong Kong lay still in peril.

Notes

1 James Legge, 'The Colony of Hong Kong—From a Lecture by the Rev. James Legge, D.D., L.L.D., on Reminiscences of a Long Residence in the East, Delivered in the City Hall, November 5, 1872', *China Review*, vol. 3 (1874): 165.

2 '1843 Principal Events', *Historical and Statistical Abstract of the Colony of Hong Kong 1841–1930*, 3rd ed. (Hong Kong: Noronha & Co., 1932), 3. The abstract relies upon E. J. Eitel, *Europe in China: The History of Hong Kong from the Beginning to the Year 1882* (Hong Kong: Kelly and Walsh / London: Luzac & Co., 1895), 191. Though this is a commonly cited set of statistics by historians, locating the origin of this important data beyond Eitel has proved elusive.

3 The National Archives, Kew [hereafter NA]; Colonial Office [hereafter CO] 129/3: 440, Pottinger to Johnston, 7 Sep. 1842.

4 *Friend of China*, 23 Mar. 1843; 'Synopsis of Events in China During the Year 1843', *Canton Press*, 6 Jan. 1844.

5 CO 129/3: 34, Aberdeen to Pottinger, 4 Jan. 1843.

6 Ibid., 44a.

7 Ibid., 3: 34a–35.

8 Ibid., 3: 36a.

9 'Synopsis of Events', *Canton Press*, 6 Jan. 1844.

10 *Canton Press*, 19 Aug. 1843.

11 'Synopsis of Events', *Canton Press*, 6 Jan. 1844.

12 Ibid.

13 *Canton Register*, 23 May 1843.

14 CO 129/2: 84a, Stephen to Stanley, 16 Oct. 1842. As marginalia.

15 *Canton Press*, 1 July 1843.

16 William Tarrant, *Hongkong Part 1, 1839 to 1844* (Canton: Friend of China, 1861), 33. I refer to the Wong Nai Chung Gap and Tai Tam Gap roads, created principally for military access to their stations at Sai Wan (north-eastern side of the island) and Chek Chue (south-eastern side).

17 CO 129/3: 31a–33, Stephen to Addington (Foreign Office), 30 Jan. 1843.

18 See CO 129/4: 201a and CO 129/4: 205 as examples.

19 CO 129/3: 24–24a.

20 Ibid., 3: 24a.

21 Ibid., 3: 25.

22 CO 129/3: 14, Stephen to Stanley, 3 Jan. 1843.

23 CO 129/3: 8a, Stephen to George W. Hope (Treasury), 5 Jan. 1843.

24 CO 129/3: 25a–26, Stephen to Addington.

25 CO 129/3: 4a, Hope to Stanley, 5 Jan. 1843.

26 Lt. Col. R. S. Hawkins R.E., 'Far Eastern Outpost', *Royal Engineers Journal*, vol. 82 (March 1968): 38.

27 *Canton Register*, 23 May 1843.

28 Ibid.

29 Hong Kong Public Records Office [hereafter HKPRO]; file: HKMS 140-1-1, 'Transcripts of Correspondence of Lieut. Thomas Bernard Collinson R.E. Dec. 1838–29 Mar. 1846' [hereafter 'Transcripts'], Collinson to Miss Cecilia Collinson, Boldon Rectory, Gateshead (Hong Kong, 21 Mar. 1845).

30 Hawkins, 'Far Eastern Outpost', 39–40.

31 Ibid., 40.

32 CO 129/4: 340–343a; CO 129/4: 344–347a.

33 As both brothers were surveyors of Hong Kong it is therefore not certain to which brother 'Mount Collinson' and 'Cape Collinson', features on the west of the island, are attributed to. Although it is

likely to be named *by* Bernard, as he certainly bequeathed 'Aldrich Bay' and 'Cape D'Aguilar' to his commanders.

34 HKPRO; *Transcripts*, Collinson to his father, Rev. J. Collinson, Boldon Rectory, Gateshead (Kilkenny, 2 Oct. 1842).

35 Ibid.

36 Hawkins, 'Far Eastern Outpost', 40.

37 Ibid.

38 Ibid.

39 Ibid., 47.

40 The only known layout plan of West Point: CO 129/2: 455ff. (map MPG 1/156).

41 James Legge, 'The Colony of Hong Kong', 164.

42 CO 129/5: 143, 'Detailed Account Disbursements of the Land Department from June 1841 to January 1844—Military and Naval'.

43 CO 129/10: 638a, Pottinger to D'Aguilar, 2 Feb. 1844. We have a snapshot of the earlier arrangement from 'Pottinger's Map' of 1842, MR 029, extracted from NA; Foreign Office [hereafter FO] 925/ 2427, which shows a scattering of less orderly barracks entitled 'Volunteer Barracks'.

44 NA; Admiralty [hereafter ADM] 1/5530, Pottinger to Saltoun, 4 May 1843 (copy).

45 Ibid.

46 ADM 1/5530, Parker to Saltoun, 15 July 1843.

47 Ibid.

48 'List of H.B.M.'s Military Forces in China', *Chinese Repository*, Jan. 1843, as recorded in the *Canton Register*, 28 Feb. 1843.

49 CO 129/7: 182a, Proceedings of the Medical Committee, 15 July 1843.

50 Ibid., 182a.

51 We know of abandoned rice-growing terraces in the vicinity through a medical-topographic report. See ADM 1/5530, Wilson, Reid, and King to Parker, 12 July 1843.

52 See NA; MR 029, 'Pottinger's Map' (1842).

53 Names of all the barracks are provided in the notice of public auction of 'the whole of the Materials of the Barracks and other Military buildings at West Point' (Commissariat, 6 Feb 1844), *Friend of China*, 10 Feb. 1844.

54 CO 129/5: 637a, Pottinger to D'Aguilar, 2 Feb. 1844. Pottinger suggested 'that a Committee should be appointed to report on the [West Point] Barracks and to decide whether the materials should be sold or kept for future Military Buildings'.

55 CO 129/5: 473, Land Department receipt, 5 Aug. 1843.

56 *Hongkong Eastern Globe*, 5 July 1843, as reprinted in the *Canton Press*, 15 July 1843.

57 *Canton Press*, 15 July 1843.

58 CO 129/7: 182, Proceedings.

59 Ibid., 183.

60 Ibid., 183a.

61 Ko Tim-Keung, 'A Review of development of Cemeteries in Hong Kong: 1841–1950', *Journal of the Hong Kong Branch of the Royal Asiatic Society* [hereafter *JHKBRAS*], vol. 41 (2001): 245.

62 Tarrant, *Hongkong*, 77. Tarrant quoting from *Friend of China* in 1844.

63 CO 129/10: 479, Pottinger to Saltoun, 18 July 1843; Tarrant, *Hongkong*, 64.

64 CO 129/10: 475, Pottinger to Vice Admiral Sir William Parker, 15 July 1843.
65 CO 129/10: 485a, Pottinger to Saltoun, 26 July 1843.
66 CO 129/10: 493–493a, Pottinger to Saltoun, 7 Aug. 1843.
67 CO 129/10: 490, Pottinger to Saltoun, 3 Aug. 1843.
68 CO 129/10: 492a–493, Pottinger to Saltoun, 7 Aug. 1843.
69 *Canton Press*, 26 Aug. 1843.
70 A. R. Johnston, 'Note on the Island of Hong-Kong', *Journal of the Royal Geographical Society of London*, vol. 14 (1844): 115. There is no sense of superiority in Johnston's text, however, one must be cautious at to the extent of knowledge conveyed on Chinese medical matters by the author.
71 Ibid.
72 *Canton Press*, 12 Aug. 1843.
73 *Canton Press*, 26 Aug. 1843.
74 *Canton Press*, 2 Sep. 1843.
75 Ibid.
76 CO 129/2: 304a, Pottinger to Stanley, 1 Sep. 1843.
77 *Canton Press*, 7 Oct. 1843.
78 *Canton Press*, 14 Oct. 1843.
79 *Canton Press*, 11 Nov. 1843.
80 *Canton Press*, 18 Nov. 1843.
81 'Leighton's Hill' to the left, and skirting the passage to the Wong Nai Chung Gap, was owned by Jardine Matheson's Bombay dealer Sir Jamsetjee Jeejeebhoy, CO 129/10: 524, Pottinger to Saltoun, 26 Oct. 1843.
82 It is with reference to this bungalow that Land Officer Gordon in his report of 6 July 1843 provides justification for reclassifying future lots for sale, as this was the only residential lot he could think of remote enough from the sea 'that should be placed in the class of "Suburban"', CO 129/2: 150–150a, Gordon to Malcolm, 6 July 1843.
83 National Maritime Museum, Greenwich, London [hereafter NMM]; CRJ/5, Private Journal of E. H. Cree, 15–20 June 1841.
84 See CO 129/10: 692a–693, Woosnam (Pottinger) to Gordon, 15 Mar. 1844, regarding the granting of permission of 'a proposed Sea Wall which certain owners of Marine Lots wish to build . . . on the clear understanding that the contemplated management shall neither be considered to alienate in any degree or shape, the rights of Government, nor to prevent any other future measures.' However, legal uncertainty remained as to whose rights revoked the other, especially with regards to the terms of the 1841 sale, providing a serious impediment to the speed of the city's growth for the next several years.
85 Cambridge University Library, Jardine Matheson Archives [hereafter JMA]; C6/3, A. Matheson to Gordon (Macau, 10 Mar. 1843)
86 JMA; C6/3, A. Matheson to A. Howell (Macau, 25 Feb. 1844).
87 CO 129/2: 138, Gordon to Malcolm, 6 July 1843.
88 Ibid., 141–141a.
89 Ibid., 141a–142.
90 Ibid., 143.
91 Ibid., 142a.
92 Ibid., 142a–143.
93 *Canton Press*, 26 Aug. 1843.

94 Tarrant, *Hongkong*, 45–46.
95 Ibid., 45.
96 Ibid., 46.
97 Ko, 'Cemeteries in Hong Kong', 242.
98 CO 129/7: 310a, Davis to Stanley, 26 Dec. 1844.
99 Ibid., 310a–311.
100 *Friend of China*, 7 Sep. 1843, as recorded in the *Canton Press*, 9 Sep. 1843.
101 Ibid.
102 *Friend of China*, 13 Apr. 1843, as recorded in the *Canton Press*, 15 Apr. 1843.
103 Ibid.
104 CO 129/4: 201–201a, E. Villiers (Colonial Land and Emigration Office) to G. W. Hope (Treasury), 31 Aug. 1843. Villiers is citing the original letter.
105 *Friend of China*, 6 Feb. 1844. This seems almost too preposterous to be true, but there appears to be no other explanation for the repetition.
106 Ibid.
107 'Art. V. Sickness and deaths in Hongkong; remarked upon by a member of the Church of England, in a letter to the Editor of the Chinese Repository', *The Chinese Repository*, vol. 12, no. 11 (Nov. 1843): 145–166. The situation was somewhat relieved by the arrival of the first official colonial chaplain, Rev. Vincent Staunton, on the *Lady Amherst* (22 Dec. 1843), *Canton Press*, 30 Dec. 1843.
108 Eitel, *Europe in China*, 192; Tarrant, *Hongkong*, 58. Tarrant, however, states that the appointments occurred on 17 August.
109 Eitel, *Europe in China*, 192.
110 CO 129/5: 461–461a, 'Accounts of the Colony of Hong Kong for the Quarter ending the 30th of September, 1843', Pottinger to Stanley, 14 June 1844. Excerpt of accounts of the Land Department, 31 Aug. 1843.
111 CO 129/10: 705a–706, Pottinger to D'Aguilar, 18 Mar. 1844.
112 CO 133/2: 137–38, Dr F. Dill, Report of the Colonial Surgeon's Department for the Year 1845, *Blue Book of the Colony of Hong Kong 1845.*
113 Tarrant, *Hongkong*, 65.
114 Legge, 'The Colony of Hong Kong', 165.
115 Ibid., 163.
116 Capt. Arthur Cunynghame, *An Aide-de-Camp's Recollections of Service in China* (London: Saunders and Otley, 1844), 75.
117 CO 129/5: 465, Land Department receipt, 4 Aug. 1843. Note that British phonetic spellings of local Chinese place names understandably varied between authors at this time. This area is now spelt in English as 'Chek Chue'.
118 Notice of tender for 'articles for the use of the Troops and Hospitals' (Commissariat, 26 Jan 1844), *Friend of China*, 27 Jan. 1844.
119 Cunynghame, *Recollections*, 77.
120 Ibid., 76.
121 Ibid., 76–77.
122 CO 129/17: 95, Dill to Davis, 14 Aug. 1846. Dill is quoting John Wilson M.D., *Medical Notes on China* (London: John Churchill, 1846), 149.

123 Ibid.

124 CO 129/5: 231a, Woosnam (Pottinger) to Capt. D'Aguilar, Assistant Military Secretary (ASM) to D'Aguilar, 18 Mar. 1844.

125 'Art. III. Religious and charitable institutions in Hong Kong: churches, chapels, schools, colleges, hospitals, &c.', *Chinese Repository*, vol. 12, no. 8 (Aug. 1843): 442.

126 Notice of public auction of 'the whole of the Materials of the Barracks and other Military buildings at West Point' (Commissariat, 6 Feb. 1844), *Friend of China*, 10 Feb. 1844.

127 Eitel, *Europe in China*, 175.

128 NA; War Office [hereafter WO] 7/118, *Hong Kong Survey—by Lieut. Collinson, R.E., 1845* (Southampton: Ordnance Map Office, 1846).

129 CO 129/17: 96, Dill to Davis, 14 Aug. 1846 (as recollected).

130 CO 129/17: 92a, Davis to Gladstone, 19 Aug. 1846.

131 CO 129/17: 98a, Dill to Davis, 14 Aug. 1846.

132 JMA; C6/2, A. Matheson to Captain Ramsey, Hong Kong (Macau, 20 Jan. 1842).

133 *Friend of China*, 14 Feb. 1844.

134 CO 129/5: 231a–232, Woosnam (Pottinger) to Capt. D'Aguilar, ASM, 18 Mar. 1844.

135 As asserted by Jonathan Andrew Farris, *Enclave to Urbanity: Canton, Foreigners, and Architecture from the Late Eighteenth to Early Twentieth Centuries* (Hong Kong: Hong Kong University Press, 2016), 16.

136 *Canton Press*, 16 Sep. 1843.

137 Ibid.

138 William C. Hunter, *The 'Fan Kwae' at Canton before Treaty Days 1825–1844* (Shanghai: The Oriental Affairs, 1882), 14.

139 Ibid., 14–15.

140 JMA; C6/3, A. Matheson to J. Jejeebhoy, Bombay (Macau, 12 Dec. 1842).

141 *Canton Press*, 16 Sep. 1843.

142 JMA; C6/3, A. Matheson to J. Jejeebhoy, Bombay (Macau, 12 Dec. 1842).

143 JMA; C6/3, A. Matheson to J. Jejeebhoy, Bombay (Macau, 19 Dec. 1842).

144 JMA; C6/3, A. Matheson to J. A. Smith, London (Macau, 4 Feb. 1843).

145 *Canton Press*, 24 June 1843 (Advertisements dated Macau, 18 Jan. 1843 and Macau, 22 Dec. 1842 respectively).

146 Colin N. Crisswell, *The Taipans: Hong Kong's Merchant Princes* (Hong Kong: Oxford University Press, 1981), 33.

147 *Canton Press*, 15 July 1843 and *Hongkong Register*, 18 July 1843 (Advertisement dated Macau, 12 July 1843).

148 *Friend of China*, 24 Feb. 1844. This recounts a carefully planned attack on Mrs. White's bungalow, an incident in which 'they beat in the inner or glass door, and in a body rushed into the House throwing in Pots of fire, one of which severely scorched Mr. Lind'.

149 JMA; C15/2, Jardine Matheson & Co. to A. Hamilton, London (27 Aug. 1846).

150 See JMA; C15/2, Jardine Matheson & Co. to A. Hamilton, London (24 June 1847): '. . . With reference to the same we beg to acquaint you that the Godowns assured under Policies No. 111,444 & 111,445 do not communicate with each other, as they are situated on different parts of Queens Road'; JMA; C15/2, Jardine Matheson & Co. to A. Hamilton, London (24 Aug. 1847): 'In reply we beg to inform you that the three first policies are in protection of Merchandize stored in Godowns, which are situated in different localities, and policy, No. 111,453 on Buildings, covers 21 Houses in Gage Street, which communicate with each other'.

151 JMA; C15/2, Jardine Matheson & Co. to R.W. Crawford, Secretary, Bombay Insurance Society, Bombay (Hong Kong, 26 Aug. 1846). The contract was to be from 1 May 1846 to 30 April 1849. The acquaintance was a Mr. B. A. Baretto who was then agent for the 'Canton Insurance Office'.

152 Jan Morris with Simon Winchester, *Stones of Empire: The Buildings of the Raj* (Oxford: Oxford University Press, 1983), 18.

153 WO 44/593, H. J. Savage to Major O'Brien, Port Louis, Mauritius, 9 Apr. 1842.

154 WO 44/593, I. A. Lloyd, Surveyor-General (Mauritius) to the Colonial Secretary, 2 Dec. 1847.

155 Ibid.

156 JMA; C6/2, A. Matheson to Captain Ramsey, Hong Kong (Macau, 20 Jan. 1842). Matheson, in offering various building advise to his acquaintance, remarks that 'Mr Ouchterlony recommends flat roofs—what is your opinion on that head?'

157 JMA; C15/5, Jardine Matheson & Co. to A. Hamilton, London (25 Feb. 1851).

158 *Canton Press*, 28 Oct. 1843; *Canton Press*, 4 Nov. 1843.

159 *Canton Press*, 25 Nov. 1843.

160 *Friend of China*, 23 Dec. 1843.

161 CO 129/5: 4, Pottinger to Stanley, 22 Jan. 1844, as recollected by the governor.

162 Ibid.

163 CO 129/3: 285a, Pottinger to Saltoun, 6 Apr. 1843.

164 *Hongkong Register*, 17 Oct. 1843; CO 129/3: 287–287a, Pottinger to Aberdeen, 5 May 1843.

165 CO 129/10: 491–491a, Woosnam (Pottinger) to Aldrich, 5 Aug. 1843.

166 CO 129/10: 498–498a, Woosnam (Pottinger) to Aldrich, 10 Aug. 1843.

167 CO 129/3: 290–291, Woosnam (Pottinger) to Edwards, 15 Apr. 1843; CO 129/3: 294–295, Woosnam (Pottinger) to Edwards, 27 Apr. 1843.

168 MR 1/381, Edwards' 'Admiralty Survey' (1843), extracted from ADM 1/5530. See also *Canton Press*, 20 May 1843.

169 Compare MPG 1/156, Edwards–de Havilland Survey (1843), with MR 1/381.

170 CO 129/2: 349, Pottinger to Stanley, 13 Nov. 1843.

171 CO 129/5: 496. He left an arrears of salary $929.95, at a monthly salary of Rs. 500.

172 CO 129/10: 473, Woosnam (Pottinger) to Aldrich, 11 July 1843.

173 CO 129/5: 496.

174 CO 129/2: 455, Pottinger to Stanley, 25 Dec. 1843.

175 Ibid.

176 Hal Empson, *Mapping Hong Kong: A Historical Atlas* (Hong Kong: Government Information Services, 1992), 160–161. For the original, see NA; Foreign Office [hereafter FO] 925/2427. Likely to be the survey of Lieut. Sargent in 1842, the dating of this map is curious as it shows the 1841 lots without any construction upon them. The pencilled title, author, and date are frustratingly blurred on the original. Portions of this survey can be seen as figs. 2.7, 2.9, and 2.17.

177 W. A. Taylor, *Crown Lands: A History of Survey Systems* (Victoria, British Columbia: Registries and Titles Department, 1975), 3.

178 CO 129/ 4: 204a, Villiers to Hope, 31 Aug. 1843.

179 CO 129/2: 357, Pottinger to Stanley, 13 Nov. 1843, enclosing copy of the government notification dated 21 Aug. 1843.

180 CO 131/1, 23 Aug. 1844, as quoted in Carl T. Smith, *A Sense of History: Studies in the Social and Urban History of Hong Kong* (Hong Kong: The Hong Kong Educational Publishing Co., 1995), 47.

181 Ibid.
182 CO 129/5: 29a, Land Grants Committee's first report, 4 Jan. 1844.
183 CO 129/5: 37–37a, Land Grants Committee's second report, 13 Jan. 1844.
184 Ibid., 37a.
185 129/10: 599a–600, Woosnam (Pottinger) to Land Grants Committee, 6 Jan. 1844.
186 Lt. Col. D. H. Oxley, *Victoria Barracks 1842–1979* (Hong Kong: British Forces Hong Kong, 1979), 13.
187 *Canton Press*, 29 July 1843.
188 For Bruce's lithograph see Hong Kong Museum of Art, cat. no. AH1964.0389.007.
189 CO 129/10: 514, Pottinger to Saltoun, 9 Sep. 1843. 'I conclude the materials of the present mat Barracks will be of more or less use in the erection of the permanent Barrack, and recommend they should be applied to that purpose.'
190 Woosnam, *Canton Press*, 29 July 1843.
191 Frank Welsh, *A History of Hong Kong*, rev. ed. (London: Harper Collins, 1997), 145.
192 CO 129/2: 102, Saltoun to Pottinger, 29 June 1843.
193 CO 129/2: 71a, Pottinger to Saltoun, 2 May 1843.
194 Ibid., 69a–70.
195 Ibid., 71.
196 CO 129/2: 120, *Memoranda*, Aldrich to Saltoun, 28 June 1843.
197 Ibid., 124a–125.
198 Ibid., 124a.
199 Ibid., 120a.
200 Ibid., 121–121a.
201 Ibid., 123–123a.
202 Ibid., 124a.
203 Ibid., 125a.
204 CO 129/2: 102, Saltoun to Pottinger, 29 June 1843.
205 Ibid., 103.
206 CO 129/2:130a, 133a, Pottinger to Saltoun, 4 July 1843.
207 Gordon lamented that 'more regularity might have been preserved in the buildings upon either side of the "Queen's Road"', and that 'along the southern side of the Queen's Road eastwards from Government Hill, as far as Town Lot marked No. 14 on the Survey (a site past the old burial ground in Wanchai) there should be lots for European shops and Dwelling Houses' (CO 129/2: 138a, 140–140a, Gordon to Malcolm, 6 July 1843).
208 CO 129/2: 131a, Pottinger to Saltoun, 4 July 1843.
209 Ibid., 132a.
210 Ibid., 133–133a.
211 CO 129/2: 98, Pottinger to Stanley, 17 July 1843.
212 CO 129/4: 216a, Stanley to Pottinger, 9 Dec. 1843.
213 CO 129/ 5: 230a, Woosnam (Pottinger) to Capt. D'Aguilar, ASM, 18 Mar. 1844.
214 CO 129/10: 525a–526, Pottinger to Saltoun, 26 Oct. 1843.
215 Dafydd M. E. Evans, 'Chinatown in Hong Kong: The Beginnings of Taipingshan', *JHKBRAS*, vol. 10 (Hong Kong, 1970): 71, 77.

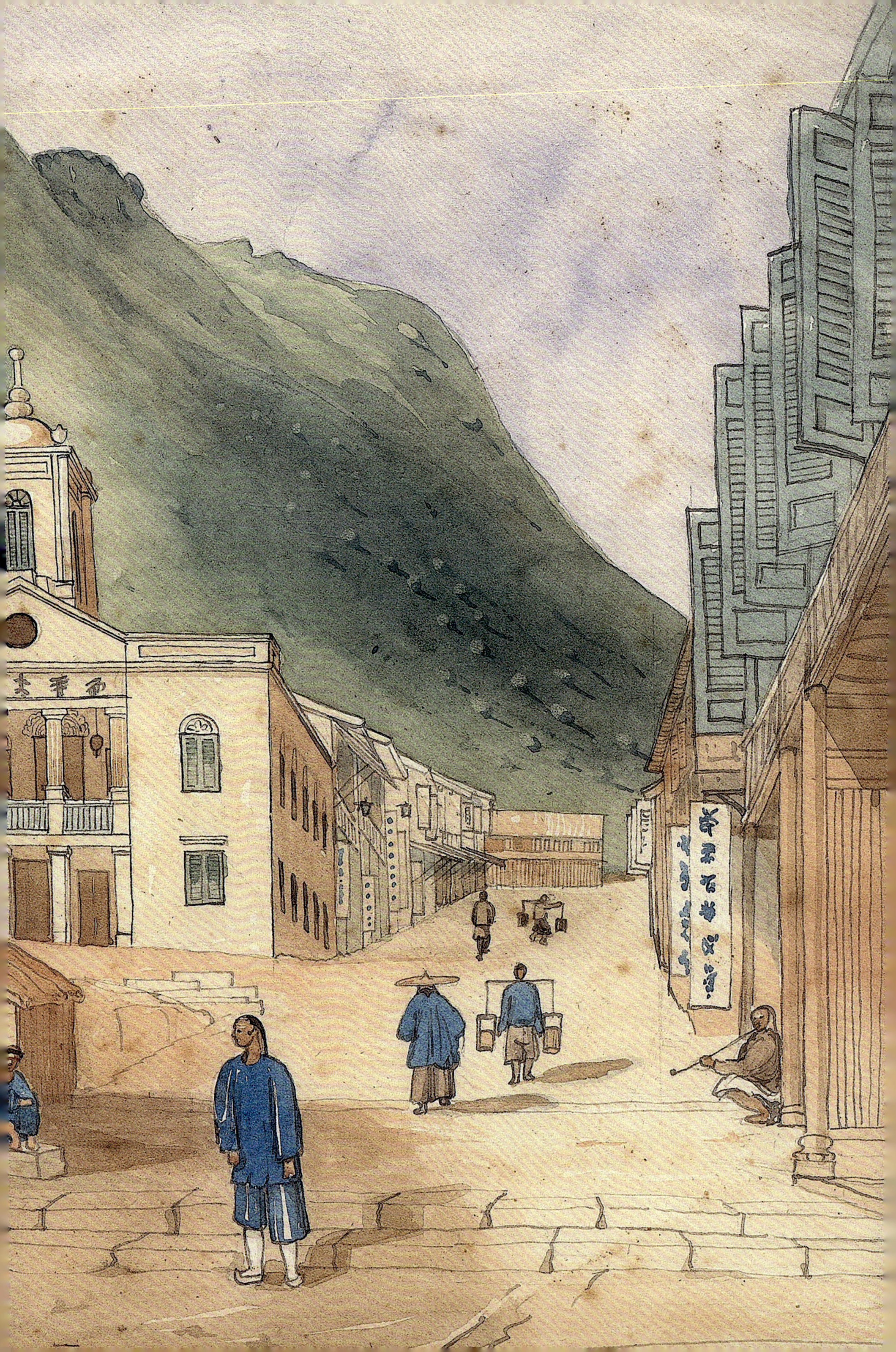

CHAPTER 4

A Labour Renewed, 1844–1846

We now know something about the European experience in dealing with life in colonial Hong Kong during the first turbulent years of its establishment. Yet, it was the Chinese who built the city of Victoria. They constructed its buildings and its roads, drains, and sewers, to eventually encircle the island and render it accessible and relatively healthy. The conjoined effects of their labour would be highly evident within these subsequent years and generate debate, complaint, and eventual pride in the outcome.

This chapter is a companion piece to the next, following in parallel as a sequence of events. It focuses on how the city was quickly constructed, acquiring its first cohesive shape and form in the aftermath of the fever of 1843. It describes the physical processes of surveying, commissioning, and building Hong Kong during the critical years of 1844 to 1846 under the relatively more proactive military and civilian governments of Major-General (and Lieutenant-Governor) George Charles D'Aguilar and the second governor, Sir John Davis. This process would, upon reflection, be credited with the general decline of malaria. At the heart of the story lies the tangled issue of human managerial relations. Apart from the comprador system, the building sites of Hong Kong were the most overt points of daily interaction between the British and the Chinese. Unable to share a common language, western overseers faced a steep education in the art of labour relations to ensure that the labour force completed building work on time and to expectations. Miscommunication and differences in cultural values manifested themselves in the works constructed and in their assembly processes. Moreover, the world of Chinese contracting was a far more complex, transient, and interdependent environment than historians might suppose. The building of Victoria was, therefore, the first tortured test of intense cross-relations—a relationship between those that commissioned and those that built Hong Kong.

The second section of this chapter will look at how labour and politics met within the domain of government public works. The focus will be on the infrastructural provisions of Davis's government. This need was, by 1844, a politically pressing issue regarding health grounds and, therefore, the actual commercial survival of the colony. The surveying of Hong Kong was essential to the success of these programmes. Consequently, it must be said that there was a genuine, cooperative involvement between the military and the civilian arms of government to ensure that such provisions were met. In essence, this history is about a definitive reshaping of the city of Victoria and a supposed *taming* of the island of Hong Kong.

Chinese Contractors and Builders

> Because I have contracted for two houses and have allowed Asseye to deprive me of $9,000, and a fire having caused me a loss of $4,500, and having in the present house[1] an amount of additional stone work being required, lost $7,000, and being obliged to put down English stone in the Verandahs, I lost $500 more, making a total of $21,000. By these means I have lost my just debts, that is why I die. I beg that the person who receives this paper will explain my losses to the English officers, and get what Asseye owes me, so that my family may not come to trouble. I beg with blood in my eyes, not tears, that some portion of the money recovered may be given to my creditors, and the rest to my family.
>
> —(Signed) ACHOU, Pen dipped in tears of blood.[2]

On 2 January 1846, a cold Friday morning, the body of a contractor was found hanging from a rafter at his nearby residence. He had worked on the new military hospital, the officers' quarters, and the barracks at Cantonment Hill.[3] Following tradition, suicide ensured that his debt was settled. His death, particularly the final note he left behind, would divide the community. It would throw into sharp relief the hardship many Chinese had endured in rapidly building Hong Kong for the British and expose the exploitative, dark practices behind the bright granite palaces now rising across the city.

As has been recounted, almost immediately after the initial landing of British and Indian troops on Hong Kong Island in 1841, there quickly grew a labour pool to feed the evolving public works, primarily in the construction of roads, ditches, and rudimentary drainage gullies. Indigenous techniques of construction, principally that of the 'mat-shed' variety, were rapidly deployed. Slowly, the Chinese workforce met their foreign clients' demands in the first, faltering works of an architecture in an unfamiliar language for the local mason. Indeed, masons and carpenters, those with broader skills, inevitably had to be sought within a wider compass, with many risking their lives under threats of bodily harm and being branded as traitors from their Canton (Guangzhou) guilds.[4] Meanwhile, the coordinating role of the Chinese contractor was necessary for this increase in buildings and infrastructure of permanence, scale, and expenditure.

At first, several English contractors applied in the newsprint for prospective clients. One such was Messrs. Carter & Co., who advertised their 'long experience in England', their 'punctuality' and their 'workmanlike manner'.[5] At around the same time, in early 1844, surveyors, mechanics, and builders from New South Wales had somehow heard that Hong Kong was a place of bounteous employment, and several enquiries were made to the local government and private individuals about their prospects. Most enquirers were respectfully dissuaded, though a number came anyway, including the architect Edward Ashworth, whom we will hear more of later.[6] The *Canton Press* described it as an 'inconsiderate immigration to Hongkong from New South Wales of English mechanics and labourers'.[7] Apart from those of a highly skilled trade it was, they insisted, like bringing coals to Newcastle. 'In no country can the importation of manual labour and, in some degree, of mechanical skill be less needed than in China, where multitudes abound, able and willing to work at a much cheaper rate than Europeans can possibly do, and where mechanical skill has attained to a very considerable degree of perfection.'[8]

Few contractors of any background could match Tam Achoy, otherwise known as Tam Sam-tshoy or Tam Shek-tsun.[9] His glory years were yet to follow as both a main contractor for the British and a philanthropist to the Chinese community. Still, he was peculiarly well placed to benefit from the initial burst in construction during the colony's first years. A native of Kaiping, he was one of the many Chinese that flocked to the Straits, settling down as a foreman at the government dockyard at Singapore before moving with the British to Hong Kong in 1841.[10] He was therefore both conversant in his employers' verbal and ideological languages and understood the ways of the British as few of his native colleagues could. Yet even he fell badly into debt on one or two occasions and was almost imprisoned—one such event being as a defaulting contractor in the construction of the Wong Nai Chung Gap in 1843.[11] However, he was among the first contractors able to move up the scale into larger, more complex work, involving the coordination of many different trades and demonstrating the ability to work in the 'British' style. At the time, this style was neo-classicism, and Tam used this in building the highly-praised Peninsular & Orient Building and, somewhat earlier, Dent's equally-admired, Regency-styled Exchange Building in 1845 (**fig. 4.1**).[12] The Exchange Building was generously offered to the Government in 1847 for the reasonable sum of £5,000 as a home for the Supreme Court.[13]

Charles St. George Cleverly, acting surveyor general, applauded the quality of the two-year-old exchange for its solidity and material quality. Teak and molave from the Philippines had been used for the structural timberwork, while the joinery was in teak and cedar of a quality 'such as is seldom seen here'. Not all the handiwork of the Chinese was praised, however. The exterior plasterwork of Roman cement, especially along the cornice, lacked drips and weathering. In contrast, the interior ceiling and cornices, recognised as of much higher quality, were noted—with assurance to the colonial secretary—as having been executed by an English plasterer.[14] Regardless, Tam's ability to hire Chinese and European artisans as needed demonstrated him to be a progressive and significant contractor.

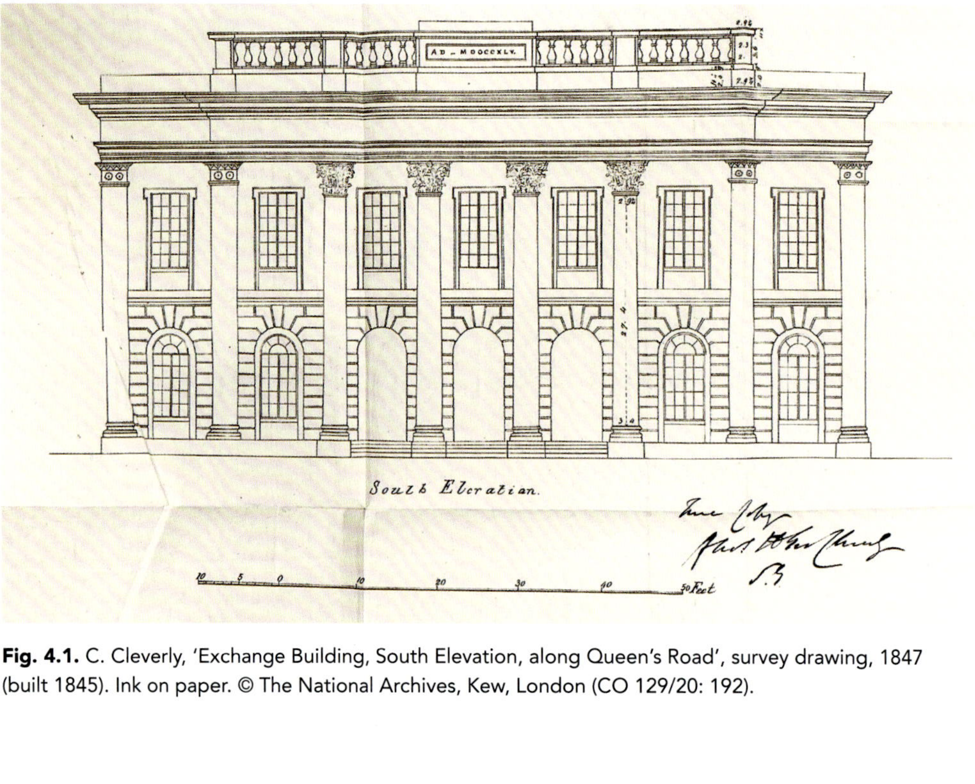

Fig. 4.1. C. Cleverly, 'Exchange Building, South Elevation, along Queen's Road', survey drawing, 1847 (built 1845). Ink on paper. © The National Archives, Kew, London (CO 129/20: 192).

At the start of 1844, Tam was just one of several contractors vying for projects from merchants, the military, and the civilian government (under the Lands Office). Government and military contracts were advertised in both the local press in English and by posted proclamations translated into Chinese.[15] Occasionally, the means of pricing for a job, as in the case of a military contract for cutting and levelling, was by way of on-site inspection. One such instance was advertised through the Commissariat—a contract offer for levelling the ground in the barrack square at Chek Chue 'according to the plan which may be seen marked out on the ground'.[16] This was a simple bid process, where each bidder was also required to confirm the number of labourers needed to complete the work within the allotted time. In general, however, most contracts were priced via 'plans and specifications' (that is, drawn and written information) or by a 'plan and sections' (drawings alone), usually displayed at limited times per day at the offices of the potential client. For example, in the case of the Surveyor-General's Office (previously the Lands Office), this was often between the hours of 10 am and 12 noon.[17] Tenderers would invariably pitch in at ridiculously low bids or were considered unqualified for the work. So, the whole tendering process had to be restarted.[18] This had the added problem, not just of shifting the programme, but of potentially jeopardising the work for that year as, by 1844, it was realised by all that the most effective period for construction was during the winter months.

The enormous teething problems in gauging bids by both sides would take some time to resolve. For the unscrupulous British procurer, it was easy to exploit the eager contractor, downplay the risks, or insert items into the contract after the award. The Chinese were often caught out in biddings related to earthworks since many of the problems were, quite literally, buried. There was also a problem in transferring vernacular construction techniques to modern multi-storied European buildings. The *Hongkong Register*, in mid-1845, noted the proposal of a tax to be levied on sand by the government of Bombay. 'What a valuable hint this might form to the Colonial Government of Hongkong,' it caustically remarked, 'if the Chinese workmen could only be persuaded to use sand like other people.'[19] This may have been a reference to a particular tragedy that had occurred two years before when, either in late 1842 or early 1843, following the death of the architect F. Langer, Jardine Matheson's magnificent three-storey office building at East Point collapsed (**fig. 4.2**). As a detailed account by the *Hongkong Almanack* of 1848 revealed,

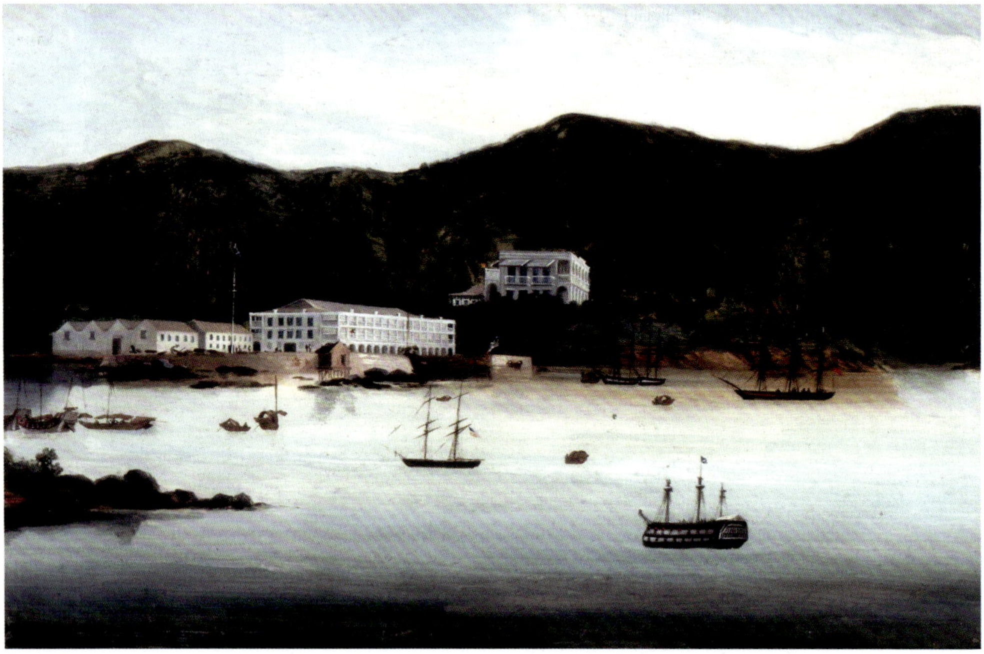

Fig. 4.2. Anon., 'East Point, Hong Kong', with the three-storey office building in the foreground, ca. 1843–1846. Oil on canvas. © Hong Kong Museum of Art Collection (AH1988.0014).

> It was just now stated that the Chinese builders were great scamps if not well looked after, in nothing are they more so than in their style of bricklaying; an instance of this occurred in the erection of the first building of any magnitude in the colony; owing to the early death of the architect who had come on with his family from India, the second and third stories were ran up with but very little inspection, and the roof was in progress of being laid, when a main wing of the building came down with a tremendous crash, killing and maiming several of the workmen.[20]

The reasons behind this, the *Almanack* recounted, were to become self-evident upon inspection of the wreckage.

> On examination into the cause, it was discovered that the brick walls of two or three feet in thickness, had been constructed by simply decorating the outer edges of the outer course of bricks with a quarter of an inch border of wet Lime, laying the bricks to about 2 feet in height of stretcher or length-wise, to one course of header or a-cross, placed on a grouting of mud and sand, whilst in the whole body of those walls which were

> still standing, the bricks had been packed dry, and were taken out as clean as when first landed for the work; how the building could ever have attained such a height, was more to be wondered at than its fall; as a matter of course the whole of the building was pulled down, greatly to the annoyance of the proprietors, who had it rebuilt under the supervision of an English overseer, but even in this instance from a want of attention, sand from the salt sea beach was allowed to be used in making the mortar, and to the present day, one of the most showy buildings in Hongkong, is in a measure incomplete from the impossibility of getting colouring to stand on the walls.[21]

Despite what appeared to be a callous act of neglect by Chinese bricklayers, the British did not generally know that this dry construction method was a typical, quite acceptable practice in constructing Chinese vernacular buildings. The problem occurred in combining an indigenous technique with an unsuited foreign typology. Except for tower and pagoda structures, buildings of such magnitude and height as the Office Building were almost unheard of by local contractors. To counter many Europeans' derogatory conceptions of Chinese craftsmanship and, by extension, of Chinese built culture, several contemporary articles appeared in journals by travellers, often missionaries, recounting their favourable impressions of cities, such as Peking (Beijing). For example, the *Semanario Filipino* described the effect of the architecture in that city as 'master performances of the Bramantes and the Palladios'.[22] 'Chinese Architecture,' it argued, 'has been so much assailed in latter times, and accused of bad taste, that much fortitude is requisite to oppose a prejudice so deeply rooted, and to claim in its favour a small page in the history of the fine arts.'[23]

Yet, many European commentators were scathing of the precise detailing of buildings. One observer, a traveller to the Chinese treaty port city of Foo-chow-foo (Fuzhou), mockingly noted that in carpentry,

> It is not considered always essential that a door be made to shut or a window to open, and, indeed, a medium between an approach to a fit between window and frame seems rather to be preferred. . . . We in building, have some narrow prejudices about the sight-lines, not to say the importance of perpendicular, horizontal, and parallel lines. These are rather beneath the notice of a Chinese workman, or beyond his reach of art.[24]

One of early Hong Kong's most significant architectural participant–observers was the English architect, Edward Ashworth. On his way back home from New Zealand via Australia and hearing of the building boom in Hong Kong, he arrived on the island in mid-July 1844 just after the second major land auction. The building boom was not the only thing he heard. He discovered a Hong Kong seething with people and filled with strange, diurnal and nocturnal noise. He first sought lodgings in the rowdy Hong Kong Inn, a shelter for drunken petty officers. That first night Ashworth suffered insomnia, awoken by 'a detachment of large rats [that] dropped from the roof upon the beds scouring, scuffling & scampering over the chests & other furniture with so much noise that they quite banished sleep'. Over the following few nights, these rodents were joined in chorus by the regular, hollowly percussive sounds of bamboo beaters. These were watchmen hired by the merchant community and 'giving testimony of their vigilance by thumping a piece of sonorous bamboo, at each of the houses boasting any importance' at two- to three-minute intervals. The new lieutenant-governor, George D'Aguilar, driven to distraction by this nightly practice, silenced it once and for all, passing a government order for its cessation some two months later.[25]

Ashworth's arrival, nevertheless, was impeccably timed. He spent two years in Hong Kong, until 1846, during which he would take part in one of the most astonishing periods of transformation in the young colony's history under the second governor, Sir John Davis. Some of Ashworth's views of Hong Kong, once thought lost, have recently come to light in Australia and since purchased by the Hong Kong Museum of Art. Significantly, these predate lithographs of the well-known architectural and urban images of his colleague Murdoch Bruce.[26] His first major studies of landscapes and streetscapes were of early colonial New Zealand (and are revered as an important collection in that nation's national library).[27] Now he was greeted by an entirely different landscape, one of peculiarly narrow and elongated intensity. Over this time, the city dramatically changed shape as new streets were added, often carved into the hillside, while older ones were erased, and the Chinese and European communities forcibly detached. The architect was keen to understand the nature of this urban topography at a glance. And so, that first winter, in 1844, once the weather had sufficiently cooled, Ashworth ventured up to Victoria Peak (or simply 'The Peak'), the high point of the island. There he surveyed far beneath 'some of the low, white-plastered dwellings & rows of houses that displayed their roofs & the straight & serpentine streets separating them with map-like distinction 2000 feet below me'. Five years later, in one of the earliest surviving views of Victoria and Kowloon from The Peak, naval surgeon Edward Cree would record, from a similar vantage point, that these streets were now lost in a tumble of a roofscape, while the city itself had significantly climbed (**fig. 4.3**).

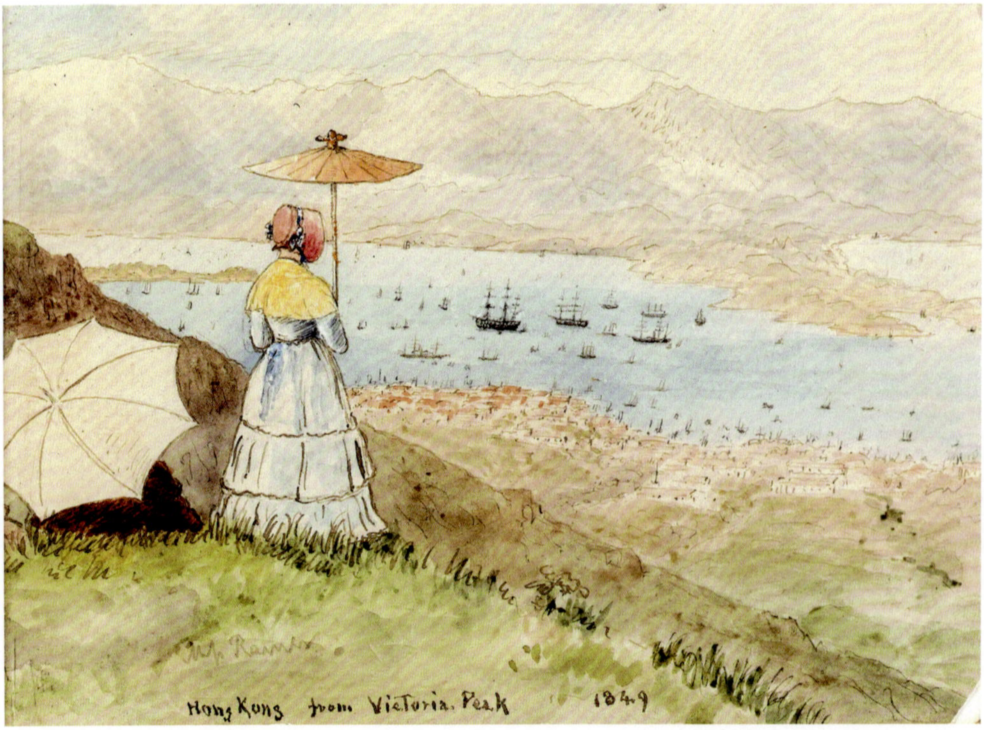

Fig. 4.3. Dr. E. Cree, 'Hong Kong from Victoria Peak' (detail), April 1849. Watercolour on paper. © National Maritime Museum, Greenwich, London (CRJ/12).

On his way back down, Ashworth was struck by the preposterousness of the young city. Set incongruously within a strange body of water, it appeared opposed by a distant mainland that he perceived as both hostile and barren.

> The effect on me was very moving. The sublime scenery, the beautiful English town at my feet, the proud men-of-war, lording it over the multitudes of junks, fast boats & sampans, . . . the ravines of the mountain that sloped so abruptly from the seashore as to induce an idea that it had on a sudden arisen "from out the azure main" to obey the rule of the female personification of England; and the red, barren, forbidding mainland of China interposing a mountainous horizon to the northward, with here and there, a lowly little village scarcely discernible at the water's edge, were not the eye led by the ever-present sampans ready to heave their wood anchors & spread their wing-like masts to flee to the haunts of the wealthy.[28]

Imperialist nostalgia had quickly overtaken fear. Hong Kong was a sudden miracle for Ashworth, its rapid urban bravado revealing how it was a creature nourished by a remote and vast maritime system of exchange that visibly included regional trade through local vessels. This adaptive hybridity was the essence of its Englishness. Buoyed by this excitement and sense of opportunity, it seems that Ashworth was more fortunate in gaining commissions in Hong Kong than he had in New Zealand. We know that he designed some commercial and domestic architecture for Europeans, though he struggled to see them constructed, having difficulties in communication with local Chinese contractors and builders.[29]

Ashworth still found time to draw and paint views of the city in the throes of development and expansion. These scenes are invaluable to us. They record, with an architect's forensic eye, though stripped of the atmosphere of, say, a George Chinnery, the everyday humdrum life of a streetscape, with the architecture acting as a dramatic backdrop. Ashworth saw these illustrations as almost anthropological in ambition. Unlike his small coterie of architectural colleagues, he grew fascinated by Chinese architecture. His objects of fascination were not just the Cantonese temples and pagodas that had so captivated the architect and supercargo William Chambers in the mid-eighteenth century but the more mundane Chinese shophouses of Macau and Hong Kong, and also, in one rare instance, the home of a wealthy Chinese merchant. In the year he disembarked, Ashworth drew three remarkable studies of one Hong Kong building, the quayside house of Chan Akuen otherwise known as Chun Chinam, a Canton opium trader and tea merchant. 'Chinam's Hong', as it was dubbed, was in Ashworth's words 'the only good Chinese mansion existing at Victoria, Hong Kong'. Chan invested in 1843, during the worst year of fever, paying a sizeable $8,000 to its European owner, Richard Oswald, for Marine Lot no. 54, and lavishing another $10,000 to entirely demolish and rebuild.[30] He built a large compound, with European-style storerooms towards the rear facing a private pier, with a more formal Chinese-style persona facing the Queen's Road, close by the new Central Market.

Ashworth was both intrigued and disturbed by this front-to-back dyslexia. His watercolour of the front portion shows a defensive screen wall constructed along the road with the house front set back and concealed (**fig. 4.4**). The wall screen, itself protected by a western-style railing, is punctuated by a pair of glazed bamboo-mullion grills between an elegant, large stone-carved crack-pattern screen. The hybrid door

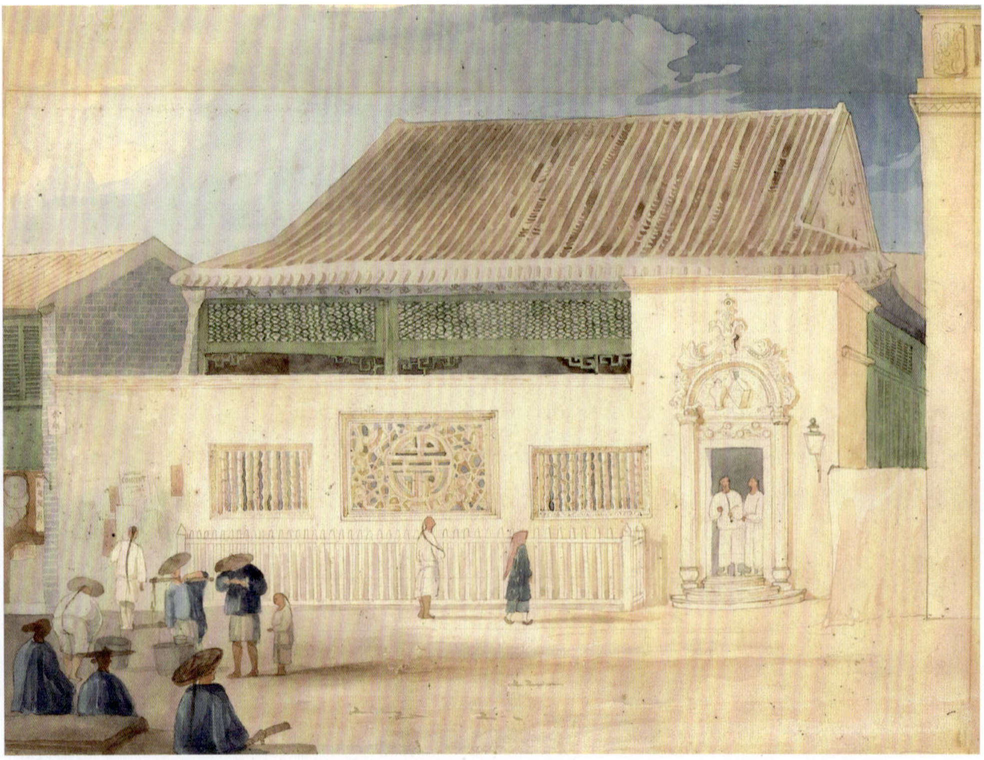

Fig. 4.4. E. Ashworth, 'Chinam's Hong, Residence Built for a Chinaman at Hong Kong', Street View from the Queen's Road, 1844. Watercolour on paper. © Hong Kong Museum of Art Collection (AH2015.0011).

to the forecourt is set back and to the right. The columnar surround has turned bases similar to the temple at Tin Hau, also studied by Ashworth. Yet the tympanum above the door is of a hybrid European–Chinese form that Ashworth found uncomfortable. A literate Chinese passer-by in white smocks and full queue studies the side wall to Chinam's Hong for news, walls being one of the only sources of print media available to local Chinese at the time. Ashworth was fascinated by the screen wall, which would soon be pulled down and the luxuriously empty forecourt filled by more valuable shop fronts the following year. 'Sometimes the screen wall is adorned on a larger scale, with mimic bamboo stanchions modelled in lime', he noted. 'In towns, the shop-fronted houses have generally these open façades, sometimes richly carved.'[31]

With Chinam's Hong, Ashworth presents the most complete painterly study of a work of early Hong Kong architecture. The three views may be seen to form an architectural promenade of sorts. The first from the front, the second within the complex, and the third looking back from the harbour. This last image is the earliest close-up view of Hong Kong from the water that we have. It is clear that the sequence of space from street to forecourt to interior to rear delighted the English architect.

The interior view (**fig. 4.5**) is a unique image of a Hong Kong Chinese domestic interior of the time, and the earliest example to survive. This was no slapdash Singapore-framed housing system, as seen along the Morgan's Bazaar (see **fig. 2.10**). Rather, a fine display of the Chinese joiner's art is revealed in fretwork upon the column brackets, rails, door-panels, and architraves. Ventilation and light permeate this architecture within a private world of courtyards linking building elements, with servants and clerks busying themselves within the merchant complex, its interiors open to the warm breezes. And, yet, transverse to the courtyard, we see the building's western pragmatics: a simple casement window, a western-style staircase with balustrade, and a side door into the compound beyond.

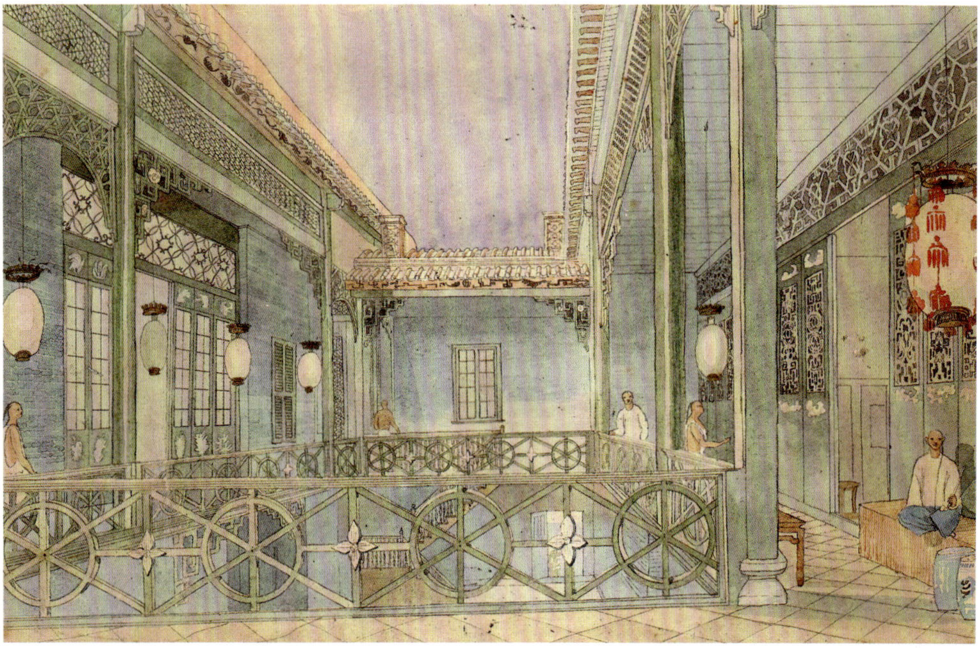

Fig. 4.5. E. Ashworth, 'View in the Interior of "Chinam's Hong"', 1844. Watercolour on paper. © Hong Kong Museum of Art Collection (AH2015.0012).

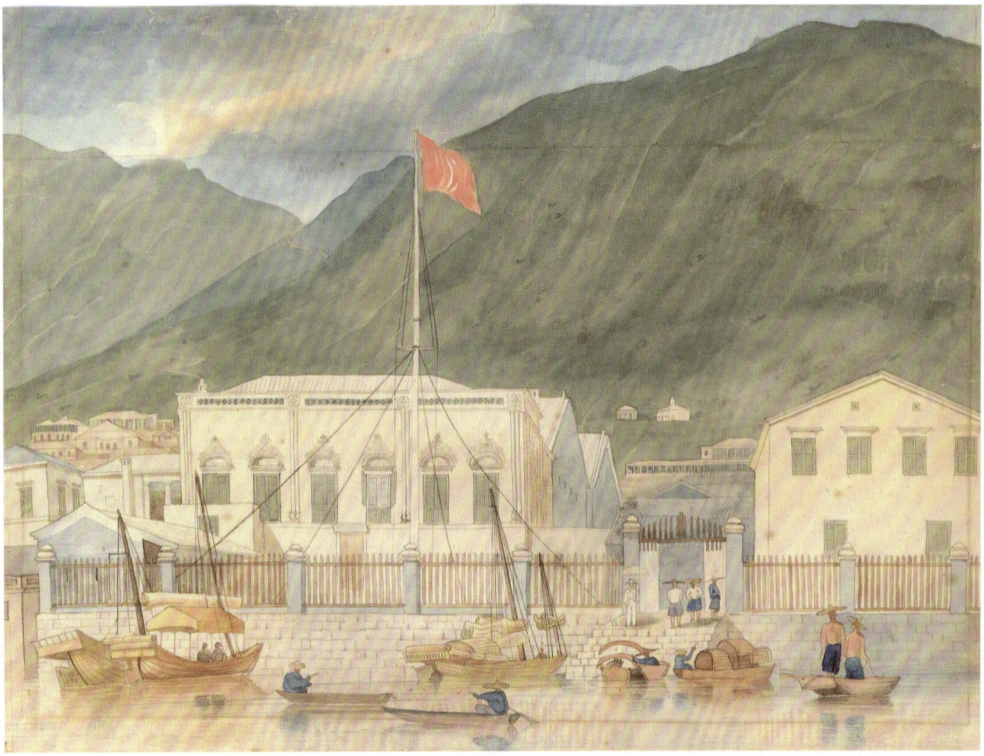

Fig. 4.6. E. Ashworth, 'Chinam's Hong, Residence Built for A Chinaman at Hong Kong', Rear View from the Harbour, 1844. Watercolour on paper. © Hong Kong Museum of Art Collection (AH2015.0013).

Meanwhile, at the rear (**fig. 4.6**), Ashworth painted one of the most remarkable early–Hong Kong harbour-front scenes to have survived. Judging by the light and position, the young architect perched himself upon a boat in the early-morning hours to have captured this. Eastwards, two properties to the left, was the new Central Market; westwards, to the right, sat the ordnance store and hospital. Between these was a small hotel that sat on Chinam's property facing the Queen's Road. To the left, upon the hillside, can be seen the Magistracy complex of Major Caine. Deep-draft ships had to be moored from mid-harbour to the Kowloon side with the relative shallower waters by the island capable of accommodating only shorter-draft vessels such as trade sampans and ferry boats.

Chinam was the only Chinese merchant of the time with such a prominent marine lot, and he put it to good use by building a quay with stepped access into his compound. Revealing as much about Ashworth's prejudices as about Chinam, the architect paid significant attention to the rear façade of the Hong complex and was disturbed by the Chinese merchant's attempts to show a western side to his tastes. The six giant windows at the piano nobile seemed to repeat the motifs found above the main street-entrance door, an outward display of respectability aimed at European merchants sailing past. The effect was a tad desperate for Ashworth. It was 'perhaps rather too civilized and comfortable to English practice to be called Chinese' he said dryly. Though admiring the level of enrichment, Ashworth considered the oddly shaped series of semi-circular tympana above the windows to be an example 'very barbarous, and seeming to caricature the style of Inigo Jones and Christopher Wren'.[32] *The Idler* had criticised the Record Office back in 1842 as 'shades of Vitruvius, Palladio, and Wren'. Now, another European was clearly stating that the Chinese—in building for themselves—ought stick to what they knew. Such reactions beg the question: how much of this criticism derived from neutral connoisseurship and how much from a fear that a mastery of the language of western classical architecture by Chinese posed a threat to European authority on the island?

After arriving back in England, Ashworth began writing for the *Architectural Publication Society* in their edition for 1850–1851, an essay account which would later form a significant entry 'Chinese Architecture' in the Society's *Dictionary of Architecture*, volume 'C to D', published in 1858.[33] Ashworth recounted some of his observations on architectural craftsmanship and, in the main, he remained unimpressed. Chimneys, for instance, were 'merely traps of tiling propped a foot or two above the general surface'. Carpentry was 'decidedly the weak point in Chinese building', while 'out-door works in carpentry . . . cannot be called engineering works, as they are executed in a very flimsy manner'.[34]

Unfavourable experiences undoubtedly coloured Ashworth's negative views as a practising architect in Hong Kong. During his two years in the colony from 1844, he had made copious notes in his diary and voraciously read the works of several European scholars on Chinese construction. One fascinating account is his experience overseeing a house-building job which led to stormy relations with the main contractor, a man called Achone. In his *Memoranda Concerning the Erection, by Native Artizans, of an English House in China, Designed and Superintended by the English Architect*, published as part of the same journal, Ashworth gives a disdainful yet detailed account of construction methods used by Chinese workmen. Through the outward manifestations of craft production on the building site, Ashworth argues that the Chinese revealed a cultural set of normative values.

For instance, he considered the builders to be neglectful of levels and tolerances. They were either too tight or too loose. 'The face of the wall was kept exactly flush with the granite below, leaving not a quarter of an inch for plastering,' he complained. Meanwhile, 'the doors, two inch double-worked doors, hung with brass butts, before the floors were laid; there was no fear, to be sure, of the doors not shutting, as there was above half an inch clear of any possible floor board'. Traditional methods of fixing were also viewed as slack or lazy. 'To avoid corbelling, the joiners nailed a single floor board close to the wall, and based the brick jamb upon it. Every means was employed to save bricks, the windows gaped inwards with splays, that placed the lintels in a critical position.' As for the king post trusses, the English architect exclaimed that 'when these were set up, the carpenters began to bed the hip pieces; four clumsy round pine logs—they were tied to nothing, had no square bearing anywhere—being just bedded in the brick walls, and the purlin spars rested on them'.[35] The strategic sequencing of the work was appalling to Ashworth, allowing him to, again, vent his familiar culturalist spleen.

> The greatest proof, perhaps, of want of civilization shewed itself in forming the access to the cellar in the staircase compartment, about fifteen feet square. Instead of contriving the descent under the staircase, they boarded the whole floor before beginning to build the staircase, and sawed out a large square trap in the centre of the apartment to get at the cellar.[36]

And yet, Ashworth, the anthropologist, could be a more sympathetic observer. 'The building operations when new to me, seemed certainly very singular, though they gave evidence of an advanced state of civilization among the Chinese.' He was impressed by Chinese labourers' on-site skills as they worked with deceptively simple tools, especially with stone. A diary entry compared the raised granite blocks for doorways, often constructed first, as being 'massive and lofty, so as almost to remind one of the marvellous stones on Salisbury Plain'.[37] He was not alone in his admiration. The naval surgeon, Edward Cree, was fascinated by the beguilingly casual manner of working with stone by the local craftsperson. His drawn study of Chinese stonemasons in 1843 is one of the very first sketches seen of Hong Kong labour (**fig. 4.7**). 'With a narrow plane,' wrote Ashworth, 'destitute of top iron, and worked with a cross handle, the workman sitting astride his work, it was wonderful to witness what true and smooth work they put out of hand.'[38]

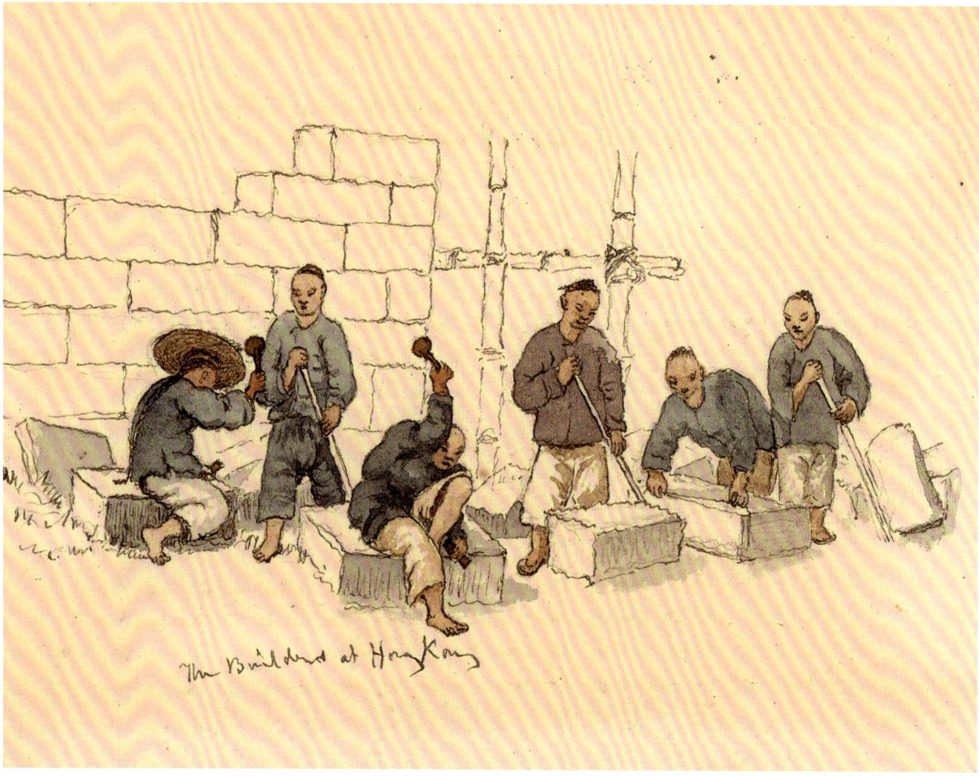

Fig. 4.7. Dr. E. Cree, 'The Builders at Hong Kong', 1843. Watercolour on paper. © National Maritime Museum, Greenwich, London (CRJ/7).

The architect gives a particularly detailed and frustrated account of the construction of a first-floor veranda, complete with Doric columns and entablature, revealing the learning curve that workmen required, in his estimation, in getting to grips with the western classical idiom.

> I had profiles cut for the rough brick work which Achone vowed should be executed to a nicety, leaving three quarters of an inch for plastering everywhere. Unfortunately, I was compelled to leave the men to their own devices for a few days, and Achone to his opium pipe. When I came back—good heavens! What was the veranda like? The pillars were right in height, but the coupled columns were stuck together; the bases, two clumsy toruses, in form something between a turnip-radish and a pumpkin; the capital was a single meagre tile.[39]

Ashworth, frustrated, instructed the work to begin again. This time, on his return to site, he found that while the intrinsic classical language remained meagre, in contrast, the surface embellishments had become unnecessarily exuberant.

> After having the columns reconstructed, the stucco work began. All the fillets and squares leaned inwards, the soffit of the architrave cut an inch deep into the abaci, the triglyphs were pentaglyphs, the cornice the masons would not project more than the half of a twenty-inch tile instead of nearly two feet (I got it eventually done in granite slabs). Instead of the plain blocking course designed, I found the industrious plasterers flourishing away in flowery enrichment, of a series of little piers projecting from other slight projections, so that each division of the attic had six arrises, and the corresponding mitres in the moulding coping, to say nothing of intervening panels, all filled with elaborate designs. It seemed a sad pity to have to abolish all this exuberance, especially as the contractor never dreamed of an extra for it.[40]

Communication between the contractor and the English overseer was invariably conducted in Pidgin English. Ashworth recounts several heated conversations that he had with Achone. These make for uncomfortable reading. The architect describes the workmen as 'roosting at night like fowls on little perch-like platforms in the roofs of the temporary workshops'.[41] Once a floor had been constructed, he was frustrated to note that they would move their belongings and their mat beds across and into the partially built house, lying down and fanning themselves during the working day.

> I said to Achone, 'Why do you let your men leave their work and smoke?' 'Cheenaman', he replied, 'not all same Inglis-man. Spose Inglis carp'nter ten minest away from walk [work], to-morrow he catchee walk, stoppee he wage—Cheenaman no all same. Dat man (pointing to one) stun may-sun, to day he got no walk, to-morrow he catchee walk, nex day spose no got—spose rain come, he catchee lice (rice)'.[42]

Ashworth learned that when it rained and all external works had come to a stop, an allowance of rice was 'paid' to the skilled craftsmen ('mechanics') in addition to their salary which amounted to one third of a dollar per day, and for unskilled workers, about seven-and-a-half cents. Achone was referring, obliquely, to the unionising power that different trades had over their members and the contractors themselves. And, as will be seen, Achone had a lot to be worried about.

Contractors and not just builders could be men with vicissitudinous habits. Many ran into debt or were involved in lending rackets. A typical solution was to flee from the island with work incomplete or once advances of fees were received. A landowner, Robert Webster, found that he had to defend his transfer of ownership to a parcel of land, a bazaar lot originally in possession of Captain Meik, a former member of the 1842 Committee for Lands and Roads. Webster argued that the Captain had been forced to sell to him as Meik had 'contracted with a Chinese for the completion of the work, and had expended about four hundred dollars in clearing the ground, and in building the walls, when the absconding of the contractor, who had received advances to a considerable amount, and the sickness of Captain Meik, put a stop for a time to the progress of the building'.[43] Contractors also abandoned each other. In the construction of the Queen's Road, one contractor, Amoon, pleaded that

> In consequence of the absconding of Assam, who entered into a contract with Government for the formation of a certain portion of the Queen's Road for the sum of $920, he has himself paid $1,200 in addition to $700 previously expended by Assam; that the Contract is not yet fulfilled, that the removal of one mass of rock will cost him $150; and in conclusion, therefore prays, that Government will defray the expense of completing the Contract.[44]

Soon, wary government officials required that contractors demonstrate their ability through past work or good references. In October 1844, an advertisement appeared, calling for builders to construct Aldrich's barracks. The work required 'a Builder of known experience or capable of producing respectable testimonials from Europeans, either of Canton, Macao or Singapore'.[45] This was the start of a new, more controlled vetting process in tendering and effectively reduced the pool of eligible applicants, thus consolidating power for the earlier, larger contractors such as Tam Achoy. In this instance, the contractor who would eventually win would be the same man, racked with debt, who would take his own life fifteen months later.

Aldrich raised the bar in information provision and construction management. He was among the first to produce meticulous measured drawings to assist in pricing instead of general instructions, the care in interpretation of which further limited the contractor's pool. We are fortunate to have some surviving pricing drawings that were made for inspection at the offices of the Royal Engineers that autumn in 1844. The building sections were labelled using a bilingual notation method, with the left-hand side of the measurement data denoting the numerical value and the right-hand side the unit of measurement in feet and inches (**fig. 4.8**). Doubtless, such drawings were intended to have the fantastical effect of producing a comfortable distance between the European engineer and the Chinese contractor, in the vain hope that all necessary information could be contained within the document.

One cause of tension between contractors and European overseers was the increasing unionisation of labour. By the end of 1844, with the start of the cooler working season in which competition for labour began again to get intense, this had started to find form. Referring specifically to the supervision of road gangs, one writer named *Viator* remarked that, compared to working for a private contractor, those labourers on government construction had found collective ways to abuse the system. 'Their system is, to go dawdling along with a few pounds . . . and having thrown this out they saunter back again as slowly as they possibly can . . . almost invariably as soon as their baskets are emptied they sit down in knots and chat away for some ten or fifteen minutes.'[46] The Chinese overseers 'asleep under their umbrellas' were part of this conspiracy of sloth apparently 'unless one of the Government Europeans makes his appearance, then all is bustle till he is past, when a general grin takes place, and a "strike" for the next five minutes to make up for it'.[47]

This behaviour was, in fact, the aftermath of an actual strike that had taken place one month before, in late October. The trigger was Davis's 'Registration Ordinance' No. 17 of 1844. The scheme had been one of a number concocted by the zealous new colonial treasurer Robert Montgomery Martin, inspired initially by Pottinger, to enable the government to tax the population and control immigration more easily. The ordinance decree was dated 21 August, but it was announced to the general population almost two months later, as if rather ashamedly.[48] It would trigger the first universal act of resistance by the European and Chinese communities, cause organised letters of protest, generate group lobbying, and ultimately lead to the closure of shops, businesses, and construction sites. For site labourers, the clause in question was the seventh paragraph entitled: 'Headmen Contractors &c. required to have the men in their employ registered.'

Section of Gallery for B. C. E. D & H Barrack

O. S. No.

28. 41. 42. 31. 32

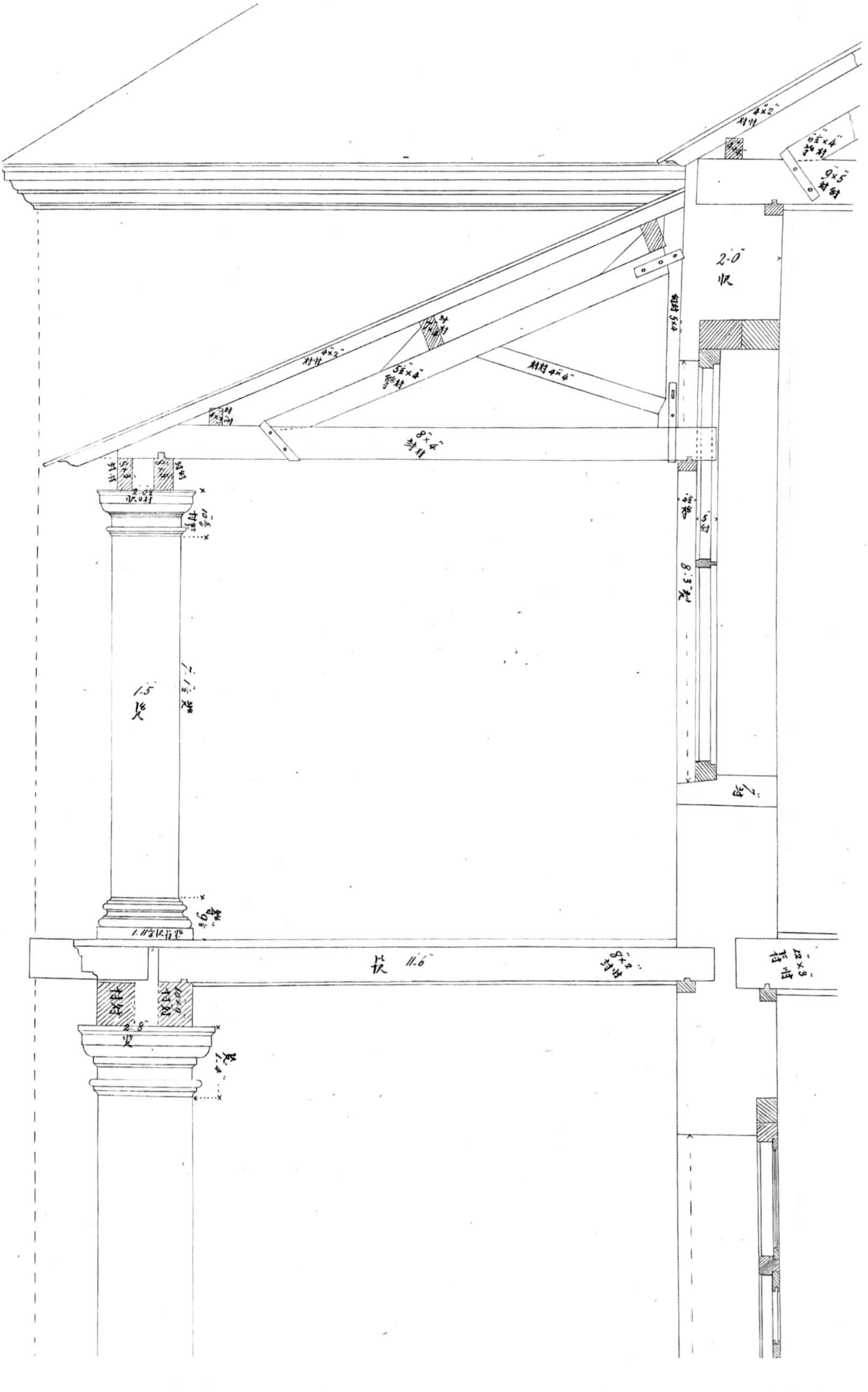

> And it be further enacted and ordained, That if any person being a Headman Contractor or other shall hire any or other persons Coolies or workmen not being previously resident in the Colony for the purpose of executing any work or service in the said Colony he shall be bound and is hereby required as soon as the said Coolies or workmen are landed in the said Colony to cause them to proceed to the said Office or such branch offices as may be appointed in the manner hereinbefore provided.[49]

Though Davis appeared blasé about the concerns of the Europeans, he was shocked by the Chinese reaction. He accused the merchant 'memorialists' of conspiring in the city strike. He then abruptly backed down, suspending the ordinance.[50] 'He has conceded to the threats of an ignorant rabble', sneered the *Friend of China*, 'what he would not grant to the petition of intelligent and influential men.'[51]

The damage to labour relations had a lasting effect. As Achone had tried to tell Ashworth, Chinese labourers, generally paid by contractors on a daily basis, had jealously guarded their working schedule, including their mobility to and from the island. Now, those of shared trades began to seek the protection of each other, even going so far as to protect their brethren from legitimate prosecution.

> In some instances, contractors are obliged to throw up contracts; the labourers refusing to work for certain individuals who have incurred their displeasure by informing upon any of their number who may have committed crime. The stone-masons form one combination, the brick-layers another and the carpenters a third. Each set appear to act independently, but either of them can impede the erection of a building by leaving off work.[52]

One case that went one step further was the intimidation of a second Chinese contractor who picked up the work of a former who himself had been the victim of union pressure. The authorities arrested the stonemason responsible for these threats and had him fined and imprisoned. The new union of stonemasons met and threatened to strike unless the new contractor backed down, paid all their arrears in wages, and ensured the release of their colleague. Unsurprisingly, he complied with all of their demands.[53]

◂ **Fig. 4.8.** E. Aldrich, 'Section of Gallery for B, C, E, D & H Barrack', 1844. Ink on paper. © The National Archives, Kew, London (WO 44/67 [9]).

However, perhaps the most peculiar case of collusion was between the Englishman George Duddell and a Chinese contractor named Youngket. This scam relied upon the belief by gullible proprietors on the testimonial (written by Duddell) of Youngket as 'a builder from Singapore well recommended by Merchants there', with Duddell brought in as a faithful 'Interpreter'. Youngket had no intention of constructing anything, but subcontracted out the work to trusting workers, siphoned off the money, and disappeared with the proceeds.[54]

Despite the occasional fraud and the more frequent acts of incompetence, the industriousness of local Cantonese workers was a trait admired by Europeans. In comparison, despite the rapid building works in Shanghai, the British noted that 'the Shanghai workmen are a very lazy set of fellows'.[55] Major Edward Aldrich, the man later to be at the centre of the suicide scandal, as chief commanding and superintendent engineer of the military works in Hong Kong, had unreserved praise for the local labour force. As Davis communicated to Lord Stanley, 'Major Aldrich informs me that in all his experience he never met with such intelligent and clever workmen as the Chinese; and that in some cases, where a less expensive mode of executing a work would have sufficed, a more expensive one has been adopted at their own charge, rather than be surpassed by other contractors.'[56] It is possible, nevertheless, that Aldrich deliberately selected a simpler 'Grecian' classical style of trabeated, that is post and lintel architecture, rather than a round-arched Roman classicism or a pointed-arched Gothic-revival form for his major works, as a consequence not just of his training but from an awareness of the experience and ability of local craftsmen. These significant works would include the Officers' Quarters (later named Murray House), the 'B' and 'C' blocks of the general barracks (Murray Barracks), the Military Hospital, and Headquarter House (later, Flagstaff House). This approach may have been taken based upon the experiments of Captain George F. Mylius and his experiences with local labour in constructing the early, solidly built barracks complex at Chek Chue—a masterwork that, though probably of brick and plaster, formed a stylistic prototype for Aldrich's efforts (**fig. 4.9**).[57] In offering his comments to Davis on the Gothic design for the colonial church (the future St. John's Cathedral) in early 1846, the governor recounted that: 'the Officers of the Ordnance declare themselves unpractised in the execution of that style, and recommend that a modern structure be authorised, as being better suited to the place, easier of execution, and to be erected on more reasonable terms.'[58]

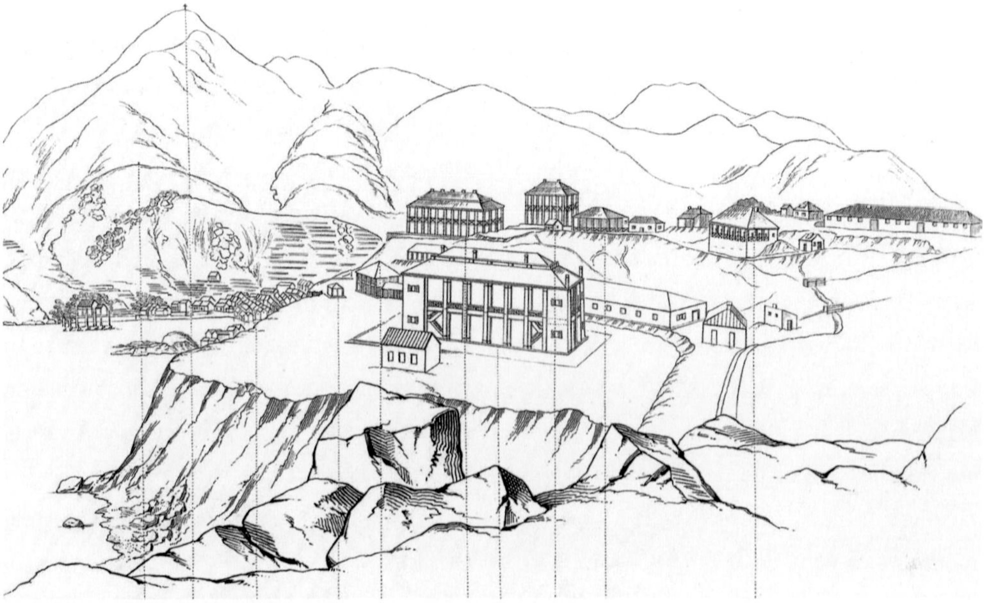

Fig. 4.9. Lt. T. B. Collinson, 'Chek-Chu[e] from the Southwest' (detail), *Ten Outline Sketches of the Island of Hong Kong*, 1846 (plate 5).[59] Engraving. © The National Archives, Kew (WO 78/115).

Aldrich, like Ashworth before him, held an almost anthropological fascination with the methods of work exhibited by local builders. In July 1846, he published a short article for his corps' annual journal: *Papers on Subjects Connected with the Duties of the Corps of Royal Engineers*, otherwise known as the 'Professional Papers'. It was entitled 'Description of the Mat Covering Sheds used at Hong-Kong in the erection of the Ordnance Buildings, and of the mode adopted by the Chinese in transporting and raising heavy Weights for these Buildings'. He enlisted the help of Collinson, his understudy, to furnish it with illustrations. Collinson had recently published his *Ten Outline Sketches* together with his ground-breaking survey—the *Ordnance Map*—a contoured survey of the island.[60] Aldrich wrote admiringly of the enormous mat-shed structures that were used as temporary outside envelopes for each building constructed, complete with a roof, which protected workers from the rain and sun. 'Not a nail is used in such a bamboo shed,' Hong Kong's commanding engineer marvelled, 'and when the shed is completed, it has the elegant appearance, representing the creditable ingenuity and ant-like labour of the Chinese for their application of manual power in its simple state.'[61]

Ashworth, two years earlier, had written on these mat-shed canopies similarly, describing the builders as 'the little men high aloft, adding stick to stick & binding them with bamboo thongs, might be compared to birds building their nests or forming cages'.[62] These men's choice of words revealed both an operational distance from the workers by British overseers and a denial of their individuality and humanity, yet conversely a feeling of sublimity in their massed, coordinated action, their bodies made smaller by the scale of their efforts. Clearly there was an autonomy to the way they were allowed to work. Aldrich was so enamoured by the raw power of organised, manual labour that he compared the combined force of the Hong Kong work gang to that of the ancient Greeks or Egyptians, and his designs, as a consequence, to vie in 'rivalry of the Temple of the Sun at Heliopolis'.[63] But labour-saving devices unfamiliar to the local workforce were rejected. He recounted that he had tried to introduce mechanisation in the form of the wheeled carriage, or 'devil carriage' as the locals had called it. Still, it went untouched for several months following an unfortunate accident in the crushing of a workman. Consequently, the Chinese devised a set of ramps made of a bamboo frame covered with China-fir planking ascending at the same comfortable incline but at differing distances from the building to carry material to the first and second floors (**fig. 4.10**). They also created a complex cradle system to enable thirty-six men to carry granite columns, each weighing 38½ cwt (or 38½ 'hundredweight', just under 2 tonnes).[64] Its ingenious weight distribution—the carrying spars orientated in two directions and distributed diagonally across the central load—evidently allowed the men who carried it to manoeuvre their burden into place without recourse to turning. The bamboo shed, constructed around what appeared to be the erection of the Officers' Quarters and the cradle system, with an examination in plan of its asymmetrical distributive layout, was painstakingly illustrated by Collinson.

It was Collinson who provided the illustrations accompanying Aldrich's study. One would be forgiven to assume that the young Royal Engineer, an empirically trained scientist, chose to arrange his two images of the carrying device based purely upon clarity of what was observed—a plan view of the bare device above an in-situ sketched view of it being carried. But Collinson, knowing he was publishing these findings for a pan-European audience, had in fact borrowed a visual quotation. Much like that enigmatic first travelogue *Hongkong and the Hongkonians*, and the hybrid borrowed styles of officials' buildings constructed in Hong Kong, nothing here can be taken at face value as merely 'observed' and scientifically detached. The visual layout is lifted directly from one of

William Alexander's famous illustrations taken during the first British diplomatic mission to China, the Macartney Embassy of 1793, and published in Sir George Staunton's account *Embassy to China* in 1797. The split image of plan and painterly view, almost identical in arrangement and entitled 'Method of Carrying Heavy Packages', had apparently become, by the 1840s, synonymous with Chinese mass labour and the carrying of large, heavy objects (**figs. 4.11a** and **4.11b**).[65]

The sight of 'ant-like labour' might have stirred admiration from their foreign overseers. Still, the relentless, daily toil of multitudes of Chinese workers generated frustration among the more religiously inclined members of the European community, though they appeared less concerned by the workers' exhaustion than by their perceived sabbatical transgressions. A commentator, signing himself 'A Free Man', wrote, 'Is this an English Colony? I should say No!!! If it was we should have the laws of England in force; and the Sabbath would be kept holy, and the Overseers of the China workmen (some of them, I believe are under Government) would then be allowed to attend their spiritual duties.'[66] A more socially-conscious writer retorted, 'we all know that the pay allowed to Chinese labourers by their countrymen—most of the jobs being contracted for by natives—is so small that it barely feeds them, and would not, were they Christians, ALLOW them to rest on the seventh day.'[67] Governor Davis, painfully aware of this dilemma, quickly decided by late June 1844 to instruct the Lands Office to desist from continuing constructing the public works on Sundays.[68] Just to be sure, he followed this with a proclamation for a 'general cessation from secular labour and employment on Sunday' in late February 1845.[69] It had the beneficial effect of creating one whole day of relative quiet in the city, where the percussive noise of mallets and the occasional blast of dynamite would be stilled. Chinese builders reacted wistfully. When it came to religion, the contractor Achone told Edward Ashworth in Pidgin that 'Cheenaman Jos let him makee walk, catch wage S'nday. Inglisman Gott say no walk S'nday'.[70]

With one day less work, contractors and their workers found it increasingly hard to meet previously agreed deadlines and cover their outlay and living expenses. Soon after the barracks and military hospital contractor Achou had committed suicide during the New Year 1846, the seedy and deadly world of debt finance within the Chinese building trade was peeled open. European readers of the *Friend of China* learned that the run-up to Chinese New Year was traditionally the time when creditors desired their loans back. It was also the season of suicides, the Chinese belief that if one took one's life, creditors

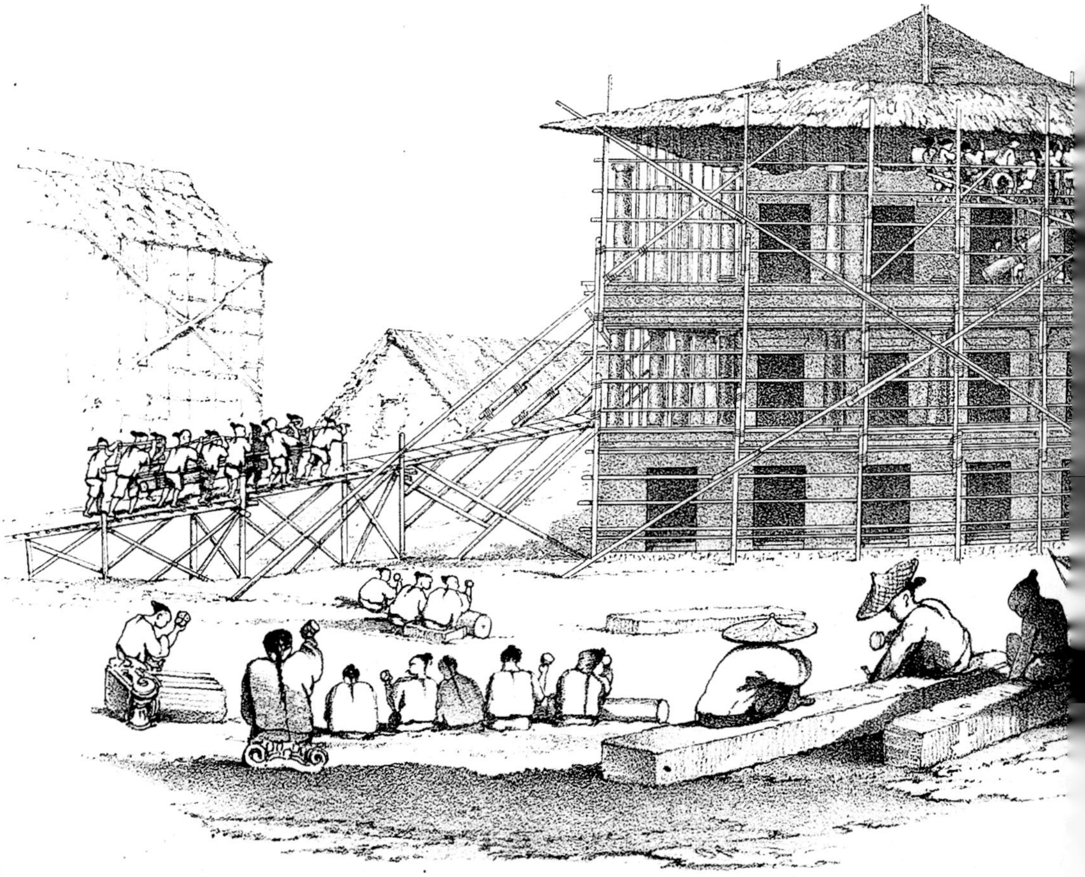

LIEUT. COLLINSON, R.E.
Hongkong 1846

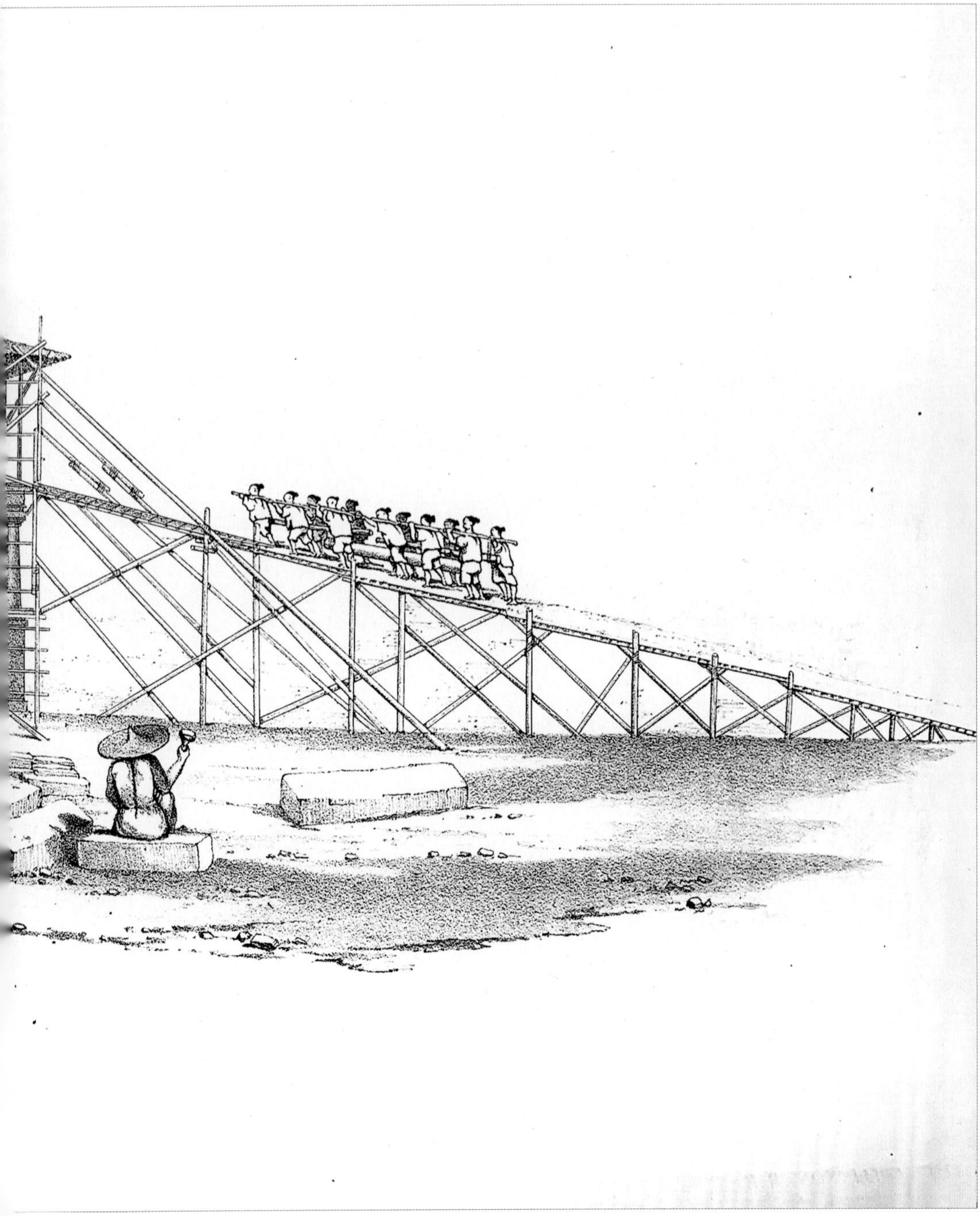

Fig. 4.10. Lt. T. B. Collinson, '"Mat Covering Sheds" Used to Construct the Ordnance Buildings', 1846. Lithograph. *Papers on Subjects Connected with the Duties of the Corps of Royal Engineers* 10, 1849 (plate 5). © British Library Board, shelfmark PP.4050.i.

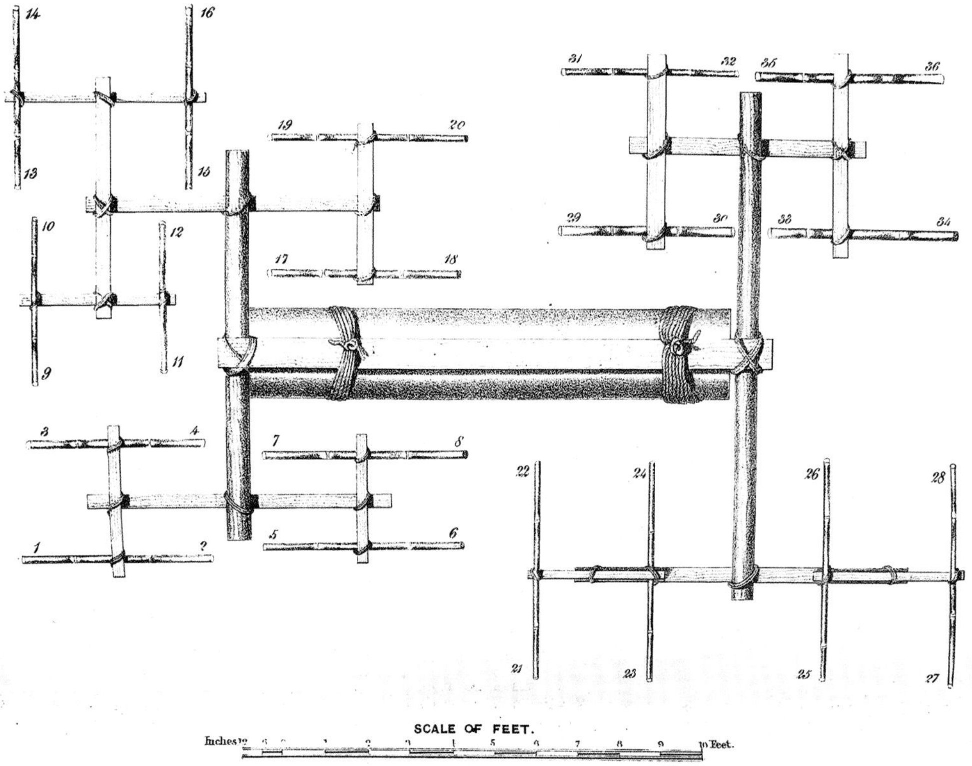

ELEVATION.

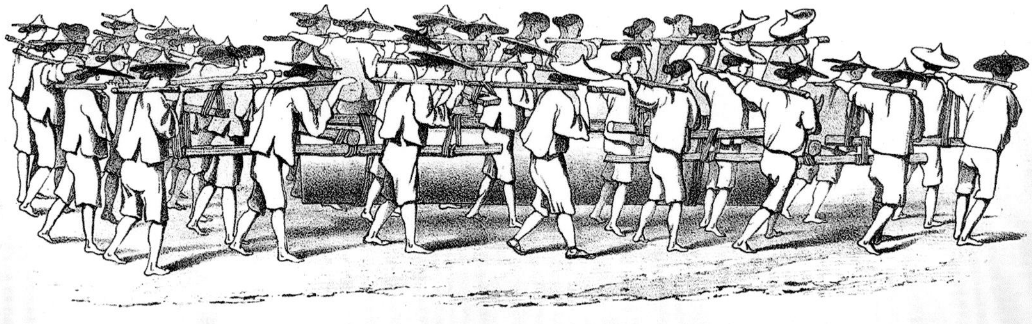

LIEUT COLLINSON, R.E.
Hongkong. 1846.

John Weale, 59, High Holborn. 1849.

C.F. Cheffins, Lithog. Southampton Buildings, Holborn.

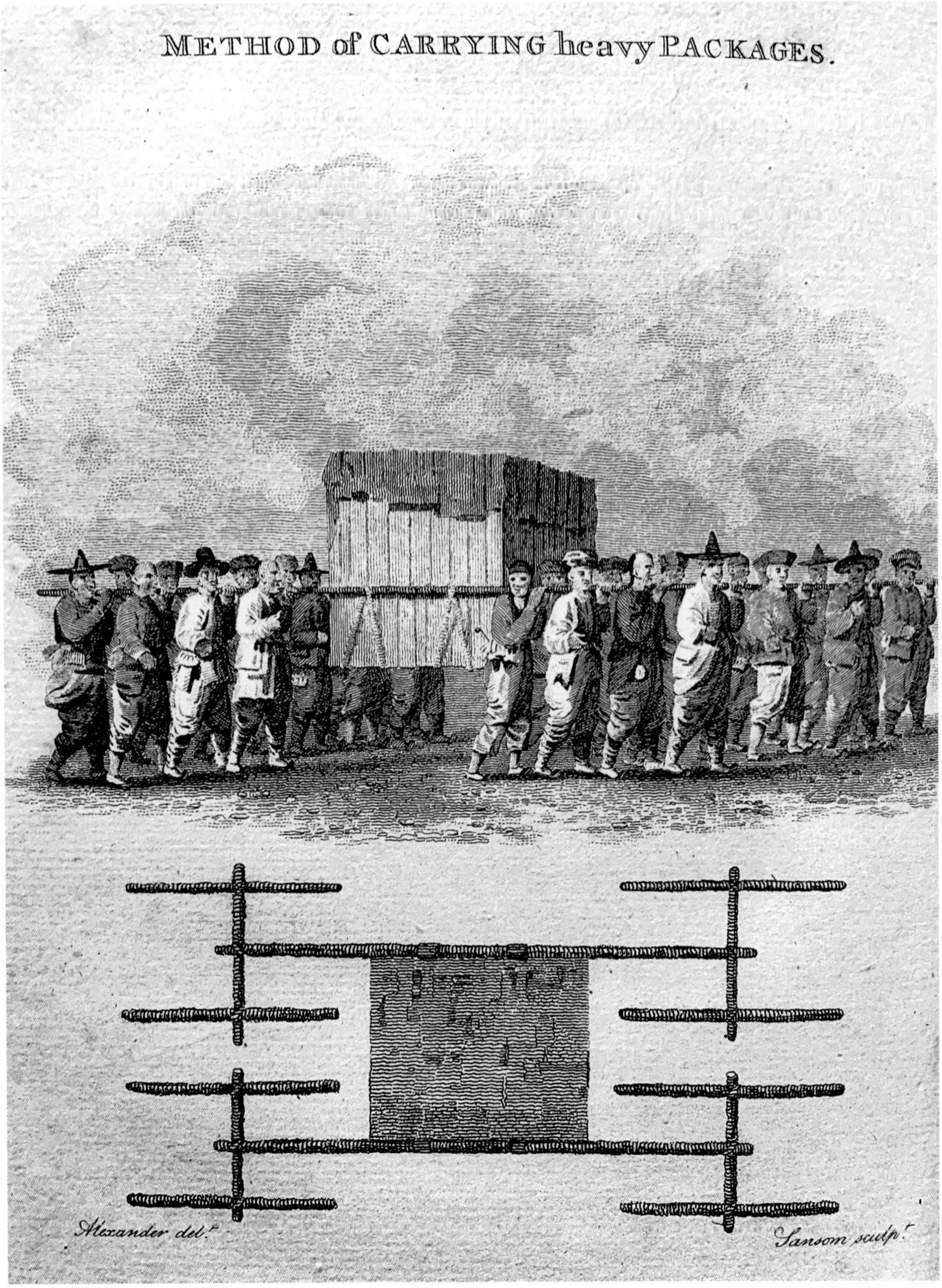

▲ **Fig. 4.11b.** W. Alexander, 'Method of Carrying Heavy Packages' (in China), 1793. Engraving. G. Staunton, *Embassy to China*, 1797. © British Library Board, shelfmark 10056.bb.15.

◀ **Fig. 4.11a.** Lt. T. B. Collinson, 'A 36-Man Bamboo Carrying Cradle System', 1846. Lithograph. *Papers on Subjects Connected with the Duties of the Corps of Royal Engineers* 10, 1849 (plate 4). © British Library Board, shelfmark PP.4050.i.

could not pursue the grieving family.[71] As if to demonstrate, the second example of this terrifying practice occurred on the same project soon after. A contractor, Low-atsoy, a stone-cutter working nearby on the Military Hospital, was kidnapped by three of his creditors, apparently, for money he owned them for work they had done for him at Chek Chue (the area now renamed by Davis as 'Stanley').[72]

However, one anonymous writer calling himself 'Alpha' laid the blame for Achou's death directly at the door of Aldrich. 'The particular building referred to is by no means an exception to the wrong the poor Chinese contractors have received at the hand of the Commanding Engineer,' he charged.[73] This personal attack had all the hallmarks of an insider with procedural knowledge of the military building works. Alpha accused the commanding engineer of 'altering the kinds of works', that is, of adding additional requirements to the previously priced contracts without an increase in the budget.[74] Achou's suicide note had described how he had been 'obliged to put down English stone [granite] in the Verandahs' of the Officers' Quarters. Alpha claimed the work had been priced for brick but that the contractor had been obliged to replace this with 'an identical stone entablature'. In addition, the bases to the 'B' and 'C' blocks behind the Quarters had been altered at the last minute by Aldrich, who now demanded a more labour-intensive rusticated finish. Achou had also been required to 'repaint and grain in imitation of Rosewood and varnish' the entire interior of Headquarter House, including 'cook, knife, shoe and servants rooms'. Alpha concluded that it was 'a matter of national humiliation and deep regret, while it begets and perpetuates among the Chinese distrust and contempt for our character'.[75] It is hard to gauge how contemptuous the Chinese felt towards the British military regarding this incident. However, it certainly did not halt or jeopardise the continued construction of further installations for the British. As will be shown, the task of building roads and drainage was another exploitative act of labour management that had attained some degree of sophistication as to the contractual methods of employment.

Despite withstanding immediate effects of the attack, Aldrich's eminent position and the considerable respect he had garnered both within the tight circle of Davis's administration and among the wider public had received a sustained blow from which he was unable to recover. Six months after the suicide, Aldrich was on his way out. 'Major Aldrich, the Royal Engineer at this place we hear has been ordered home by the Board of Ordnance', the *Friend of China* announced without a hint of pity. 'It is attempted from some reason to be kept a profound secret. From all that we can understand, it would have been a benefit to the service at large with which he is connected had his recall taken place a year ago.'[76]

Roads, Drains, Sewers, and the Taming of Hong Kong

Despite Edward Aldrich's prickly personality—and indeed evidence suggests him to have been a profoundly disagreeable man for many of those who worked alongside him—he was crucial to the successful development of Hong Kong. Beginning his tenure with proposals for a central military cantonment under Major-General Alexander Fraser, Lord Saltoun in 1843, Aldrich, between 1844 and 1846, was able to realise a hospital, a set of barracks, and a military headquarters under Saltoun's successor, Major-General George Charles D'Aguilar, in addition to the construction and repair of several buildings within the military stations at Sai Wan and Chek Chue. But this was not all. The new governor, John Davis, quickly possessed a poor opinion of the state of the Lands Office left by Pottinger, and his view of Alexander T. Gordon, Pottinger's cousin and the surveyor-general in charge, was little better. Davis might have received this low opinion from any number of unsolicited advisors. 'It appears,' Ashworth noted, 'that the Colonial Engineer [Gordon] & his assistant [Cleverly] found a more pleasant and creative occupation in planning houses for private individuals than in fulfilling the duties of their office & expediting the formation of streets *pro bono publico*. . . . these engineers in spite of their pretentions, know as much about architecture as cows, though they knew very well how to charge for their worthless drawings.'[77] And so, Davis would come to rely increasingly upon the military professional for assistance. He would, in effect, depend on both the skills and advice of Major Aldrich for almost every branch of the public works and especially concerning the vital matter of infrastructure provision for the island.

This programme for the development of the infrastructural public works of Hong Kong, namely the government's programme for the provision of roads, drains, and sewerage, may be split into two distinct territories and, therefore, objectives. The first objective concerned the urban districts of the city itself. This would be driven both by private market obligations of the government to ensure that the land it sold was adequately accessible, and alongside, a drainage and sewerage system that basic, modern hygiene provision demanded, especially within a dense habitat. The second objective was to build an extensive road network to link the rest of the island. This urge was driven by the military and navy, enabling the connection of their dispersed installations. Subsequently, this ambitious second project became Davis's proud yardstick of progress in his communications with Whitehall.

For all his boasting to London, Pottinger's January 1844 land sale proved an unmitigated disaster for public relations within the colony. Not only had he disenfranchised much of the Chinese population with his draconian measures to forcibly relocate the entire population of Upper Bazaar to the new, lower, fringe neighbourhood of Tai Ping Shan, but he also alienated most of the European landowners. Those that had already purchased in 1841 under Elliot were known dissenters. To these were added the new European landowners who had replaced the Chinese, and to whom had been promised roads and other amenities that would provide an adequate connection from their elevated properties down to the rest of the city. As they grew impatient, a flurry of frustrated letters was placed in the local press. As one disgruntled owner complained,

> SIR,—Being a Purchaser of Two Lots of Land at the late Sale, . . . I feel, naturally, very anxious to know, when I shall be able to approach the Lots I have purchased.
>
> I see little or no preparation towards making the Roads, and I believe such was the express stipulation, on the part of the Government, at the Sale. It was asserted that they would bear the expence, and until they are formed it is practically impossible, to carry up building materials to many of the allotments—mine I regret are so situated.
>
> I am Sir,
> Your Obedt Servant,
> & COSMOPOLITE.[78]

Hong Kong's urban landscape was a mess. By mid-1844, houses under construction were perched in absurd positions adrift of a road system, 'where no man would risk his limbs by approaching after dark—which is quite inaccessible to any vehicle or the foot of a quadruped less firm than a mule'.[79] The *Friend of China* sarcastically suggested the government's current road programme to be 'the poetical creation of an imaginative draftsman, for anything approaching to the appearance of those streets which in the original are laid down parallel with the Queen's road, would defy the industrious search of the most inquisitive. We see ravines, with intervening ridges, covered with huge stones and rocks, making an approach to them somewhat difficult—but streets or roads none.'[80]

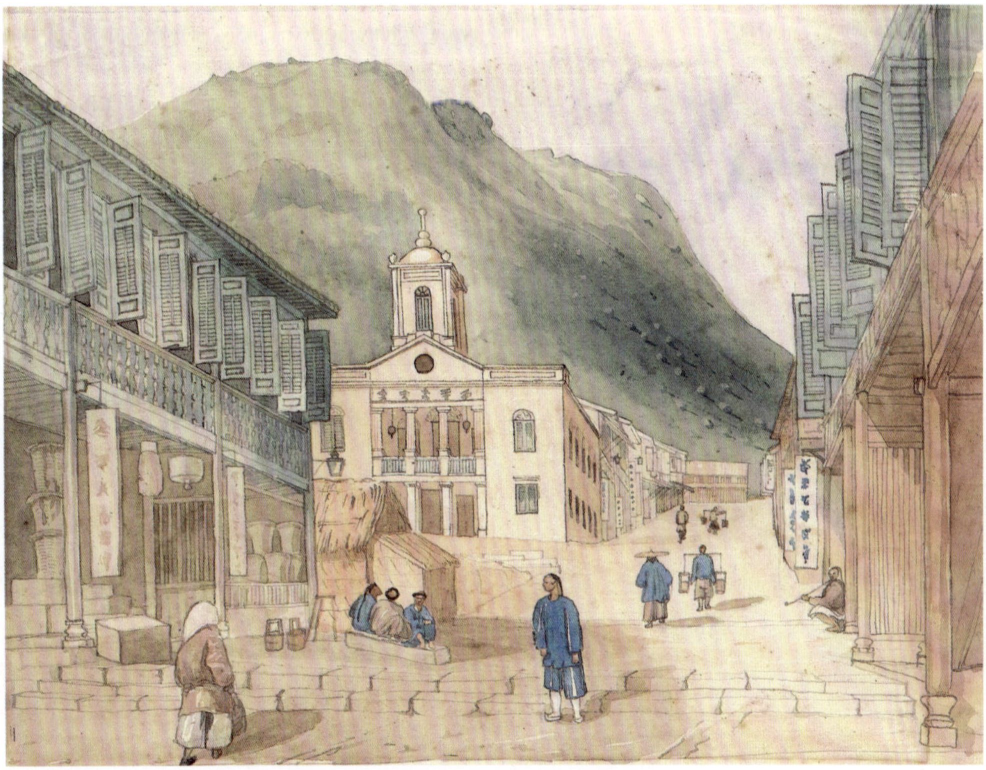

Fig. 4.12. E. Ashworth, 'Chinese Street in Victoria, Hong Kong, with the "Tae Ping Shan" American Baptist Mission Chapel Erected 1844', ca. 1845–1846. Watercolour on paper. © Hong Kong Museum of Art Collection (AH2015.0017).

Ironically, the relocated Chinese initially fared much better with their new topography. Tai Ping Shan was quickly laid out in series of tight parallel roads climbing up the hill, adopting characteristics of the old Upper Bazaar many in the community had been forced to abandon (**fig. 4.12**). Here, at the very borders of the newly configured Chinese and European settlements sat Reverend J. Lewis Shuck's American Baptist 'Tai Ping Shan' mission school and chapel, on the corner of Gough Street and Shing Wong Street, while the actual mountain of Tai Ping Shan baldly loomed above.

It is hard to imagine now, but the Central District as we now call it (then known as part of the wider 'Western District'), as with most of the other sections of the mountainous island, consisted of a series of connected ridges and troughs.[81] These furrows had aided Davis in administratively splitting the city into three portions: the 'Western', 'Central', and

'Eastern' Districts. The 'Western' extended from West Point up to the (Harbour Master) Pedder's Hill (now opposite to Pedder Street); the 'Central' from the stream immediately west of this to the eastern edges of the Cantonment (that is, to the boundary of the old cemetery within Ha Wan); and from then on, through and beyond the Wong Nai Chung Valley (Happy Valley) and East Point, was the 'Eastern District'. For Davis, still, the centre of the city was the Cantonment area of the Ordnance District and Cantonment Hill (now Admiralty), the original portions of the first settlement. Without a proper height-related survey, the consequence for new development in the Western District was an ill-fitting street plan. Nevertheless, despite the wait for Collinson's contoured island map, the simple grid layout to the south, above the line of the new Hollywood Road, would work if the correct levels and gradients could be struck to provide the optimum effort (and reusable soil) in cutting and filling.

Once the roads were rudimentarily complete within the new district, in late 1844, many purchasers faced the rather comical situation of having their front doors either 'accessible by a short flight of steps, perched some ten or a dozen feet above the road' or 'shocked to discover . . . that the usual order of things is reversed—the door being gained by a descent of several feet'.[82] Poor surveying was blamed, and that a correct base line at the lowest point had not been struck prior to the setting out of all the subsequent elevated roads.[83] Cleverly, the acting surveyor-general, 'observed that several lots could not be built on, owing to the want of means of access to them'.[84]

Two years later, in mid-1846, the same stretches of road would be complained about. A significant dip still existed between Caine's Magistracy–Prison on the ridge beside Old Bailey Street, the old 'Magistracy Hill', and across a short distance towards the west at the end of Elgin Street, within the new district. A writer calling himself 'Sewer' was frustrated as to the inconvenience of unfinished drains and the consequent remains of large stones and pools of water. 'From the Old Bailey to end of Elgin Street, or the whole breadth of the valley, every road is in this state, and it is impossible to take a large package up either of the streets, so that you are necessitated to go round to the other valleys East or West, at double expense.'[85]

Another problem was the parcels of land created by some of the bisecting streets, such as Lyndhurst Terrace and Elgin Street. 'Roads are actually being made!' celebrated one writer caustically, 'But oh-ho—these small lots, triangular, rhomboidal, trapezoidal, pentagonal, hexagonal, and what not. And houses built to suit the lots! Think of living in a triangular house!'[86] One such ungainly triangle was the parcel of land created between Lyndhurst Terrace, Cochrane Street, and Wellington Street, as illustrated by the overseer of roads, Murdoch Bruce, drawn in 1845 and published in 1846 (**fig. 4.13**). Here, a descending platoon of troops unable to pass eastwards into Wellington Street are obliged to make a sharp turn to the left.

If anything, however, the provision of drains initially proved to be a more politically sensitive issue and was undoubtedly at the forefront of Pottinger's mind as he prepared to leave office in early 1844. The Wong Nai Chung Valley, a significant location of outbreaks of the previous year's fever, had become totemic of the link between stagnant freshwater and miasma, and an extremely delicate issue. Mists had been seen to hang in the early morning within the gullies and ravines and were particularly thick within the valley itself.[87] Despite his scepticism, therefore,[88] Pottinger initiated a comprehensive programme under Gordon to drain the Wong Nai Chung Valley (together with the nearby So Kon Po Valley) and raise its level at considerable expense.[89]

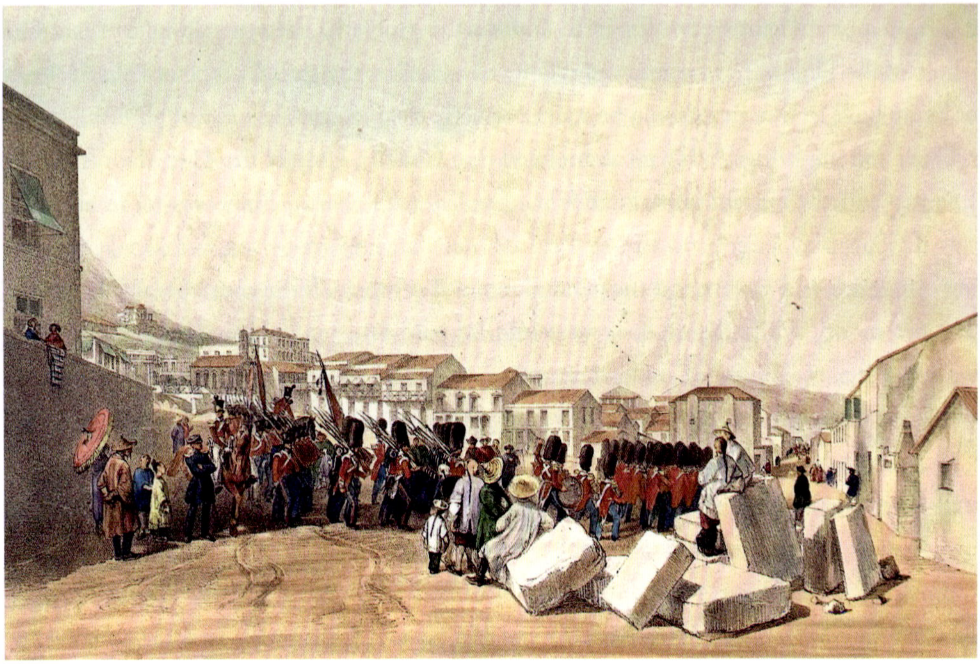

Fig. 4.13. M. Bruce, *View of Lyndhurst Terrace, Wellington Street, and Cochrane Street*, 1846. Coloured lithograph. © Hong Kong Museum of Art Collection (AH1964.0389.005).

its course.[104] It would take a considerable amount of time to repair the damage; meanwhile, malaria season was looming for residents. Fortunately, sanitary workers manually drained the water in time. Yet, one difficulty remained: a lack of natural escape points for torrential surface water as it passed across the shore-hugging Queen's Road. No hillside streets had been planned to traverse that road to the sea. Only one wharf was open to the public, belonging to the Harbour Master, William Pedder.[105] Because of this unique access, Pedder Street would eventually come into existence. The second transverse street, some distance further west, was laid out on the site of the Central Market close to Chinam's Hong.

The narrow widths of the streets above the Queen's Road had always been a source of criticism. After the annual storms had commenced back in 1844, the *Friend of China* recalled the recommended street widths proposed by Colonel Malcolm during the first Lands Committee of 1842. These were to be sixty-foot wide for the principal highway, the Queen's Road, and fifty-foot in width for all the cross streets that ran down the hill and formed the inevitable sluice routes for rainwater. As the new city grew across and above the obliterated site of the Upper Bazaar, Gordon decided to halve these dimensions for all road widths.

> Colonel Malcolm's experience of tropical climates satisfied him of the necessity of the streets being wide, to admit a free circulation of air; Mr. Gordon, however, fresh from home, knowing nothing of the tropics, has altered Colonel Malcolm's plan, and the streets—gullies they would call them in India—are now to be twenty-five feet wide. We trust it is not too late to rectify this error fatal to the health and comfort of the inhabitants.[106]

However, the newspaper, still smarting from its loss of gazetted status, hoped that a new governor would dispense with this miserly approach to investing in the city's future. 'We believe he [Davis] will not be influenced by any paltry fuelling of the policy of narrowing the streets, on purpose to obtain a few more building allotments, and thus add a trifle to the colonial exchequer.'[107] Unfortunately, if there was a governor who revelled in advertising his frugality in the use of the colonial purse, it was Davis. The road widths would remain narrow above the Queen's Road and permanently affect the relative positions of business areas against residential neighbourhoods.

By July 1845, two months after the great storm, the smell emanating from the drains was dreadful, according to one writer to the *China Mail* calling himself 'I Carry A Snuff Box'.[108] In his letter, the new resident complained that Aberdeen Street (a north-south, steeply sloping street connecting Caine Road to Wellington Street below) remained a gaping excavation. Workers had opened its central drain a month before leaving a six-foot-wide, twelve-foot-deep trench uncovered and unprotected. The 'slight bamboo fence' that had been hastily constructed one or two weeks before, presumably near Snuff's front door, 'was speedily broken down and carried away', leaving a narrow verge for pedestrians to balance upon 'whose extreme width is to be reckoned by inches'.[109] One victim of the trench was a pony, who fell headlong into the pit and was hauled out with incredible difficulty.[110] Murdoch Bruce's lithograph shows this street in its recently completed state, with all the ventilatory benefits of a direct sea-view and breeze, the sunnier southern façades of its buildings fitted with shade-giving awnings and jalousies (**fig. 4.14**). The slow pace in providing good drainage proved a nightmare for the government, particularly within the new upper Western District (today's Central District) neighbourhood. The government may have successfully relocated the more pliant Chinese merchants from their homes in this area of the old Upper Bazaar, but a vocal and demanding set of European residents rose in their place.

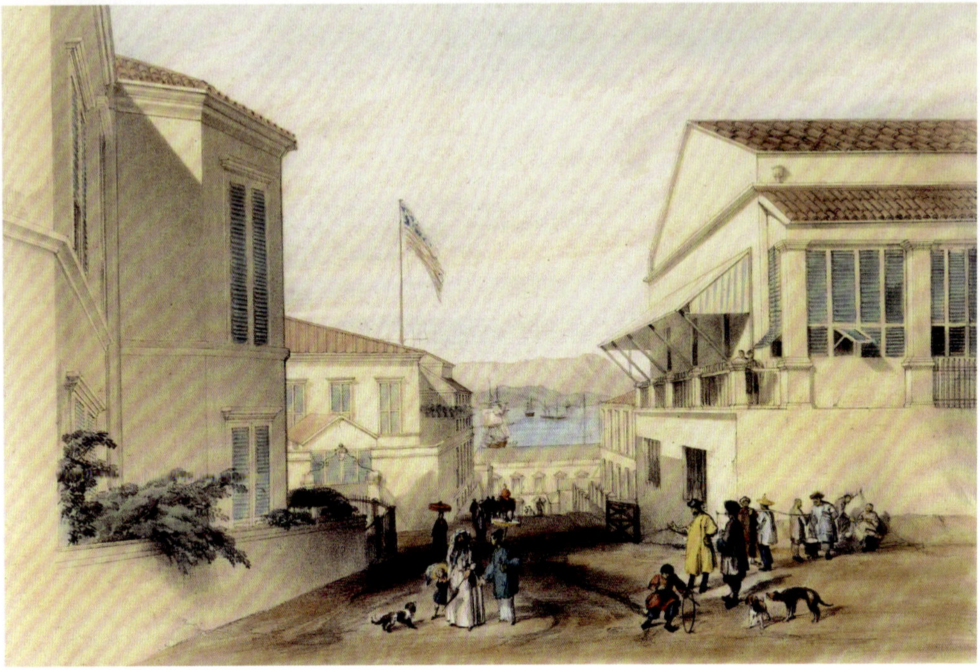

Fig. 4.14. M. Bruce, *Aberdeen Street, Looking North, Hong Kong*, 1846. Coloured lithograph. © Hong Kong Museum of Art Collection (AH1964.0389.002).

In his remaining few months in office, Pottinger focused his efforts on the development and maintenance of Victoria itself. On the other hand, his successor, Davis, was additionally influenced by military and naval interests in expanding the scope of the public works into an island-wide programme of improvements. The new commander of British forces in China exerted the most significant early influence on Davis. Major-General D'Aguilar, soon after his arrival in late December 1843, was intent on establishing a regular postal courier link between the military establishments of Sai Wan and Chek Chue with the city. This mail service would take effect from 1 February 1844, with outbound letters despatched by runners on Mondays, Wednesdays, and Fridays, and inbound, back to Victoria, on Tuesdays, Thursdays, and Saturdays.[111] Consequently, he requested that Pottinger instruct his land officer (now surveyor-general) to examine the line of bridle paths that connected these installations to prepare an estimate for their reconstruction as suitable roads for the increased military traffic.[112] As all construction of roads since the ratification of the Treaty of Nanking (Nanjing) rested in the civil domain, the governor held the purse strings. Gordon made a tracing of the initial stretch, a new line towards East Point. But Pottinger, baulking at the expense and the uncertainty of the area's future use (still contemplating that the seat of government might move across to the Wong Nai Chung Valley), decided to wait upon London.[113] He did sanction the construction of a twenty-five-foot-wide temporary road in the vicinity, pending estimates.[114] Whether due to the poor roads or the widely accepted incompetence of the deputy post master, Thomas J. Scales, the messenger scheme failed, and five of the seven original runners were dismissed.[115]

Davis first entered the colony's waters on 7 May 1844, approaching the island from the southwest. The new governor later claimed to Lord Stanley that he was surprised by the sight of 'a depression of the ridge of mountains, which at once struck me as the proper point, on first making Hongkong in Her Majesty's Steamer "Spiteful"'.[116] He was speaking about the ideal position from which to connect the southwestern fishing village of Shek Pai Wan to Victoria along the north by the construction of a new western road. This observation may have been a true account by Davis or a post-rationalisation brought about through the influence of Rear-Admiral Sir Thomas Cochrane.[117]

Cochrane had stubbornly refused to remove his naval stores and coal depot (called the 'Middle Stores'), currently located directly at the foot of Government Hill, frustrating Pottinger. The site of the stores had been intended for a relocated military parade ground, the current elevated position of which, together with an adjacent 'acclimatising barracks', were obstructing the area designated for a colonial church—the future St. John's Cathedral. The Rear Admiral deliberately blocked the anticipated moves in an urban chess game. Cochrane cheekily suggested that the governor forcibly evict Jardine Matheson & Co. from East Point but was slapped down. Off the cards, too, was the bottlenecked entrance to the harbour at Lei Yue Mun, further east. As previously mentioned, the Admiralty had already drawn up plans by Captain Clement Edwards in mid-1843 to take over Shek Pai Wan as a naval base. It only remained for the governor to give the nod. Pottinger's replacement by Davis soon provided this opportunity.[118]

It was as if one was hearing Cochrane's own words in Davis's mouth. The new governor described taking

> a circuit of the Island which I made with that Officer. It was impossible not to be struck by the admirable locality and general advantages of Shek-pai-wan (Chuck-py-wan) a sheltered position on the south side, lying due south of the middle of Victoria town and of a gap in the central ridge to which a good bridle road has been constructed.[119]

This is the first mention of a preliminary route that would become the Pok Fu Lam Road, forming the first link in Davis' ambitions to encircle the island in a ring of connected roads. With his fondness for anglicisation in cultivating his connections, Shek Pai Wan would later be renamed 'Aberdeen' by Davis in honour of British foreign secretary, Lord Aberdeen. Cochrane had told him that a small number of troops placed there during the 1843 fever had been extremely healthy. But what probably played upon Davis's fears the most was that the rear southwestern flank of the island lay unprotected.[120] 'The plans and estimates for this most desirable road,' wrote Davis to Stanley, '. . . will open out by the shortest way the south side of the island, and give value to many a building site in pleasant and healthy positions, which are now worthless from want of approach. Indeed it is much to be wished that a road entirely round the island were completed for Military, Police and all other purposes.'[121]

This road, however, had not been accounted for. When Davis arrived, he soon received a letter from Lord Stanley attaching the entire estimated budget for the public works. Gordon had provided these that February at a total of $718,500, of which the estimate for all future roads, streets, sewers, drains, and land drainage came to $214,500 or just over one-quarter of the total budget.[122] For roads and streets, these included: the completion of the Queen's Road from the site of the West Point Barracks to the east side of the Wong Nai Chung Valley ($28,000 including bridges); continuing the same road to East Point ($15,000); the construction of a bridle path to Sai Wan ($3,000); repairs to the road to Chek Chue ($1,500); and within the urban area the formation of new streets, principally to the west of Magistracy Hill ($35,000); and the necessary demolition work in removing the houses from the Upper Bazaar to re-plan the area ($25,000)—a total of $107,500. Almost equal in expenditure, drainage and sewerage were budgeted under constructing sewers to the city ($100,000) and for draining the two valleys ($7,000).[123] Stanley attached a simple instruction that had originally been formulated and conveyed to him by Charles Trevelyan at the Treasury.[124] Only three reasons were permitted for Davis to order works to commence without prior authorisation from the Colonial Office. 'In like manner you will of course not authorise any expenditure which is not required for the transaction of the public business or for preserving works and buildings already in progress or for securing the public health until you shall have received the express sanction of Her Majesty's Government.'[125] Davis would quickly absorb these rules and use them to successfully justify the extensive road and drainage network he would propose. 'The Works,' he would later write to Stanley, 'which have been undertaken with my authority, exclusive of a few secondary buildings of absolute public necessity, are Drains and Roads, that is, such as pertain either to the health or the internal communication of the Colony.'[126] This included his pet project, his road from West Point to Shek Pai Wan—the Pok Fu Lam Road—which would be approved by his executive council late in 1844.[127]

Aldrich's involvement in Davis's schemes happened quickly. D'Aguilar, as head of the military, had wanted a speedy repair to the road system he had complained to Pottinger about. However, the construction and maintenance of roads since the Lands Office was established fell under the Governor's civil jurisdiction.[128] Nevertheless, as lieutenant-governor, D'Aguilar felt able to influence the situation and asked Aldrich if he would be willing to undertake the repair works.[129] In addition, the surveyor-general, A. T. Gordon, fell ill and was transported back to England from where 'it is rumoured he will not return to Hong Kong'.[130] Aldrich was quite put out. As always, when pressed, he complained to Lieutenant-General Sir Frederick Mulcaster, Inspector-General of Fortifications (IGF). He relayed that he was unable to spare his workforce at the Royal Engineers' Office to undertake additional work and that his health, after two attacks of fever, would restrict him from expanding his workload to include a colonial appointment.[131] In addition, Davis had pestered him to quickly examine the plans and sections that the departing Gordon had drawn up for the new Government House and 'to note at the foot whether you approve or not'.[132] Aldrich obliged and thereupon, whether he wished it or not, won the admiration of Davis, from whom he would continue to receive all significant documentation from the Lands Office–cum–Surveyor-General's Department for his approval and comments before the execution of any of the public works.

Davis's high regard for Aldrich was balanced by his low regard for Charles Cleverly, the assistant surveyor-general and man in charge of the public works following Gordon's departure. Cleverly had, in early 1845, miscalculated the necessary level of the military road to Tai Tam, east of the island, raising the level without Davis's approval by a further four feet to avoid the high-water mark.[133] Davis would later, in March 1846, write to Gladstone (then British colonial secretary) comparing 'the narrowness of the capabilities possessed by the former [Cleverly] . . . and the superior knowledge of Government Works possessed by the Royal Engineers'.[134] Cleverly was considered so immediately lacking in experience that Aldrich had already provided him, in early August 1844, with a basic template for drawing up reports and estimates for the various government works. Though this template was for a particular context—teaching Cleverly to prepare documents for the building of a police station at Chek Chue—they provide a general insight into how Aldrich addressed most of his civil works.

> The Report after explaining the necessity of the Service, and how it originated, should give a description of the nature and extent of the work, or repair intended, accompanied with Plans and Sections and Scantlings, and a short specification of what is proposed. It should afford every explanation for the full understanding of the nature of the Service contemplated, and when necessary, be submitted with a sketch showing the relative situation of the proposed work, with the adjacent ground and buildings.[135]

In particular, Aldrich suggested that Cleverly ought to consider three options for executing the work: either by 'day work' (the direct payment of labourers on an ad-hoc, daily basis), by 'measurement on agreed prices', or by a fixed-sum contract.[136]

Cleverly applied this newfound freedom to construct the street system within the Western District. Eight streets of an aggregate length of about 6,130 yards had, in the usual manner, been put to tender that autumn. The lowest bid 'per street' came in at $15,000 for a stretch of 700 yards, and Cleverly advised Davis's Executive Council to reject this.[137] Instead, he suggested that the work be achieved in small, independent contracts if adequately supervised, estimating that the bids would most likely work out at a rate of about $2 per linear yard.[138] The total bids eventually came in at $13,080.68 for a run of 6,000 yards or just under $2.20 per linear yard.[139]

The assistant surveyor-general was aided by John Pope, who had been an articled pupil since the age of sixteen to William Cubitt, the leading master-builder of London.[140] Pope had subsequently worked on the South Eastern Railway in England as an assistant engineer and came with 'the highest testimonials'.[141] Davis elevated him to the dual position of 'Civil Engineer and Clerk of the Works' and he turned out to be essential in maintaining the credibility of the Surveyor-General's Department and in contributing to Cleverly's survival. Pope shared Aldrich's flexible approach to procurement, recounting his experiences in applying various methods in the execution of the roads. Pope recorded his personal experiences in a lengthily entitled *Memoranda of the relative cost of Public Works in the Surveyor General's Department, when executed under Contract and when carried out by day work*. This treatise was submitted to Davis via the government's auditor Adolphus Shelley under his *Annual Report on the Civil Expenditure for the Public Works* submitted at the close of the tax year, on 31 March 1845.

Pope's general view was that contract work, whether a single contract or a set of smaller ones at measurement prices ('piece-work jobs'), operated most effectively when the 'work contracted for, is of an ordinary and simple description such as buildings and all ordinary Works in Masonry'.[142] Whereas those best let under day work were when the nature of the commission was 'of an uncertain or unusual description as the new lines of Roads'.[143] Exceptions were the simpler stretches of road, such as a length from the Wong Nai Chung Valley to the So Kon Po Valley, undertaken by fixed contract by the English contractor Mr. Cunninghame for $2,000, and masonry work in the construction of the Harbour Master's Sea Wall, again by another English contractor.[144] It was either these contractors' use of European overseers or in the possession of greater acuity at cost control that made them the exceptions in a trade by now heavily dominated by the Chinese. Three Chinese contractors, Atoong, Affong, and Atim, had been employed along the So Kon Po Road. Upon submission of their day-work receipts they were paid based on the daily rate of $1 per seven coolies and $1 per three masons. This choice of procurement was because the nature of the work was uncertain: earthworks and 'tide work' (presumably road-foundation digging involving labourers working in water).[145] The work on the Shek Pai Wan Road (later named the Pok

Fu Lam Road) was another project best suited for day work due to the 'extreme irregularity of the ground'.[146] Interestingly, Pope noticed that as workmen under contract were paid higher salaries they, as a consequence, tended to perform more effectively, while those under day-work wages required constant and vigilant supervision, thereby offsetting any savings both in terms of lower productivity and the additional cost of hiring an overseer.[147] By April 1845, Davis was able to write to Stanley boasting of his success in the island-wide road construction programme and that 'nearly every public work essential to the prosperity and uses of the Colony has now been undertaken or completed, with the exception of some drains and water courses', and 'five remaining miles of road to complete the circuit of the island'.[148]

Aldrich continued to provide a stream of advice and assistance, with some of his staff of Royal Engineers seconded to the public works.[149] By 1846, the commanding engineer was a fully integrated, though a voluntarily unpaid, component within Davis's administration. Gordon, still stuck in London and on half-pay, sat aggrieved. Writing to Gladstone, he expressed his firm opinion that 'whatever works are attached to the civil department should be wholly and solely under the control of the Surveyor General'.[150] The Colonial Office saw it differently. 'The fact is,' one official countered on the reverse of Gordon's letter, 'that it is not unusual. Military Engineers are employed as often as possible to verify or correct the estimates of Colonial Engineers. It is an highly convenient practice because the Military Officer is far more exempt than the other from local influences and prepossessions & is therefore better guardians of the Public Purse.'[151]

Aldrich not only provided advice for the road system and its construction, he was also consulted on drainage and water provision. To address the latter, Davis called upon his assistance to help respond to the Health of Towns Commission's Report. Gladstone had forwarded this substantive document to Davis at the request of the Colonial Land and Emigration Office in Whitehall.[152] The 'Royal Commission on the Health of Towns', set up in 1843, was created in response to the Utilitarian Edwin Chadwick's Poor Law Commissioners' findings on the health of the poor within the metropolis of London. Those results had been presented to Parliament in July 1842. The Duke of Buccleuch, as chairman of the new commission, headed this further enquiry which expanded the investigation 'into the *state of large towns and* populous districts' across the country.[153] The project took two years to complete with the results of this 'arduous and unremitting investigation into the causes affecting the general sanatory condition of the community' published in such professional journals as *The Builder* in the summer of 1845.[154] Five areas on drainage and ventilation issues were focused upon, namely: street and house drainage; the paving of public streets, courts and alleys; the cleansing and removal of refuse; the supply of water for public and private use; and the construction and ventilation of buildings.[155]

The timing of the release of the report was perfect, leaving the Commissioners relatively free to be enlisted to share their thoughts on the state of Hong Kong and Davis's recommendations under a recent ordinance for the improved sanitation of the city, and to recommend any further measures. At the beginning of 1846, they submitted a short report entitled *Observations on the Hong Kong Ordinance for the Drainage to the Town of Victoria*. Their initial premise was that 'the difference in climate will make no difference in the measures necessary', and noted that assuming this, 'for preserving the health of the population, . . . the ordinance does not embrace all the operations that are necessary for that purpose'.[156] Several measures were offered, including the proper drainage of houses (later echoed by Osbert Chadwick's investigations into 1880s Hong Kong housing), and the rapid removal of refuse. However, at the top of their list of recommendations was a proper supply of water for the effective sluicing of the city, for 'where so much gross matter finds its way into the sewers, [drains] cannot be made effectual without a copious supply of water to carry off the heavy substances'.[157] They cited London, 'the best Sewered Town in the World', as being dogged 'with instances of accumulations in the Sewers'.[158] For municipal purposes, Davis had also desired to split the city into three districts, and the Commissioners commented that the meaningfulness of this administrative division could only succeed if it was based upon 'an accurate survey of the whole natural area for drainage with a plan shewing the relative heights of the ground'.[159]

There had always been outbreaks of fire within Hong Kong. Now that the city was evolving into a multi-stacked environment of terraces and streets, it was becoming increasingly clear that tanks and wells built above the town level were needed for this and to address the Commissioners' primary recommendation. By June 1846, Davis, with the assistance of Aldrich, was able to submit a report and estimate to Gladstone that would address this deficiency. The basic premise was to provide a water catchment zone above and behind the city's limit. Cleverly had proposed four drains (culverts) to be placed west of the magistracy–prison. However, Aldrich believed that the scheme was insufficient to ensure that the culverts would remain filled with water at all times. He proposed drawing a supply from a ravine west of 'The Albany', a long row of new houses built for junior government officials, 'and brought to the summit level of Caine Road between the

Arbuthnot and the Old Bailey Roads—from whence it can easily be turned as it may be Required on the stone channel drains . . . to fall into either of the four culverts West of this point, and into the Tanks'.[160] It was an elegant and practical solution in the spirit of what had come to be expected of the commanding engineer. Aldrich also agreed with the Commissioner's *Observations* that fire prevention was not necessarily the greatest need in using these tanks. Instead, a greater capacity and spread were required. 'The necessity of more wells being provided for the wants of the Town appears to me so apparent not only for the Required supply of the Town but also by such means of supply to add to the salubrity of the Town by draining the substrata.'[161]

Aldrich's indispensability as a teacher also persisted. By March 1846, he was still aiding Cleverly. This time he helped him prepare estimates for the various drains and sewers, whether open or closed, constructed across the city. He suggested to Cleverly that an estimate could be more accurately targeted through an accompanying report of work already completed. This could be shown graphically 'for each street shewing opposite to each in a Tabular Form, the Number of the Estimate (the years expressed in different inks) on which such services have been executed'. 'Such Return,' Aldrich concluded, 'will afford at a glance, the full information required under each head, as to the extent of the work actually provided for, with what may remain to be included in further services.'[162] Cleverly followed this explicitly at the end of that month, providing Davis with his coded map of the open drain and culvert system entitled 'Return of services executed or in progress in the construction of Drains and Sewers in the Town of Victoria' (**fig. 4.15**).[163] At about the same time, Cleverly submitted two substantial, interrelated reports. The first was his *Report on the Construction of Roads and Buildings, and the State of the Public Works* for 1845–1846, and a second, his *Report . . . upon the Progress of this Department* [Surveyor-General's Department]' for the same period.[164] Of note in his road report is his description of the construction of the western artery, the Pok Fu Lam Road, linking West Point to the newly named 'Aberdeen' (Shek Pai Wan). The project proved more expensive than anticipated owing to the difficulty of excavation and an unexpectedly rockier substratum. On all roads, the government had attempted to locate nearby areas for stone extraction, thereby saving the cost of labour in transporting road paving. Unfortunately, only one stone quarry was discovered along the line of the Pok Fu Lam Road, with most of the rock having to be transported at great expense from So Kon Po, on the east side of the island.[165]

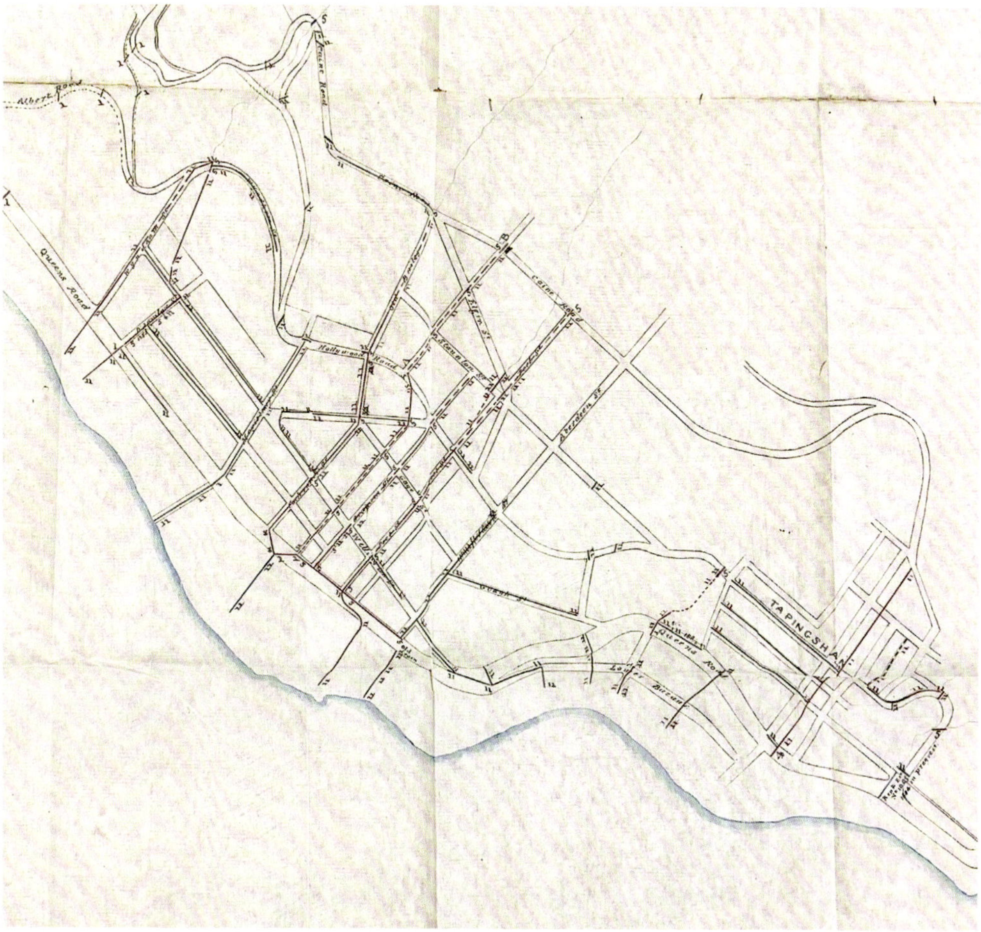

Fig. 4.15. C. Cleverly, Open Drain and Culvert Layout Map, Western (now Central) District, 1846. Ink on paper. © The National Archives, Kew (CO 129/16: 153).

In the second progress report for his department, Cleverly noted that his first estimates of both the western and eastern roads (the Pok Fu Lam and Tai Tam roads) had been inaccurate due to poor preliminary surveying. These estimates had demeaned him in the eyes of Davis. 'I was induced,' he complained, 'to make the Estimates without the necessary Surveys and levelling to enable me to judge of the nature of the ground, the actual amount of cutting and filling, and the detail of the drains and bridges.'[166] This problem was unexpectedly resolved by the long-awaited published appearance, in 1846, of Royal Engineer Lieutenant Thomas Bernard Collinson's survey masterpiece of Hong Kong

Island (**figs. 4.16a** and **4.16b**). It was a work of extraordinary skill, drawing from the young Collinson's technical experiences in working on the Ordnance Survey of Ireland (1824–1842) some years before when he was just twenty. His map would beat the same to become the first published ordnance survey in the British Empire to make extensive use of the contour line (or isobath) in determining uniform degrees of height.[167]

Collinson's work to survey the entire Island of Hong Kong took him almost two years to complete, from late 1843 to late 1845. He published his map in four quarters—northwest, northeast, southwest, and southeast. *The Ordnance Map of Hong Kong*, as it was entitled, was proudly signed off by his superior, Edward Aldrich, on 30 October 1845, before being sent for engraving and printing at the Ordnance Map Office in Southampton a year later.[168]

Davis, ever the 'orientalist', provided Collinson with all the approved spellings, the 'orthography', of both the English- and Chinese-named locations, which the young cartographer diplomatically acknowledged on his title quarter. The survey also included some neighbouring territories not yet under British control, including the tip of Kowloon and Lamma Island (of which Collinson must have covertly surveyed). Rather methodically, he surveyed Hong Kong in a clockwise or counter-clockwise manner, as he would recount to his mother. 'I am at present quartered at Chuck Chu, which is the last station of the survey; and I have finished it just in time; for the hot weather is recommencing, after one of the pleasantest winters ever known in Hong Kong. I find Chuck Chu the same as I left it last year, but the 98th have all gone and the Barracks are nearly empty.'[169]

For Hong Kong's developmental history, the *Ordnance Map* demonstrated the fortunate marriage of an individual with a terrain. Charles Hutton, a British mathematician, invented the contour line for his now lost 1774 survey of Schiehallion, a mountain in the Highlands of central Scotland. Soon after, the French first systematically used the contour line to establish fortifications. But it was the Royal Engineers in the 1830s who adopted this technique in a more comprehensive and extensive approach to the mapping of large expanses of land. Collinson was one of the first to turn this into a practical reality, his Ireland posting having been in the superintendence of 'Hill Drawing'.[170] Though just twenty-two years old when he commenced his survey of Hong Kong Island, Collinson was one of the most accomplished surveyors using this technique. Judging by his equally ground-breaking method in combining this plan with carefully labelled landscapes in his accompanying *Ten Outline Sketches of the Island of Hong Kong*, issued by the Royal Engineer's Office in Hong Kong a year later, he linked

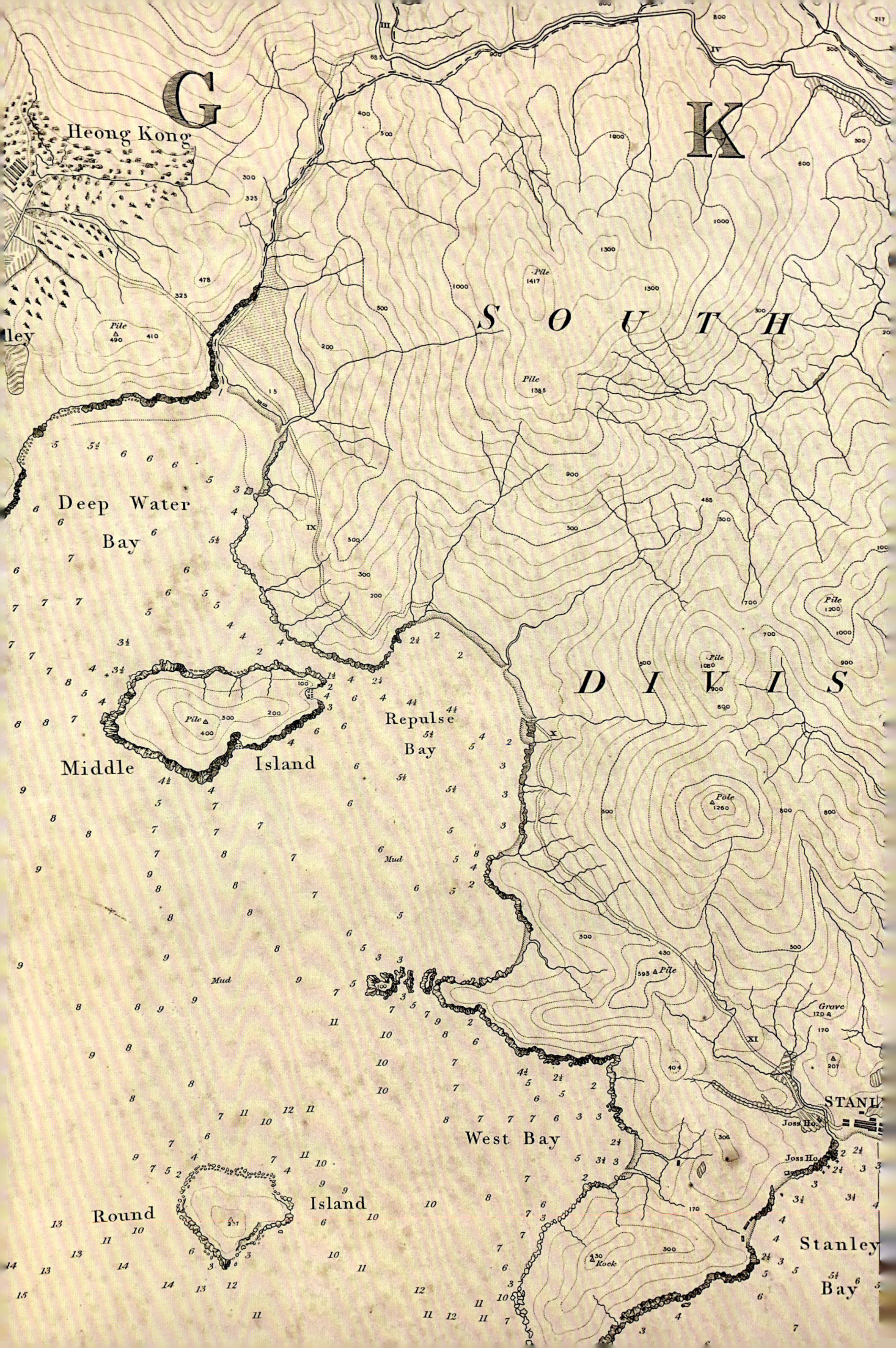
G
K
Heong Kong
SOUTH
DIVIS
Deep Water
Bay
Middle
Island
Repulse
Bay
Mud
West Bay
Round
Island
Stanley
Bay
STANL
Joss Ho.
Grave
Pile
Pole
Rock

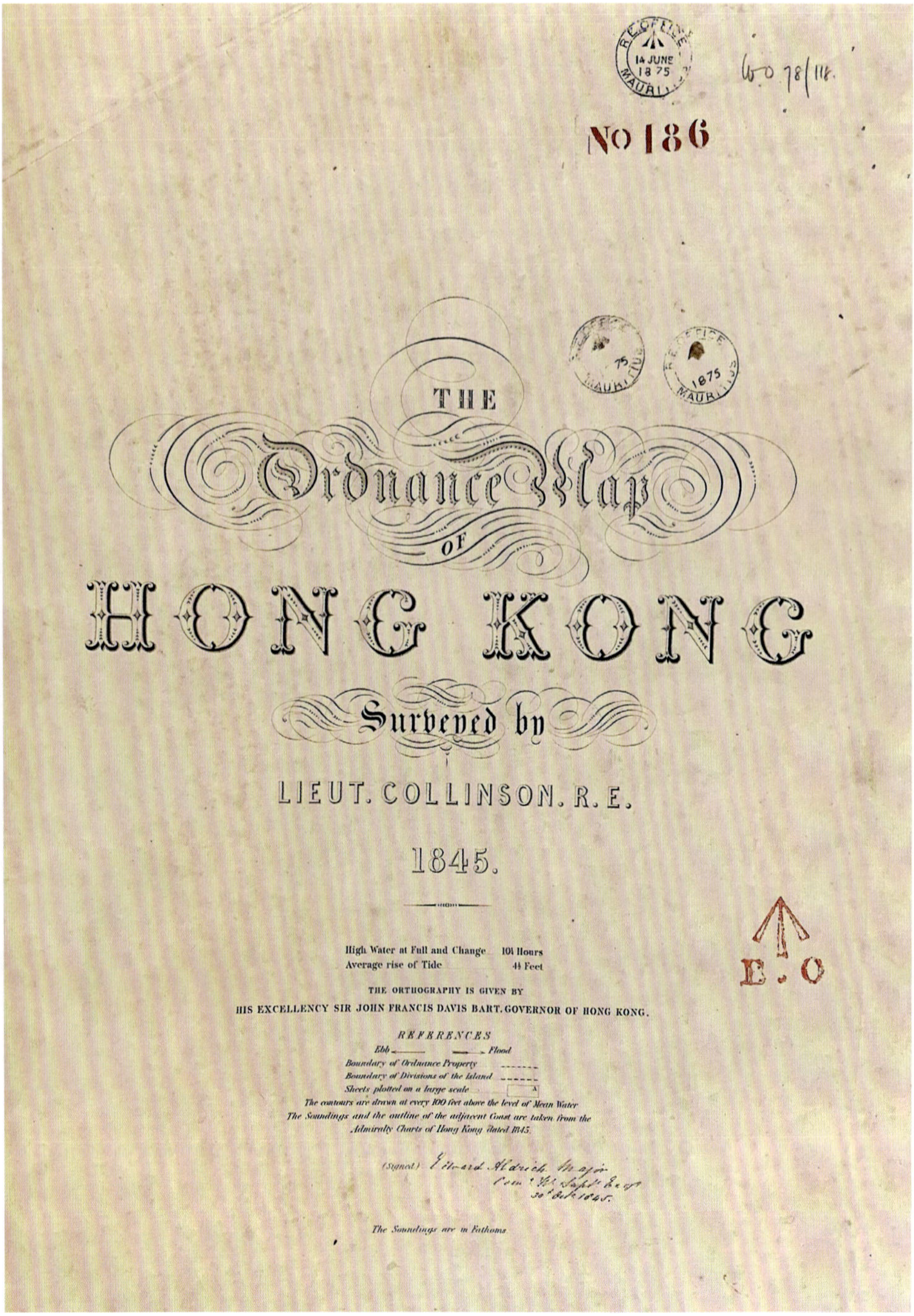

◄**Figs. 4.16a** & **4.16b.** Lt. T. B. Collinson, *The Ordnance Map of Hong Kong*. Detail and inscription, 1845. Engraving. © The National Archives, Kew (WO 78/118).

this with a visually fertile imagination. For example, his audacious panoramic view from above Causeway Bay and East Point proved to be a powerful visionary device for motivating the city's growth both across surface and in elevation. At about the same time as Collinson made these altitudinous views, Edward Ashworth first climbed up to The Peak. But where the architect had, from his perspective, described the isolation of the settlement walled in by a threatening mainland beyond, the surveyor, arranging his view to the side, placed island and mainland in equipoise. Collinson's image made it clear that the perceived heart of Hong Kong was, in fact, its harbour. The forked snake tongue of Tsim Sha Tsui penetrating the view to the right merely showed how inevitably necessary, to a security-minded surveyor such as he, the future taking of the Kowloon Peninsula appeared to be (**fig. 4.17**). Collinson would not-so-secretly survey this desirable China side of the harbour as part of the study. It would take merely fifteen more years and another bloody war to fulfil this vision.

Collinson's superiors in England recognized the spatial brilliance and perceived accuracy of his approach in linking a map with almost 'picturesque' perspective views, as if the

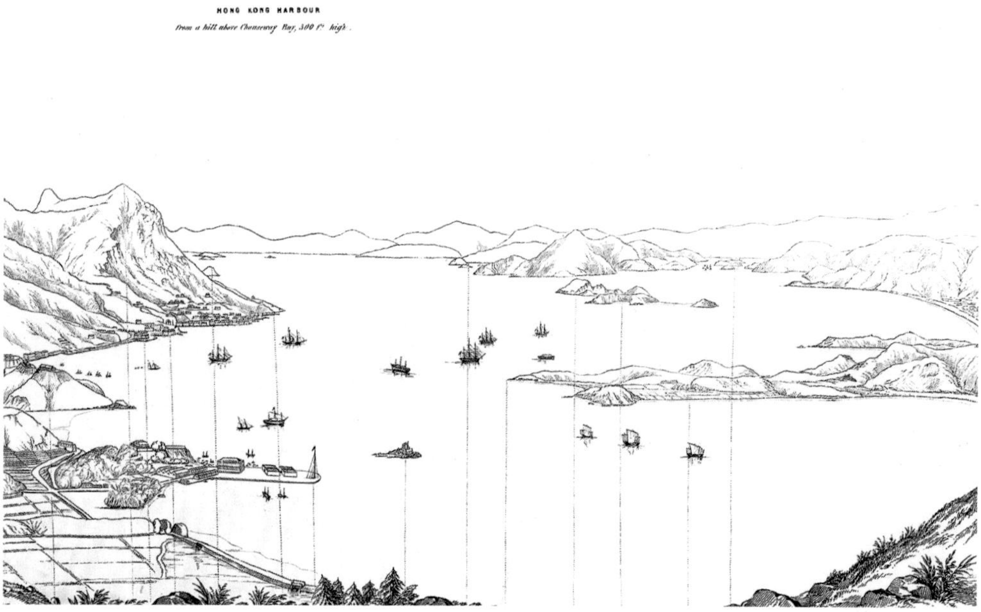

Fig. 4.17. Lt. T. B. Collinson, 'Hong Kong Harbour, from a Hill Above Chausway [sic] Bay' (detail), *Ten Outline Sketches of the Island of Hong Kong*, 1846 (plate 9). Engraving. © The National Archives, Kew (WO 78/115).

island's visually constructed appeal lay as a sequence of viewpoints strung across a gigantic English landscape garden. His work on Hong Kong became an exemplar for the rest of the internationally spread Corps of Royal Engineers to follow. One Board of Ordnance officer in 1847 hurriedly wrote on the cover margin of one set, 'These outline Sketches to illustrate the accompanying Contoured Survey of Hong Kong are to be deposited in the Royal Engineers' Office at Mauritius, for the information and guidance of the Junior Officers of the Corps, as the Maps and Sketches, together are considered to exhibit an excellent method of giving a correct idea of a Country.'[171]

The other partner in this fortunate marriage, with its limited scale and challenging topography, was Hong Kong Island itself. Hong Kong was small enough to cover accurately and with sufficient detail in the short time available to Collinson. Yet, as we shall see, no other method of surveying could have delivered the taming power that the contour line offered in mapping Hong Kong. For example, it provided the perfect guide for determining the heights of future reservoirs and in completing Davis's peripheral ring of necessarily level roads. Belcher's 1841 map, his *Navigation Chart* of Hong Kong, remained an enduring template, repeatedly reprinted to record the colony's development. But its etchings of height belonged to an older pictorial tradition, redolent of a brooding sensibility, its shaded hatchings capturing the dark uncertainties of settler life as if upon a blasted lunar surface. Collinson's 1845 *Ordnance Map* flattened and made every change in level empirically comprehensible. Information was at the service of measurement. Pinnacles were no longer differently represented from low-lying coastal edges (**figs. 4.18a** and **4.18b**).

Collinson's work proved to be essential for both military and civilian interests. And while, for the military's purpose, the map intended to accurately measure the distances and dispositions of their stations within the island's landscape, the *Ordnance Map* also shaped the physical layout of Davis's road programme, helping to connect the island into a complete, navigable circuit. It would also provide decades of valuable service as a background reference as the colony incrementally grew and developed. Davis ordered copies of the *Ordnance Map* to be sent to different branches of the Hong Kong Government. From this, it is clear that the line of the Pok Fu Lam Road benefited from Collinson's technique, as for much of its length, it was constructed to precisely follow the contour lines he had generated. The symbiotic relationship between the survey as it was being carried out and the building of peripheral roads is shown by the fact that Collinson could add the path of the Pok Fu Lam Road into the survey as it was being built (**fig. 4.19**).

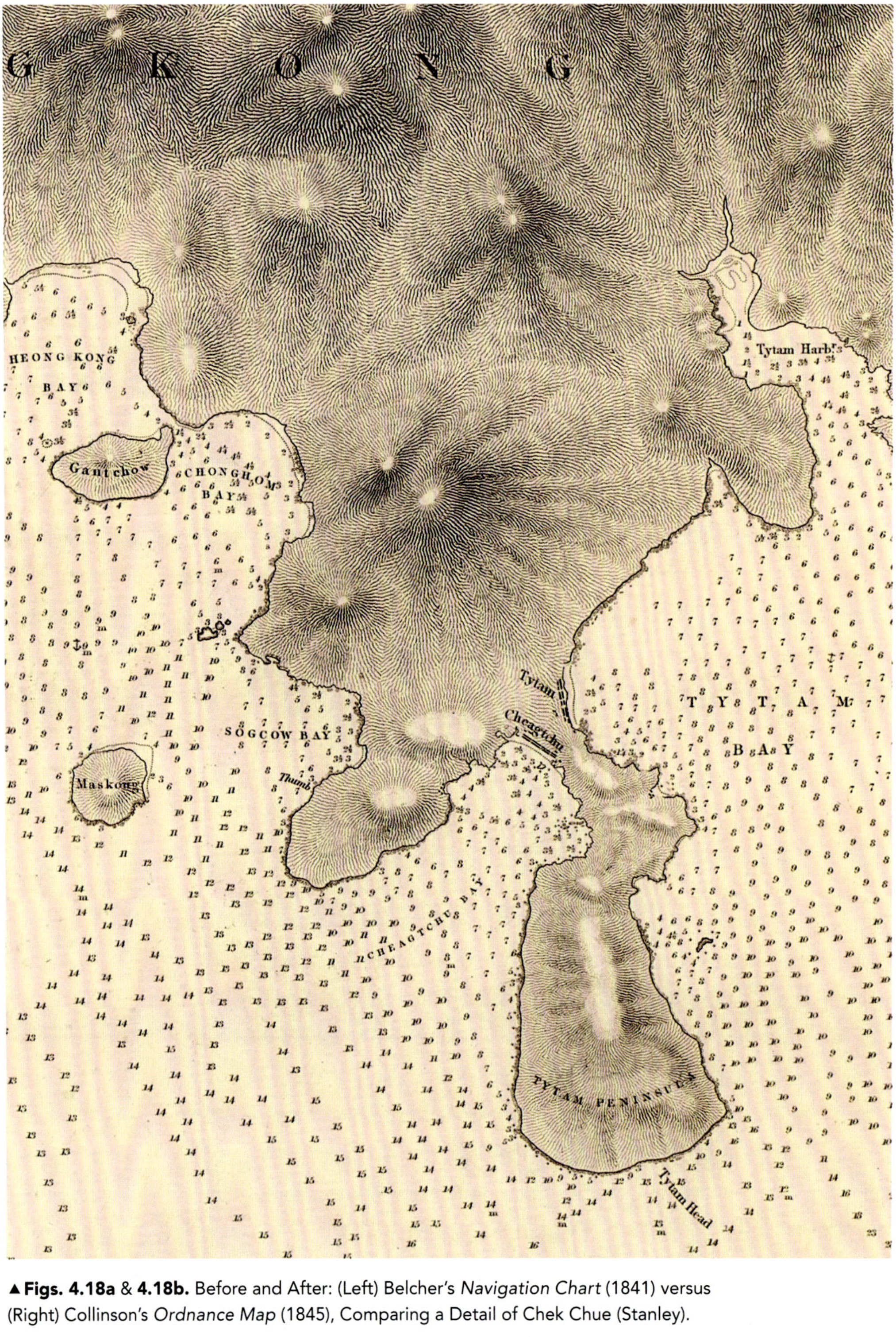

▲ **Figs. 4.18a** & **4.18b.** Before and After: (Left) Belcher's *Navigation Chart* (1841) versus (Right) Collinson's *Ordnance Map* (1845), Comparing a Detail of Chek Chue (Stanley).

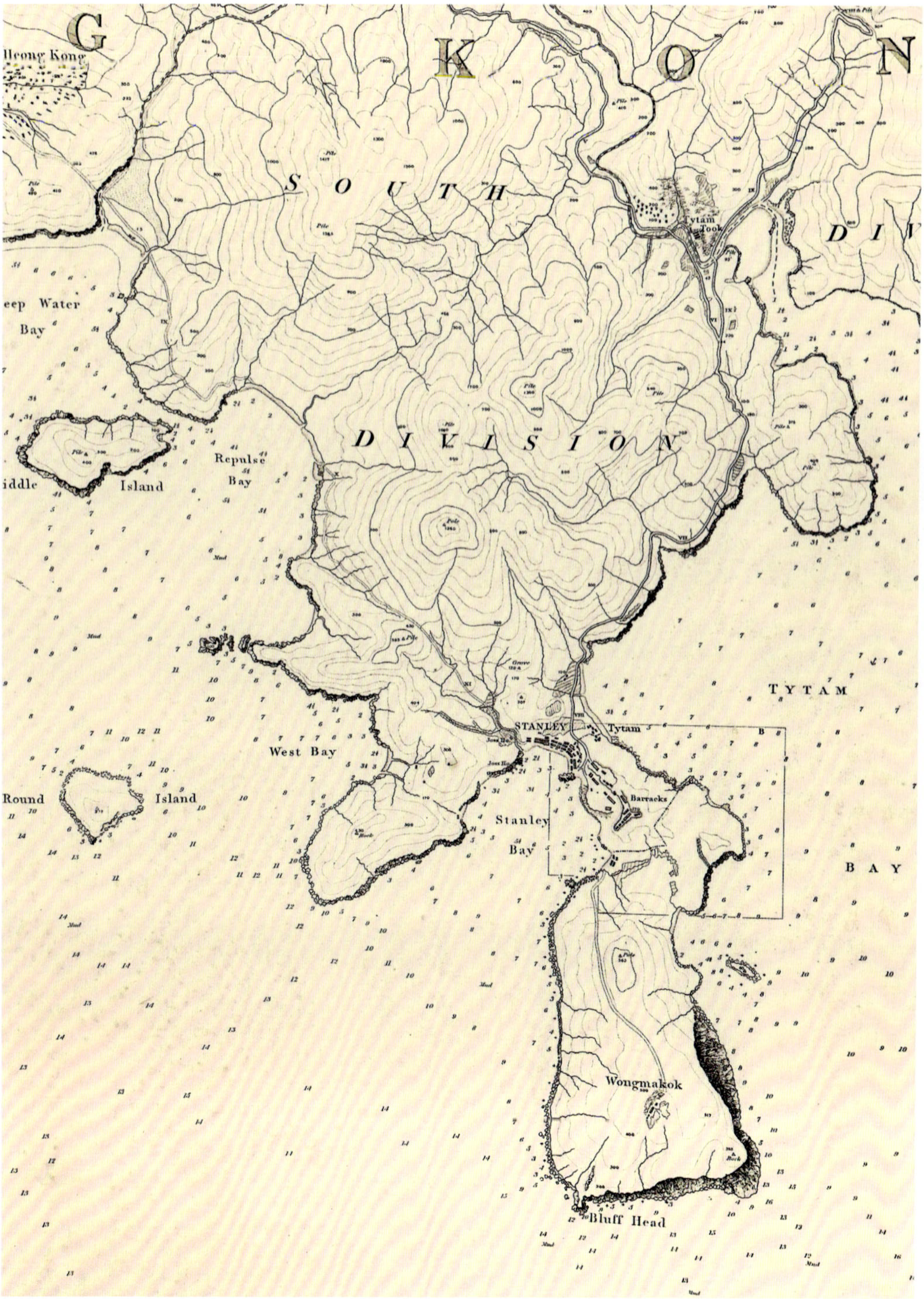

(Left) Engraving. © The Barry Lawrence Ruderman Map Collection, Stanford University.
(Right) Engraving. © The National Archives, Kew, London (WO 78/118).

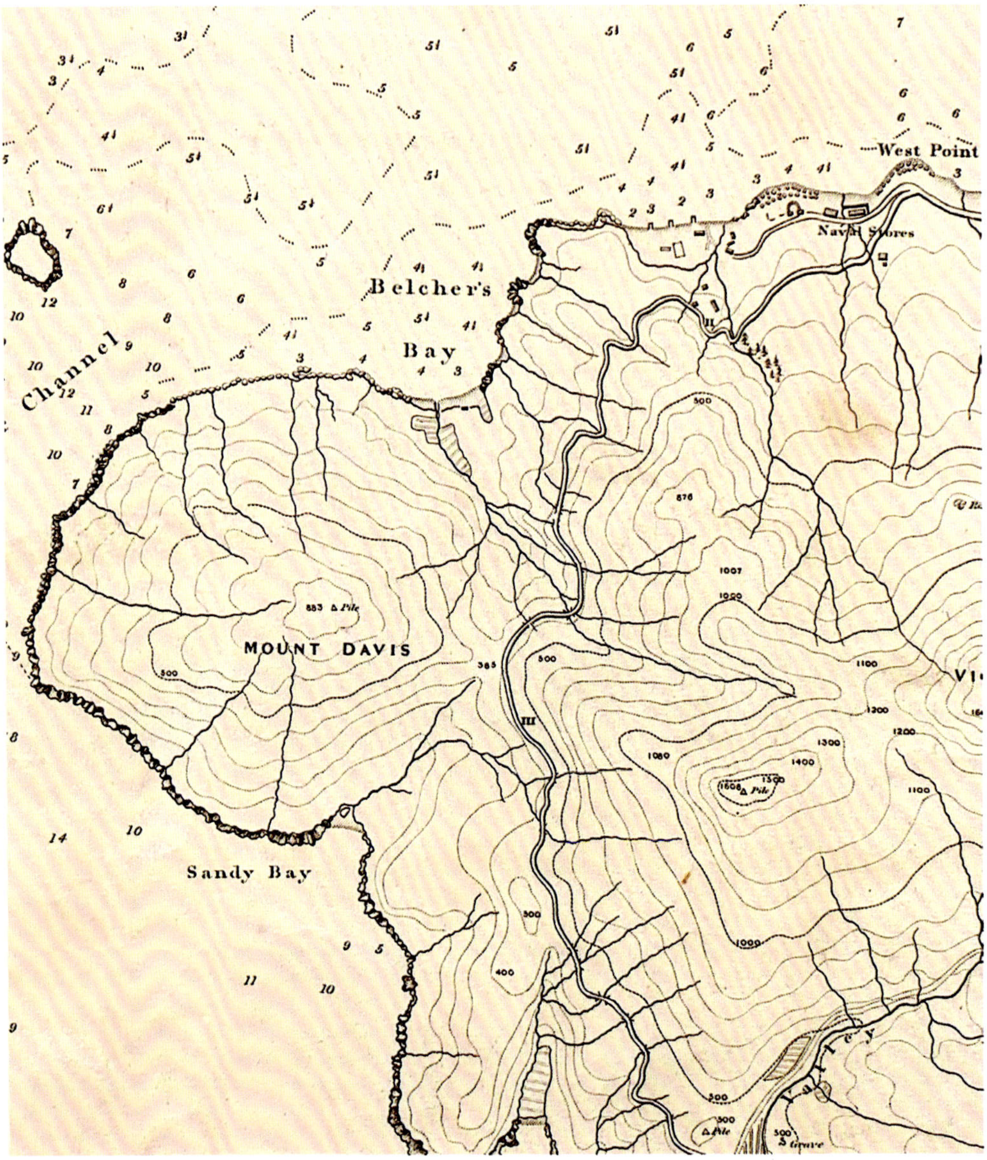

Fig. 4.19. Lt. T. B. Collinson, *Ordnance Map*, the Route of the Pok Fu Lam Road (detail), 1845. Engraving. © The National Archives, Kew, London (WO 78/118).

Davis, enjoying access to an ongoing contoured-survey project, noted to Gladstone that when new roads in their 'unfinished and loose state' were laid at an incline, they were more affected by torrential rains.

> It is only in the case of rapid declivities that much injury is experienced from the rains, and with this view care has been taken to preserve the level as much as possible. This has been effected with great success in the road round the island, where, notwithstanding the abrupt rise of some hills more than 1,500 feet above the sea, the highest point of the road which skirts them does not exceed 500 feet. This will appear from the Ordnance Survey Map forwarded home.[172]

After completing his ordnance map, Collinson was instructed to undertake additional, specific survey work to assist in the correct striking of Davis's perimeter road system. An excerpt from a letter to his mother in September 1845 also reveals his novel, nocturnal mode of working.

> I have just returned from a small surveying expedition—now don't be alarmed I did it all without going once in the sun. But the Governor required a new road to be laid down on my map & the Civil Engineers had made the road without making a survey of any kind at all of it—It was to be ready for this mail—so I embarked with my man & 4 Chinese coolies, in one of the moveable houses they call fast boats, and surveying it by candlelight—an improvement in surveying in the Tropics; that I take the credit of inventing to myself. I began at sunset every evening & finished at sunrise every morning & slept all day in the boat.[173]

Collinson had not invented night surveying, even if his candlelight method was novel. Royal Engineers had established this approach for the Ordnance Survey of Ireland to avoid the distorting effects caused by warm air during the day. Argand lamps proved ineffective over the long distances linked by traverse, so a torch was invented in 1825 using what became known as 'limelight'. Of course, Hong Kong's survey points could be fixed more closely than for Ireland, allowing Collinson to invent a humbler approach. In addition, candlelight surveying also helped Collinson avoid sun exposure, as he reassured his mother, since it was believed to be a catalyst of the recent malaria outbreaks.

Such long-distance surveying also required constructing a set of trigonometrical stations notionally linked to form a skeletal framework of triangles or a 'geodetic control network' within which to survey. In Ireland, these stations or 'trig points' were stumpy obelisks formed in hand-cast concrete. Collinson followed suit. He set up twenty-seven such trig points, of which just one survives, in stone, tucked away in Lei Yu Mun Park and only discovered in 2015.[174] These stones and their position likely influenced Collinson's views for his *Ten Outline Sketches*. Collinson and his method ensured the final, more accurate line of road linking Stanley (Chek Chue) to Aberdeen (Shek Pai Wan) and thereby realised Davis's long-term ambition to circuit Hong Kong Island with one complete ring road.[175]

The heavy, labour-intensive, yet relatively predictable work of cutting and filling steep sections of the streets within the city limits had been considered best undertaken by measured and priced work, or 'piece-work jobs' as John Pope called it. To effect savings, Davis began using convict labour on these stretches. Part of the reason was the increasing difficulty in adopting transportation as a means of punishment, since favoured destinations such as Van Dieman's Land (Tasmania) had halted the policy.[176] As he wrote in late 1846 to Earl Grey, Gladstone's replacement as colonial secretary, 'I regret that the inability to send European Convicts to Van Dieman's Land will, in their case, render it necessary to substitute imprisonment with hard labour as the only secondary punishment available. To an European constitution, imprisonment for any time in this climate becomes a much more severe infliction than transportation.'[177]

This excuse was likely just a pretext for Davis. The governor, anxious to build streets as quickly as possible, had been keen to use gang labour much earlier. In September 1845, he had asked his magistrate William Caine to draft a proposal to use convict road gangs and offered Aldrich the chance to comment. 'I consider the proposal contained therein to be a very advantageous appropriation of the Convict labour,' Major Aldrich replied.[178] 'The convicts are getting into a good style of working under the superintendence of Mr. Bruce,' wrote Cleverly in his March 1846 report, 'but their labour might be much more effectively arranged if the Gang could be divided from time to time as occasion required.'[179] Cleverly was referring to Murdoch Bruce, architect and illustrator, who was about to release his collection of lithographic views of Hong Kong.[180] Bruce was also the government 'Overseer of Roads'. Indeed, one can clearly see from the running motif of road excavation and labourers illustrated in a number of his 'urban' lithographs that Bruce prepared his original sketches while he supervised. He also had a fiery temperament, as demonstrated by his later arrest on the charge of 'horsewhipping' a Chinese man.[181] If there was a person who could bring fear into the heart of a working convict, it was Murdoch Bruce. Cleverly was also pleased to note that a watchful guard of Indian police assisted Bruce as he believed

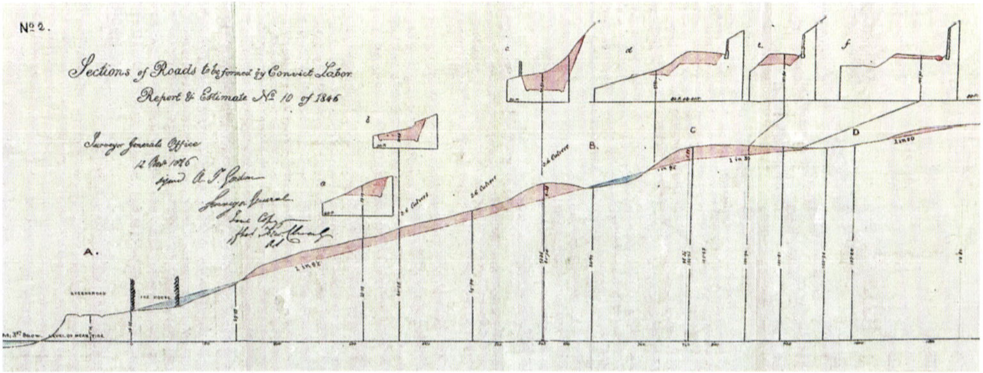

Fig. 4.20. C. Cleverly, 'Cut-and-Fill' Section for Constructing Ice House Street, 1846. Ink on paper. © The National Archives, Kew (CO 129/17: 350).

the Chinese police to be 'an idle set of men, and careless in their duty', having failed to prevent some previous escapes.[182]

One of the stretches of road that used convict labour in its forging was a conduit linking Wyndham Street (just below the magistracy–prison) to the Queen's Road below, emerging against the new ice house built at the junction—soon to lend its name to this new connection (**fig. 4.20**). Ice House Street was carved at the steep gradient of 1 in 9½, argued as 'being the least incline that can be obtained in the length, and to bring it to this there will be about 6 feet of cutting between the Harbour Master's and Mr. Stanton's House'.[183] A sizeable enclosed culvert drain was placed down its centre, and the surveyor-general (a recuperated Gordon) provided detailed sections showing the optimised slope that involved intensive cutting and filling. Gordon priced as if for private contract work and could show the amount as a saving. As a consequence, convict labour saved the government purse a total of £209. 6d.[184]

As the streets and roads within the colony reached some degree of civic completeness, they began receiving their names. Davis enjoyed giving names to places; he even bequeathed his own to the soon-to-be-constructed cathedral. Chek Chue in the southeast became 'Stanley' after the British colonial secretary. Shek Pai Wan in the southwest became 'Aberdeen' after the foreign secretary. Even the dreaded Wong Nai Chung Valley was appealingly renamed the 'Happy Valley'. However, names for streets within the city were proving more contentious, though they first appeared randomly and by stealth. 'I am surprised that neither you nor the other local papers, have taken any notice of the names which have been recently bestowed upon our streets,' complained one writer to the *Friend of China* in April 1845.

> The streets of Victoria have very properly been named after those who will pass down to posterity in connection with the late war with China, or after the leading members of Her Majesty's government; thus we have Pottinger Street, Gough Street, and Caine Street, (but why not Parker Street and Saltoun Street?) of the one class, and Wellington Street, Aberdeen Street, Peel Street, Graham Street & Stanley Street of the other. . . . but Mr. Editor, judge of my astonishment to observe *Cochrane Street* stuck up on a corner near the centre of the town!!! Surely this must be an April fool's joke; who is the Cochrane thus immortalised? Can he be the Rear Admiral of that name who was sent to China when the war was over? I sincerely trust not.[185]

Alexander Matheson, head of Jardine Matheson, had grown increasingly resentful towards Davis's administration for their disinterest in cultivating the opinions of leading merchants on the island. The new street names proved to be his breaking point. Writing from Macau to his cousin Donald, now in charge of daily operations on the island, he ranted:

> I am disgusted beyond measure just now at finding from Cleverly that Davis has named all the streets in Victoria after his personal friends—many of whom have never been to China—never perhaps out of England—and not even a lane has been called after a merchant, tho' the merchants have been the makers of the place. Just fancy "Shelley Street" named after a swindler etc. etc. How much more natural Jardine Street, Dent Street, Gibb Street, etc. would have sounded. Not the devil of a dollar shall I lay out in Hong Kong except for the sake of a profitable investment.[186]

However, despite their lack of influence on the naming of streets, the merchant elite of Hong Kong would decisively shape an equally important component of the new city—its building stock.

This account has shown that the construction of Hong Kong following the 1843 malarial epidemic was far from smooth. In the process of this development, it reveals a fractious yet interdependent set of relationships maintained between the British and the Chinese, and within the colonial government itself, between its civil and military operations. Yet, the impulse for the private investor to contribute and construct his architectural portion towards an increasingly cohesive and healthier built environment was compelling, despite Matheson's complaints, as it was for the second governor, despite his penny-pinching reputation, to provide the infrastructural framework against which to do so.

But just as malaria seemed to be receding as a threat to Hong Kong's prospects, a new politically manufactured crisis was looming. Paradoxically, against a backdrop of vigorous building activity, a newcomer launched the most vicious and relentless intellectual assault upon the very purpose and existence of the colony of Hong Kong since its inception. And it would, despite the emotional investment of many, lead the young city's community to question the viability of their future health and, therefore, survival upon the terrain they were attempting to control.

Notes

1 Major Aldrich's design for the Officers' Quarters.

2 As translated by Daniel Richard Caldwell, then translator for the Supreme Court, *Friend of China*, 17 Jan. 1846. Despite the Eurasian Caldwell's subsequent notoriety in having mixed allegiances within the colony, there is no reason to doubt the authenticity of the translation.

3 The first notice of this appears in the *Friend of China*, 7 Jan. 1846.

4 *The Builder*, vol. 5, no. 230 (3 July 1847): 318.

5 *Friend of China*, 9 Jan. 1844.

6 For example, see The National Archives, Kew [hereafter NA]; Colonial Office [hereafter CO] 129/10: 594, Woosnam (Pottinger) to James Warren, Assistant Surveyor, Moreton Bay, Sydney, NSW, 2 Jan. 1844.

7 *Canton Press*, 17 Feb. 1844.

8 Ibid.

9 Carl T. Smith, *Chinese Christians, Elites, Middlemen, and the Church in Hong Kong* (Hong Kong: Oxford University Press, 1985), 114.

10 Ibid., 115. Originally from the *Friend of China*, 5 Jan. 1856.

11 William Tarrant, *Hong Kong Part 1, 1839 to 1844* (Canton: Friend of China, 1861), 33.

12 Smith, *Chinese Christians*, 115.

13 CO 129/20: 185–191a, Davis to Grey, 24 July 1847.

14 CO 129/20: 196–198, Cleverly to Caine, 23 July 1847.

15 For examples of these invitations to tender proclamations in Chinese, see Foreign Office [hereafter FO] 233/185 passim.

16 *Friend of China*, 23 Jan. 1844.

17 For example, two contracts advertised by the civil government in the *Hongkong Register*, 6 Aug. 1844. The 'plan and sections' was a preferred method of Major Aldrich R.E., *Hongkong Register*, 20 Aug. 1844.

18 For example, the government contract to construct a police station at Chek Chue, whereby 'The Tenders for the undermentioned works not having been accepted, additional Tenders will be received at the Surveyor General's Office…', *Hongkong Register*, 27 Aug. 1844.

19 *Hongkong Register*, 12 Aug. 1845.

20 Attributed to William Tarrant, 'Brief Description of the Town of Victoria, with Remarks on the various Trades, Institutions &c. prepared as an accompaniment to the Hongkong Almanack and Directory for 1848', *The Hongkong Almanack and Directory for the Year 1848* (Hong Kong, 1848), 9 (of the article).

21 Ibid.

22 As recorded in the *Hongkong Register*, 26 Aug. 1845.

23 Ibid.

24 'The Chinese Port of Foo-chow-foo', *Hongkong Register*, 31 Mar. 1846.

25 National Library of Australia [hereafter NLA]; Mfm M602, Papers of Edward Ashworth (File 3), Notebook from 8 May 1844, entry dated 12 July 1844.

26 Christopher Cowell, 'The Drawings and Watercolours', *Edward Ashworth, Artist & Architect: Fourteen Original Watercolour Studies of Hong Kong & Macau, 1844–46* (Sydney: Hordern House, 2014).

27 Ashworth, finding it difficult to get work as an architect in Auckland, instead became the drawing tutor to the children of the first governor of New Zealand, Captain William Hobson. See the biographic entry 'Ashworth, Edward, 1814–1896', in Nineteenth Century New *Zealand Artists: A Guide & Handbook* by Una Platts (Christchurch: Avon Fine Prints, 1980), 26.

28 NLA; Mfm M602, Ashworth (File 3), Notebook from 8 May 1844, entry dated 29 Dec. 1844.

29 E. Ashworth, 'Memoranda Concerning the Erection, by Native Artizans [sic], of an English House in China, Designed and Superintended by the English Architect', under 'Chinese Architecture', *Detached Essays and Illustrations Issued During the Years 1850–51* (London: Architectural Publication Society, 1853), 16–18; and NLA; Mfm M602, Ashworth (File 3), Notebook from 8 May 1844, various entries.

30 Smith, *Chinese Christians, Elites, Middlemen*, 111–112, citing the first colonial treasurer Robert Montgomery Martin's recollections, as recorded in G. B. Endacott, *An Eastern Entrepôt* (London: Her Majesty's Stationery Office, 1964), 96. See also Tarrant, *Hong Kong Part 1*, 40. Tarrant names him 'Chun Chinam', and describes him as a 'tea merchant' only.

31 Ashworth, 'Chinese Architecture', 18.

32 Ibid., 7.

33 Arthur Cates, 'The Dictionary of Architecture, A Retrospect, 1848–1892', *Dictionary of Architecture* (London: Architectural Publication Society, 1892), 2.

34 Ashworth, 'Chinese Architecture', 6.

35 Ibid., 16–17.

36 Ibid., 17.

37 NLA; Mfm M602, Ashworth (File 3), Notebook from 8 May 1844, entry undated (ca. July 1844).

38 Ashworth, 'Chinese Architecture', 17.

39 Ibid., 16–17.

40 Ibid.

41 Ibid., 17.

42 Ibid.

43 CO 129/3: 190–191, Webster to Aberdeen, 12 Jan. 1843.

44 CO 129/10: 643a, Woosnam (Pottinger) to Gordon, 5 Feb. 1844.

45 *Friend of China*, 26 Oct. 1844 (Advertisement by the Commissariat 'to contract for Building two ranges of Barracks', dated 25 Oct. 1844).

46 *Friend of China*, 16 Nov 1844.

47 Ibid.
48 'An Ordinance for establishing a Registry of the Inhabitants of the Island of Hongkong and its Dependencies', *Friend of China*, 19 Oct. 1844.
49 Ibid.
50 'Some of the more ill-disposed of the English community had been busy among the Chinese population, and got up a sort of passive resistance in the shutting of shops, and the suspension of labour, which lasted throughout the first day [30 Oct. 1844]', CO 129/7: 200, Davis to Stanley, 6 Nov. 1844. This accusation was strenuously denied.
51 *Friend of China*, 2 Nov. 1844.
52 *Friend of China*, 11 Jan. 1845.
53 *Friend of China*, 22 Jan. 1845.
54 *Friend of China*, 17 Dec. 1845.
55 *Hongkong Register*, 29 Sep. 1846.
56 CO 129/12: 137a–138, Davis to Stanley, 11 June 1845.
57 We can deduce the quality of Capt. Mylius's output from both the relative costs of the various military works under his tenure, such as CO 129/5: 143, 'Detailed Account Disbursements of the Land Department from June 1841 to January 1844—Military and Naval'; and from two views of the Chek Chue barracks drawn by Lt. T. B. Collinson as part of his *Ten Outline Sketches*, probably drawn in 1845 (and published in 1846). See NA; War Office [hereafter WO] 78/115.
58 CO 129/16: 135a, Davis to Stanley, 24 Feb. 1846.
59 Note, this was drawn to be read in conjunction with fig. 4.18b, Collinson's earlier *Ordnance Map* detail showing Chek Chue, 1845.
60 Edward Aldrich, 'VI.—Description of the Mat Covering Sheds used at Hong-Kong in the erection of the Ordnance Buildings, and of the mode adopted by the Chinese in transporting and raising heavy Weights for these Buildings', *Papers on Subjects Connected with the Duties of the Corps of Royal Engineers* 10 (London: John Weale, 1849), 153–155.
61 Ibid., 153.
62 NLA, Mfm M602, Ashworth (File 3), Notebook from 8 May 1844, entry undated (ca. July 1844).
63 Aldrich, 'Description', 155.
64 Ibid., 153–154.
65 Christopher Cowell, 'Borrowed Verses Borrowed Verses: Code and Representation Within the First Travelogue of the City of Hong Kong, 1841–42', in Eleonora Sasso, ed., *Late Victorian Orientalism: Representations of the East in Nineteenth-Century Literature, Art and Culture from the Pre-Raphaelites to John La Farge* (London: Anthem Press, 2020), 133–162.
66 *Friend of China*, 24 Apr. 1844.
67 *Friend of China*, 1 May 1844.
68 *Friend of China*, 3 July 1844.
69 CO 129/11: 206, Davis to Stanley, 14 Mar. 1844.
70 Ashworth, 'Chinese Architecture', 17.
71 *Friend of China*, 7 Jan. 1846.
72 *Hongkong Register*, 20 Jan. 1846.
73 *Friend of China*, 17 Jan. 1846.
74 Ibid.

75 Ibid.
76 *Friend of China*, 24 June 1846.
77 NLA; Mfm M602, Ashworth (File 3), Notebook from 8 May 1844, entry undated (ca. July 1844).
78 *Friend of China*, 2 Apr. 1844 (letter dated 31 Mar. 1844).
79 *Friend of China*, 6 July 1844.
80 Ibid.
81 For reference to the 'Western District' see: CO 129/16: 451, Aldrich to Davis, 11 May 1846; for the 'Central District' see: CO 129/13: 156, Cleverly to Bruce, 14 Mar. 1846.
82 *Friend of China*, 7 Dec. 1844.
83 Ibid.
84 CO 129/7: 174a, Davis to Stanley, 2 Nov. 1844.
85 *Hongkong Register*, 9 June 1846.
86 'Senex', *Hongkong Register*, 1 Oct. 1844.
87 *Hongkong Register*, 31 Dec. 1844.
88 'Whether this idea is correct [to drain the valleys of stagnant freshwater] or not remains to be proved and must be considered at least doubtful, since the cultivation of Rice Grounds of precisely the same description all round the City of Tinghai in the Island of Chusan has been found not to affect in the slightest degree the extraordinary salubrity of that place . . .', CO 129/10: 677a, Woosnam (Pottinger) to Gordon, 29 Feb. 1844.
89 From February to April (excluding contingencies), the cost for drainage works to the two valleys was 'upwards of Six Hundred Dollars per month', CO 129/10: 740a, Woosnam (Pottinger) to Gordon, 15 Apr. 1844.
90 *Friend of China*, 6 Feb. 1844.
91 CO 129/10: 639a–640a, Woosnam (Pottinger) to 'The Editor of the *Friend of China*', 6 Feb. 1844.
92 CO 129/10: 632a–643, Woosnam (Pottinger) to 'The Editor of the *Friend of China*', 8 Feb. 1844; CO 129/10: 697a, Woosnam (Pottinger) to 'The Editor of the *Hongkong Register*', 15 Mar. 1844.
93 CO 129/10: 659a, Woosnam (Pottinger) to Caine, 15 Feb. 1844.
94 Ibid.
95 CO 129/10: 664a, Woosnam (Pottinger) to Caine, 19 Feb. 1844.
96 CO 129/10: 671a, Woosnam (Pottinger) to Caine, 22 Feb. 1844.
97 *Friend of China*, 30 Mar. 1844.
98 *Friend of China*, 24 Aug. 1843.
99 Ibid.
100 *Friend of China*, 23 Mar. 1844.
101 *Friend of China*, 22 Mar. 1845.
102 *Hongkong Register*, 13 May 1845.
103 *Friend of China*, 10 May 1845.
104 Ibid.
105 *Hongkong Register*, 17 June 1845.
106 *Friend of China*, 1 June 1844.
107 Ibid.
108 *China Mail*, 24 July 1845.
109 Ibid.
110 Ibid.

111 CO 129/10: 633–634, Woosnam (Pottinger) to Captain D'Aguilar (Military Secretary to D'Aguilar), 29 Jan. 1844.

112 Ibid.

113 CO 129/10: 756, Woosnam (Pottinger) to Gordon, 18 Apr. 1844.

114 Ibid., 756a.

115 CO 129/10: 781a, Woosnam (Pottinger) to Scales, 4 May 1844.

116 CO 129/7: 311a–312, Davis to Stanley, 26 Dec. 1844.

117 Davis suspiciously recounts the same story twice over, using similar words to describe the area in his circuitous trip around the island with Cochrane a short time later. See CO 129/7: 2a, Davis to Stanley, 5 Aug. 1844.

118 Ibid., 2–3a.

119 Ibid., 2a.

120 Ibid., 3.

121 CO 129/7: 311a, Davis to Stanley, 26 Dec. 1844.

122 CO 129/5: 138a, Stanley to Davis, 4 June 1844.

123 CO 129/5: 146–146a, 'Estimate of the probable expense of Works to be erected in the Colony of Hongkong during the Year 1844 and subsequent years', Gordon to Woosnam, 10 Feb. 1844.

124 CO 129/9: 166a, Trevelyan to Stephen, 27 May 1844.

125 Ibid., 139–139a.

126 CO 129/12: 61a, Davis to Stanley, 10 May 1845. In agreement, Stephen at the Colonial Office urged the Treasury, saying 'I am to express to you Lord Stanley's opinion that Sir. J. F. Davis' proceedings in this matter have been very judicious and should accordingly receive the approval of H.M. Govt.', CO 129/12: 64–64a, Stephen to Treveylan, 11 Sep. 1845.

127 CO 129/7: 311a, Davis to Stanley, 26 Dec. 1844.

128 'These Roads are considered as coming exclusively under the Civil superintendence whenever there is a Land Officer's Establishment', CO 129/13: 224a, Charles D'Aguilar (Assistant Military Secretary to D'Aguilar) to Caine, 25 Sep. 1845.

129 CO 129/9: 100, Aldrich to Mulcaster, the Inspector-General of Fortifications (IGF), 21 June 1844.

130 Ibid., 100a.

131 Ibid., 100–100a.

132 CO 129/9: 102, Bruce (Colonial Secretary of Hong Kong) to Aldrich, 19 June 1844.

133 CO 129/9: 226a–227, Davis to Stanley, 9 Apr. 1845.

134 CO 129/16: 154a, Davis to Gladstone, 22 Mar. 1846.

135 CO 129/7: 36a–37, Aldrich to Bruce, 3 Aug. 1844.

136 Ibid., 37.

137 CO 129/7: 174, Davis to Stanley, 2 Nov. 1844.

138 Ibid., 174a.

139 CO 129/16: 173a, 'Report', Cleverly to Bruce, 14 Mar. 1846.

140 CO 129/9: 470, 'Testimonial of William Cubitt', Jonas Hall Pope to Stanley, 17 Sep. 1844.

141 CO 129/6: 98a, Davis to Stanley, 20 May 1844.

142 CO 129/11: 243a–244, 'Memoranda' (of Pope), Shelley to Davis, 9 Apr. 1845.

143 Ibid., 244.

144 Ibid., 241, 243a.

145 Ibid., 242–242a.

146 Ibid., 243.
147 Ibid., 243a.
148 CO 129/11: 228a, Davis to Stanley, 9 Apr. 1845.
149 CO 129/13: 62–63, Aldrich to Charles D'Aguilar (Assistant Military Secretary to D'Aguilar), 20 July 1845.
150 CO 129/18: 383a, Gordon to Gladstone, 27 Feb. 1846.
151 Ibid., 385 (marginalia added to Gordon's letter).
152 CO 129/18: 260–271, Colonial Land and Emigration Office [hereafter CLEO] to Stephen, 4 Feb. 1846.
153 *The Builder*, vol. 3, no. 130 (2 Aug. 1845): 363.
154 Ibid.
155 Ibid.
156 CO 129/18: 266a, CLEO to Stephen, 4 Feb. 1846.
157 Ibid., 267.
158 Ibid.
159 Ibid., 269a–270.
160 CO 129/16: 451a, Aldrich to Bruce, 11 May 1846.
161 Ibid., 452a.
162 CO 129/16: 151, Aldrich to Bruce, 6 Mar. 1846.
163 CO 129/16: 152–153, 'Return of Services . . .', Cleverly, 31 Mar. 1846.
164 CO 129/16: 156–168,169–175, Cleverly to Bruce, 14 Mar. 1846.
165 Ibid., 165a.
166 Ibid., 172a.
167 A. I. Diamond, 'Major-General T. B. Collinson, Royal Engineers' (File Note), *Hong Kong History Workshop* (Hong Kong: Department of History, The University of Hong Kong, December 1984). As Diamond explains, 'His map was published by the Ordnance Map Office, Southampton in 1846, prior to any contoured map of the United Kingdom, the first not being printed until December, 1847.'
168 WO 78/118, Lt. Collinson, R.E., *The Ordnance Map of Hong Kong, Surveyed by Lieut. Collinson R.E., 1845* (Southampton: Ordnance Map Office, 1846).
169 Hong Kong Public Records Office [hereafter HKPRO]; file: HKMS 140-1-1, 'Transcripts of Correspondence of Lieut. Thomas Bernard Collinson R.E. Dec. 1838–29 Mar. 1846' [hereafter 'Transcripts'], T. B. Collinson, Hong Kong, to Mrs Collinson, Boldon Rectory, Gateshead, 29 Apr. 1845.
170 Diamond, 'T. B. Collinson'.
171 Margin note dated '84 Pall Mall, 12 March 1847' found on WO 78/115, *Collinson's Ten Outline Sketches to Accompany the Ordnance Map of Hong Kong* (Southampton: Ordnance Map Office, 1847).
172 CO 129/16: 265a, Davis to Gladstone, 23 Apr. 1846.
173 HKPRO; *Transcripts*, T. B. Collinson, Hong Kong, to Mrs Collinson, Boldon Rectory, Gateshead, 20 Sep. 1845.
174 This squat obelisk, measuring just over two feet in height, has the words 'B.O. No.4' carved into it, meaning 'Board of Ordinance, pillar number 4'. The Board, as a military body, was fully responsible for mapping Hong Kong up until 1855. See Kris Cheng, 'HKU Urges Heritage Status for Oldest Boundary Stone Ever Discovered in Hong Kong', *Hong Kong Free Press*, 17 Dec. 2015.
175 See CO 129/16: 468–475a, 'Report and Estimate to complete the circuit of the Island . . .', Davis to Gladstone, 15 June 1846.
176 'The interval of two years which had elapsed without an authorized place of exile caused the number of

Convicts under sentence of transportation, besides those who died in the mean time, to mount up to 39', CO 129/17: 459a, Davis to Grey, 22 Dec. 1846.

177 Ibid., 459–459a.

178 CO 129/13: 222a, Aldrich to Caine, 11 Sep. 1845.

179 CO 129/16: 171a, Cleverly to Bruce, 14 Mar. 1846.

180 *Hongkong Register*, 14 July 1846 (advertisement for 'HONGKONG ILLUSTRATED, In a Series of Lithographs' dated 6 July 1846).

181 *Hongkong Register*, 13 Oct. 1846. For evidence of his supervisory duties, see the framing of views in *The Officer's Quarters looking towards Victoria* (fig. 5.11), *View of Wyndham Street from the Post Office* (not shown), and *View of Lyndhurst Terrance, Wellington Street and Cochrane Street, looking West from the Roman Catholic Church* (fig. 4.13), all dated 1846, Hong Kong Museum of Art.

182 CO 129/16: 171a, Cleverly to Bruce, 14 Mar. 1846.

183 CO 129/17: 348a, 'Report and Estimate', Gordon to Davis, 12 Nov. 1846.

184 CO 129/17: 345, Davis to Grey, 18 Nov. 1846.

185 'An Englishman', *Friend of China*, 5 Apr. 1845.

186 Alexander Matheson, Macau, to Donald Matheson, Hong Kong, 13 Dec. 1844, in Maggie Keswick, ed., *The Thistle and the Jade: A Celebration of 150 Years of Jardine, Matheson & Co.* (London: Octopus Books, 1982), 26.

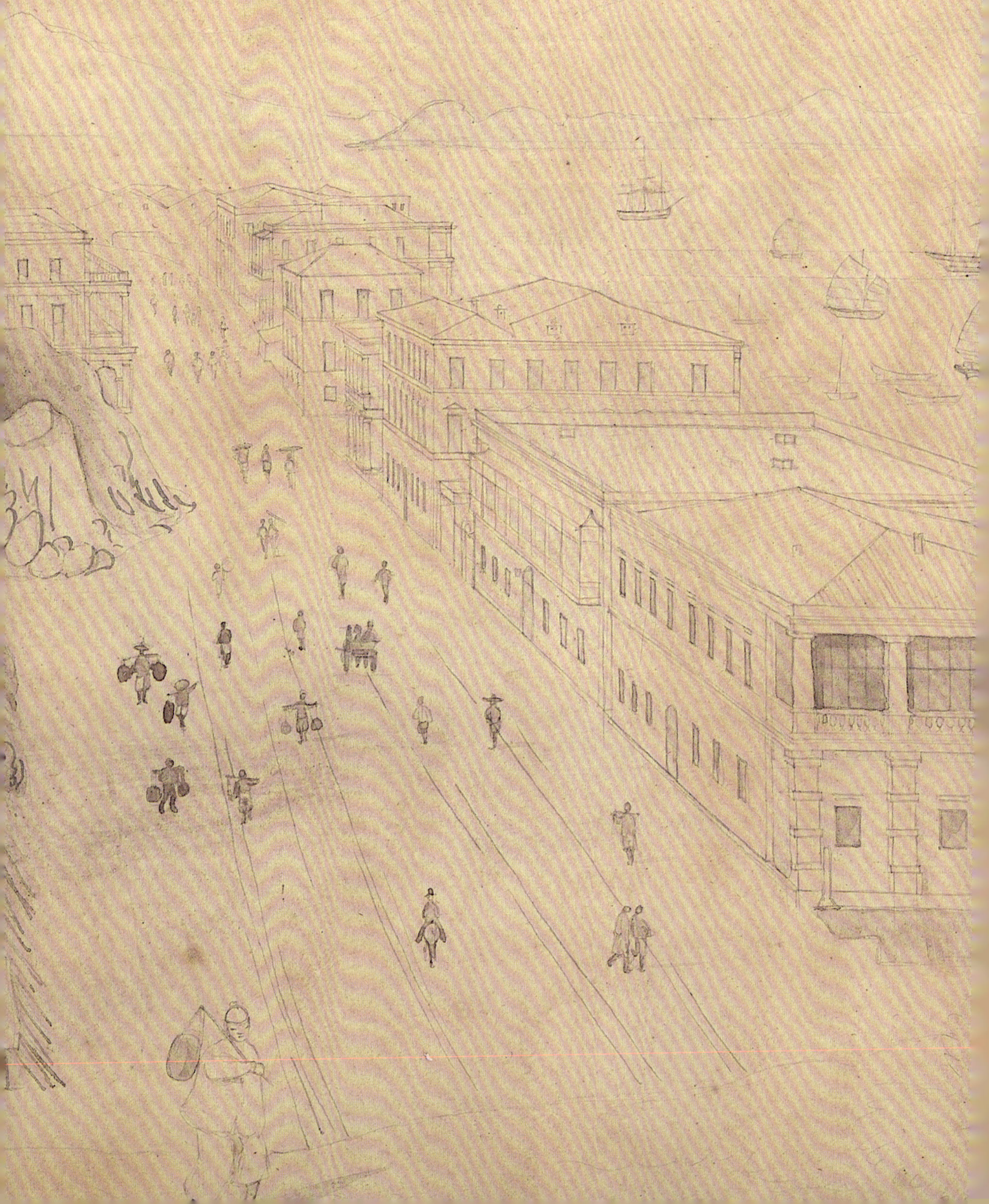

CHAPTER 5

A City Remade, 1844–1846

> A serpentine road here & there cut out in the hillside is partially formed into a street for some 2 miles, partly by godowns (warehouses) with dwellings in the upper storey, large solid edifices of granite & brick with colonnades & balconies, partly by Venetian-blinded Chinese shops stilted up upon poles & brick piers, partly by barracks & a few European shops. The steep slopes of the hill above 'the Queen's Road' are studded with veranda-covered villas of one-story terraced bungalows.
>
> —Architect Edward Ashworth's diary entry, July 1844.[1]

Over the three years following 1843, Hong Kong had dramatically expanded, with mat-shed accommodation virtually done-away with, a substantial road network created, and the city remodelled. The transformation was so noticeable even for those who resided there that the young Royal Engineer, Lieutenant Thomas Bernard Collinson, writing to his father in January 1846, could say with relief that

> The most wonderful change has come over Hong Kong. It used to be in the summer a boiling hot [city] where fever, ague and dysentery reigned . . . but ever since the West wind set in in December, the inhabitants have become quite lively . . . blooming; and Victoria is beginning to assume the station of Queen of the East, [which] place, from her merchants' palaces, & her long rows of Grecian barracks & [a] beautiful bay, I think she is entitled to.[2]

Agreement on this matter had been growing among the young officers of the colony. The slightly older Royal Navy surgeon Edward Cree would be among the first to reflect in his diary quite similar observations almost one year earlier.

> *Tuesday 21 January (1845)*
>
> Walked through the town to see the new buildings, which are wonderful considering what Hong Kong was only two years ago.

Unlike Collinson, Cree was a sojourner, though a frequent visitor, able to see the changes more sharply. A year later on a return visit, Cree would paint the very 'Grecian barracks & beautiful bay' Collinson was now proudly witnessing (**fig. 5.1**).

> *Tuesday 3 March (1846)*
>
> What changes have taken place in Hong Kong since I have been in China: when I first saw it, 1841, it was then a desolate rock with a few fishermen's huts on the beach; now the handsome town is spreading all over the place.[3]

Groups actively responsible for the city's rapid transformation—the Chinese contractors and labour force, the military engineers, and the Surveyor-General's overseers—have been discussed. This parallel study over the same period will chart the shifting canvas of executive and public opinion that attended this metamorphosis. Through a single government official's short but dramatic tenure on the island, an entire section of the English-reading public within the colony, together with their masters at Whitehall, in unifying against him, were forced to come to terms with Hong Kong's recent unhealthy past and to look forward together towards a better future. Meanwhile, with the denigration of the mat-shed typology and the emergence of a variety of well-built commercial and residential buildings, colonial Hong Kong was reshaped. And through this reshaping, it transfigured from mat-shed to mansion and from fever to form.

'A Perpetual Blister'

Robert Montgomery Martin, a prolific writer of some repute, a founding member of the Statistical Society of London (1834) and the Colonial Society (1837), became Governor Davis's first colonial treasurer in 1844. He lasted just over one year in the job. During this brief time, he played a crucial role in galvanising public opinion about the long-term healthiness and viability of the colony of Hong Kong. Unfortunately for him, but fortunately for Hong Kong's future, the tide of opinion would eventually rise not for but against him. Had he been posted to the island government a year earlier, he would have caused tremendous damage. But almost single-handedly, Martin's protestations and lengthily drawn-out diatribes against Britain's continued occupation of Hong Kong, when placed against simultaneous improvements on the island, would lay to rest the spectre that had been the perceived *inherent* and *irredeemable* unsuitability of the terrain. Malaria remained a threat. But, through the painful process of countering Martin, it was finally seen by the community as a containable one. Martin also re-opened a British national wound: the agreement to return the northern island of Chusan (Zhoushan) to China under the Treaty of Nanking (Nanjing) in 1842. He would conjure up the large island, favourably juxtaposing it with smaller Hong Kong, and giving it an almost mythical, salvific quality in comparison.

Britain's claim over Chusan had been short-lived, but its loss remained an issue of poignant regret to many who had fought or traded in China. It had preceded Hong Kong in occupation and was, at one point, the trading post of first choice. 'The island of Chusan has already been tried as an emporium of commerce,'[4] wrote the *Canton Register* on 12 January 1841, just seven days before the same broadsheet was among the first to announce to the world 'Hong Kong to be ceded to the English, terms not known: probably in exchange for Chusan!'[5] Weeks before the taking of Hong Kong, the occupation of Chusan had become an event of national pride to be instilled in British children, its capture re-enacted on stage at the annual Covent Garden Christmas Pantomime in London in 1840. 'The taking of Chusan, very prettily managed,' recalled the *Canton Press* cheerily, 'some *wee-wee* soldiers ascending the walls with ladders.'[6] Its capture and occupation would feature prominently and favourably in London conversations on relations with China over the next few years. Martin, therefore, felt he was playing to the crowd, having ample time to formulate his attacks in anticipation of his secondment to the colony.

Martin, an Anglo-Irishman from County Tyrone, had spent ten years of his formative youth travelling across many British colonies, from Ceylon (Sri Lanka) to the East African coast and Mauritius to New South Wales.[7] He returned to Britain and, as the historian G. B. Endacott notes, 'devoted himself to writing on colonial questions and to their further study'. There he produced a prodigious range of works as diverse as a five-volume *History of the British Colonies* (1834–1835) and a *Statistics of the Colonies of the British Empire* (1839), the latter combining his love of number-crunching and imperialism.[8] The job of the colonial treasurer of Hong Kong was to be his reward. It was to be the first and, for reasons that would soon unfold, the last public appointment he would receive.[9]

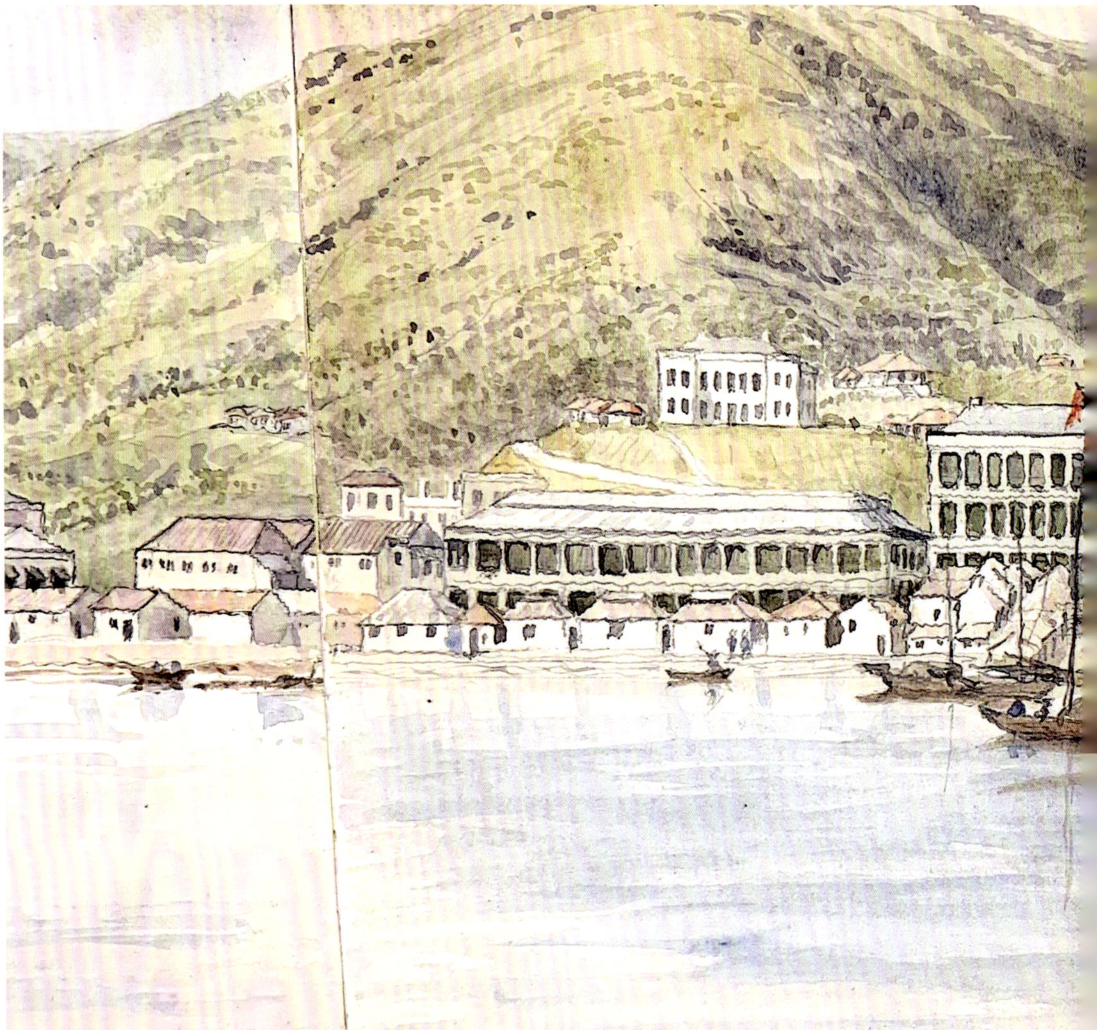
The Generals Quarters
Officers Quarters

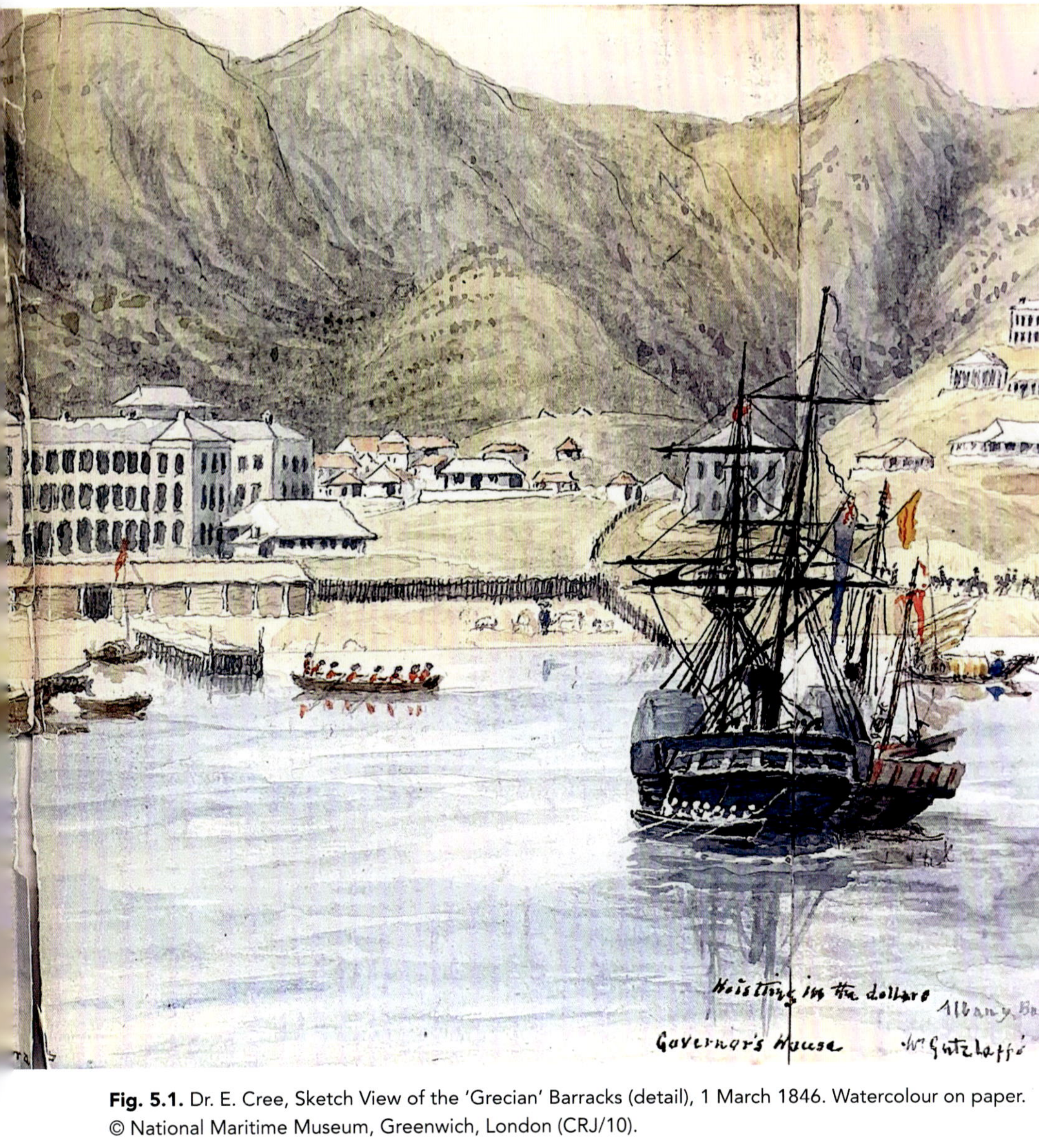

Fig. 5.1. Dr. E. Cree, Sketch View of the 'Grecian' Barracks (detail), 1 March 1846. Watercolour on paper. © National Maritime Museum, Greenwich, London (CRJ/10).

Martin arrived at Hong Kong on 7 May 1844 onboard H.M. Steamship *Spiteful* as part of Governor John Davis's retinue.[10] His first salvo against the island began just a few weeks later. Yet one must ask: how could Martin have drawn lengthy, definite conclusions over such a short space of time? Was there an element of premeditation? Might Martin have been an agent provocateur sent by those whose interests lay in discrediting Hong Kong and championing Chusan? Three weeks before his arrival, an anonymous writer calling himself 'No Geologist' sent an article to the *Friend of China* entitled 'Observation on the Hill Fevers of the Southern Peninsular of India; with some Remarks on Magnetism and Electricity as a probable Cause of Fever and other Disorders'. The author of the original article was a Dr. Heyne of the Madras Artillery. 'We have ever considered the geological nature of the soil,' the introduction stated, 'as one of the most powerful causes of the physical climate.'[11] The senior editor of the journal in which the article was first published had been assisted by none other than Robert Montgomery Martin.[12] It seems likely that Martin—a man skilled in playing within printed media—had planted the seeds of attack before he arrived in Hong Kong. At the heart of Heyne's thesis was a belief that terrain containing 'a great proportion of ferruginous hornblende, which by disintegration or separation from the rock, becomes highly magnetic', was the cause 'which produces this fever'.[13] Worse, all the rivulets, public roads, and hills hollows were washed with sand particles from this disintegrated magnetic ore and infected with miasma. Apart from the infrequent rains that produced a damp-enough atmosphere to cool the rocks and 'remove the sickness which is the consequence of it', there was no antidote except through total avoidance of the area.[14] The point made in reproducing this article in the local press was that the similarity of hill fevers in Southern India with fevers in Hong Kong was alarmingly self-evident.

There were, nevertheless, remedies to counter this fear. In its earliest years of scientific application, electromagnetism was considered as much a mysterious force of nature as the miasma it seemed linked with. The Ancient Greeks believed that the human body held, in miniature, energies at play within the broader sphere of the world, such as the four elements or humours. It was discovered that the human body reacted to electro-impulse and was therefore similarly thought to act as a modern microcosm to this universal force. Electricity, it seemed, could be both a source of harm and, if carefully managed, a force for health. One advertisement appeared over a considerable length of time in the Hong Kong newspapers from mid-1845. Hyam's 'Patent Galvano-Electric and Magnetic Ring' boasted of its

> efficacy of which in curing those diseases consequent upon a derangement of the nervous system is attested by numerous testimonials. The Galvano-Electric principle is the strongest agent in nature—it rends rocks asunder, melts metals, and is one of the same character as lightning—such a tremendous power would cause death if applied injudiciously. . . . the lower the Galvanic current is reduced in intensity the greater will be its curative effects on the human system.[15]

The device was claimed to rely upon the inherent, mild electrical power generated by the human body's circulatory system. The patented bracelet was composed of zinc and copper and could be shaped to fit fingers, arms, and legs. It was even offered as a belt for any nervous client. The advertiser promised that it was able to fight off a myriad of complaints and diseases. 'The system being supplied with the Galvano-Electric fluid is so much invigorated, that it will be capable not only to resist the power of contagion but likewise to expel the elements of disease, thus forming what Hippocrates termed the *vis medicatrix naturas*.'[16]

Barely two weeks after Martin's arrival in Hong Kong, the same anti-government newspaper that had published the findings of Dr. Heyne published another similar article. This time it was under Martin's authorship, a work originally written in 1829 and entitled 'Effects of Climate upon Man'. 'The principle, which is the object of this essay to unfold is that man is, to a certain extent, the creature of circumstances, over some of which he has no control, that his corporeal strength and mental development depend partly on birth but more especially on localities, viz the nature of the soil he inhabit, and of the air he respires.'[17] In this fascinating early work, Martin proposes such remedies as the use of elevation and distance, as these 'form excellent safeguards against marsh miasma, which apparently possess such a gravity and density, that it never rises high or travels far in the atmosphere'.[18] He uses the example of the army medic Dr. Hunter who 'found that an elevation above the ground floor of a barrack, enjoys a considerable exemption from disease'. Martin also observed that during the sickly season, the indigenous natives of Asia, Africa, and America liberally applied 'oleaginous substances, as a prevention of disease'. Martin concluded this fifteen-year-old treatise with a straightforward, general remedy for the well-being of a young colonial town: The constant cleaning of gutters and drains, the widening of streets, the digging of wells, and the clear, unobstructed flow of watercourses, combined with the unimpeded circulation of air, would ensure that 'health is secured'.[19] This begs the question: why then did the somewhat older Martin quickly and entirely dismiss Hong Kong as an irredeemable place for Europeans to reside?

On 17 June 1844, Martin gave Governor Davis his first official report as colonial treasurer on the various options for generating increased public revenue in Hong Kong. Davis forwarded the report to Colonial Secretary Lord Edward Stanley on 29 June. He agreed with Martin about the delicate and challenging task of raising revenue from 'an infant Colony' such as Hong Kong but added, 'I do not by any means entertain the same desponding news as to the future'.[20] Martin began his report in the vein of a treasurer to the Crown. He calculated the revenues collected from July 1841 to the end of the fiscal year 31 March 1844 to be only £2,789. Yet, the annual expenditure he estimated at £50,000, exclusive of the cost of public works.[21] Martin proposed a tonnage duty on imports, to be rejected by Davis. However, he noted that the Reverend Dr. Karl (Charles) Gützlaff, the Chinese secretary, had produced a recent census begun that April, which calculated the Chinese inhabitants at 20,000 persons and suggested a registration system to raise revenue. He also proposed that the government could issue a plethora of licenses to both the shop merchants and the building trades.

> Butchers, Bakers, Fishmongers, Grocers, Greengrocers, Confectioners, Hawkers, Rice Dealers, Tobacconists, Chandlers, Carpenters, Boat builders, Masons, Bricklayers, Brickmakers, Stone masons, Blacksmiths, Silversmiths, Bamboo workers, Tailors, Drapers, Shoemakers, Rope makers, Tanners, Barbers, Washermen, Stationers, Pawnbrokers, Compradors, and all other trades whether exercised in a shop or boat, or ashore or afloat.[22]

The registration tax and the trade licenses would be stringently adopted by the Davis government, inevitably leading to mounting conflicts between disaffected European traders and the government, and with Chinese labour and commercial forces actively shaping Hong Kong.

On the eighth page of this seventeen-page report, Martin began to address a matter that would dominate his future energies to the detriment of his work as colonial treasurer, questioning the very viability of Hong Kong's future. He wrote, 'So long as there are five Consular ports open to our Merchants, it is not likely that Hongkong, which is a mere harbour of refuge at the most distant extremity of the Chinese Empire, will ever become a trading Emporium.'[23] Chinese officials, he argued, were blocking the sale of provisions to Hong Kong and thereby raising the prices. The lack of land tenure in fee simple was likewise disenfranchising the Europeans and Chinese from investing their capital in building work—a fact that was now blatantly untrue. By this logic, Martin could bridge neatly across to the real issue on his mind.

> Ill-constructed dwellings render the ungenialness of this trying climate more severely felt by all classes and must necessarily tend to retard the progress of the Colony. . . . Hong Kong is a barren island composed of rotten granite and decomposing sandstone with scarcely sufficient pasturage for a few goats . . . and with a surface so rugged and unpracticable for the establishment of a large town; that there is not a sufficiently level spot on the island to put even a few Companies of Marines through their martial exercises.[24]

Martin knew that Davis was obliged to forward his report to London. It would become evident that he was not addressing it to the governor. Besides, Martin expected their views and those of others in the colony to differ. Instead, he aimed at a much wider audience—his general British readership—this time within the limited circles of Whitehall. Martin continued his first tirade, describing Hong Kong as a 'small, barren, unhealthy, valueless island at one extremity of the vast Chinese Empire on which it operates as a perpetual blister'.[25] Historians have subsequently missed the main point of Martin's initial attack by focusing on the extreme health concerns he conveyed while forgetting the greater purpose and remoter audience for which the document served. This report must be understood as a cleverly stage-managed piece of writing, where all the parts lead to a single conclusion, his ideal alternative, that the colony must move to Chusan. 'Were Chusan instead of Hongkong the Colony of England then its size, fertility, healthfulness and important geographical position midway between the Northern and Southern extremity of the Chinese Coasts opposite the great Girdle and vulnerable frontier of China . . . might justify an expense' (**fig. 5.2**).[26]

Martin's thoughts by then had become public fodder in the Hong Kong press. 'We pick up a rather amusing paragraph regarding Hong Kong,' wrote the *Friend of China* in early June.

> Who the veracious writer of the letter may be we are at a loss to guess. But the high official—the gentleman of superior attainments—who has written home to the government recommending the abandonment of the island, may blush to see his statements published in a Hongkong paper. Where is the swampy land in front of Victoria? God help the dotard, there is nothing but good salt-water. . . . It is very true that, for two years the mortality among the troops had been great—and deeply deplored. But where is the tropical climate where this is not invariably the case, when troops are badly lodged, exposed to the rains and dews, and in addition to this are landed from shipboard in a sickly state?[27]

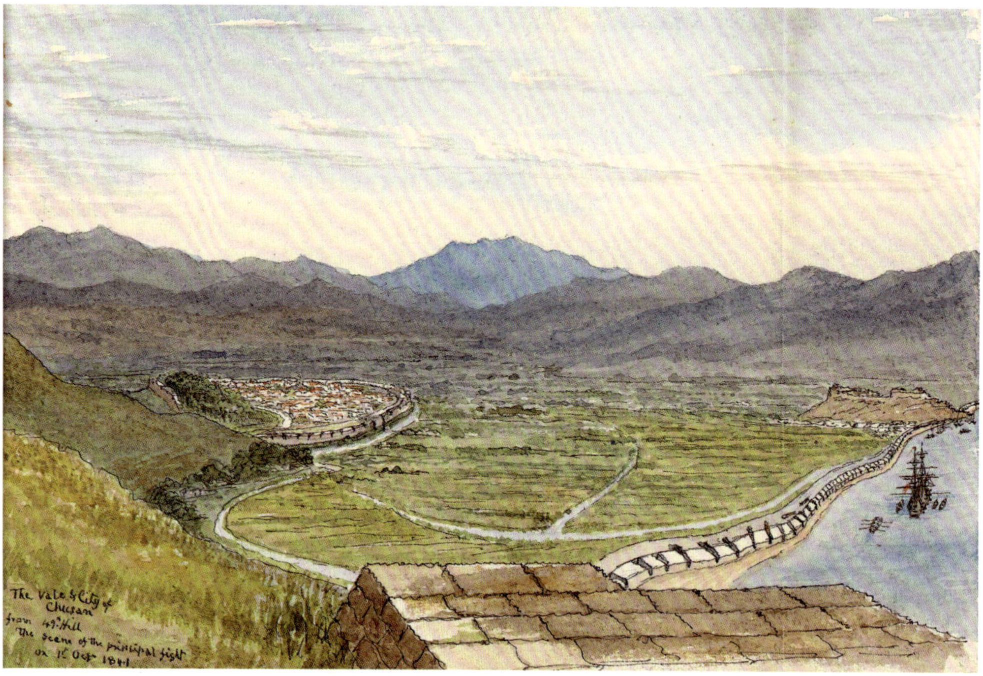

Fig. 5.2. Dr. E. Cree, 'The Vale & City of Chusan from 49th Hill', 1 October 1841. Watercolour on paper. © National Maritime Museum, Greenwich, London (CRJ/5).

Davis suspected a deliberate leak. He wrote angrily to Lord Stanley asking for precise instructions for dealing with officials who consorted with the press, 'and especially that low and needy class of newspapers that exists in Colonies'.[28] Ironically, by the end of June, Colonial Treasurer Martin was sick, unable to finish the colonial accounts and on a six-week leave of absence. Struck down too was D'Almada, the Portuguese chief clerk in the Colonial Secretary's Office.[29] Davis lamented that 'the continuance of the unhealthy season until next October, may perhaps to a great degree cripple the working Civil Establishment'.[30]

Martin may have been sick, but he was certainly not idle. He was able to use his time compiling a massive eighty-nine-page report, which he signed and dated 24 July 1844.[31] Succinctly entitled a *Report on the Island of Hong Kong*, Martin presumably was fit enough to roam out of his sickbed interviewing such local dignitaries as Major-General D'Aguilar and Dr. Gützlaff. He also gathered several physicians' testimonials or had already compiled them from his earlier notes. Martin divided this second report into ten lengthy subchapters. The first four were framed as a factual analysis of the inherent features of the physical environment under the headings 'Locality', 'Physical Aspect', 'Geology', and 'Climate'. The fifth was a large section entitled 'Diseases and Mortality', drawing upon the material of the former to take account of the statistics of the latter. The last five headings, 'Population and Progress', 'Commerce', 'Financial Point-of-View', 'Religious and Social Influence', and his summing up 'In a Political Point-of-View', argued that, as a result, the commercial and social failure of Hong Kong was inevitable.

Of all the documents that stunned Whitehall and caused a momentary lapse of confidence in their appointed government in Hong Kong, this was the most significant. The report has too much damning material to expand in sufficient detail. Suffice to say, Martin made a meal out of his language, relying heavily on a lexicon of disease imagery in the metaphors he used. The hillsides of Hong Kong after the heavy monsoon rains of midsummer were said to 'assume somewhat of a greenish hue, like a decayed Stilton cheese'. The mountainous peaks and sides of the island 'presenting the appearance of a Negro streaked with leprosy'.[32] The granite was described as 'rotten, and passing, like dead animal and vegetable substances, into a putrescent state', while the excavated earth, churned in the construction of houses, 'appeared like a richly-prepared compost, emitting a fetid odour of the most sickening nature, and which, at night, must prove a deadly poison'.[33] He continued under 'Climate',

> The clouds pour down one vast sheet of water washing away hills and rocks, furrowing the Island with deep ravines, and saturating the soft, porous, putrescent strata to the extent of many feet with daily renewed moisture. In the intervals of rain, the vertical sun acts with an intense evaporating power and a noxious steam or vapour rises from the fetid soil yielding a gas of a most sickly and deleterious nature, exactly such as I experienced on the coast of Africa in 1824 when I was seized with an 'Earth Fever' while in His Majesty's Service . . .[34]

Under 'Diseases and Mortality', Martin echoed a writer at the death of John Robert Morrison—Pottinger's beloved Chinese interpreter—in considering the disease in Hong Kong to be a peculiar blend 'combining the character of the African and West Indian fevers'.[35] Martin gave some frightening statistics of troop depletion during 1843, the year of the Hongkong Fever. He compared Hong Kong to Chusan and Koolungsoo (Gulangyu), an island close to Amoy (Xiamen), placing troop strength against mortality rates. In 1843, the 'European and Native' troop strength per annum for Hong Kong was 1,526. 7,893 men passed through the hospital, as Martin noted 'more than five times in the year!'. In total, 440 men died, the majority succumbing to fever, dysentery, or diarrhoea. This figure formed a horrific statistic of 1 in 3½, compared to 1 in 12½ at Koolungsoo and 1 in 29½ in Chusan.[36]

The year 1844, though Martin acknowledged it as less severe, was 'equally destructive to the troops' and a sign, he argued, that the disease had changed from being an *epidemic* to an *endemic* problem. D'Aguilar was quoted to say that 'the maintenance of a Garrison at Hong Kong would cost the crown one Regiment every two years'. Chinese, too, were falling victim in large numbers. Dr. Gützlaff recorded that 'of 100 Coolies with whom I was acquainted, there died between the 20th May and 15th June 1844, ten men, and thirty left the place diseased'. Martin was sure that this had nothing to do with settlement teething problems. 'The Australian colonies were perfectly healthy when founded; so also Mauritius, and St. Helena. I cannot name a single colony that was originally unhealthy, and that subsequently became salubrious.'[37]

Davis forwarded the report to Lord Stanley merely adding 'his remarks were written after only a few weeks residence under circumstances of every indifferent health'. This tolerance can be explained by Davis's closing statement. 'Much of it,' he noted defensively, 'must be viewed as applying to the proceedings and representations of my distinguished predecessor Sir Henry Pottinger.'[38] However, if Davis thought he could use Martin as a tool of one-upmanship, then it backfired. The influential James Stephen, Lord Stanley's permanent under-secretary, was unnerved. Shaken by the report and especially by Davis's non-rebuttal, he added in a devastating margin note to Stanley:

> But there remains a long and circumstantial detail of alleged matters of fact which, except on the hypothesis of the more absurd & extravagant exaggeration or the falsifying of official documents would seem almost to demonstrate that Hong Kong is a possession utterly worthless—expensive beyond comparison—and more destructive of human life than Sierra Leone at its very worst of times. . . . If he is inaccurate it seems very strange that Mr Davis should send his Report without contradiction.[39]

This was a moment of grave political peril for the colony. Stanley's response was to refuse any further British support for Hong Kong until Davis could provide him with 'a specific Report as to the points on which you dissent from Mr Martin's facts and opinions'.[40] The Colonial Office had effectively turned off the spigot to much-needed civil and military funds. So, Davis had to contrive a set of refutations against Martin.

Within the interval between despatches, relations between Davis and his colonial treasurer had worsened. By late August, Martin remained indisposed, and Davis was obliged to place the Treasurer's Office in the hands of his colonial secretary Frederick Bruce and Adolphus Shelley, the colony's auditor.[41] But, by the beginning of September, Martin was back at work, and Bruce and Shelly were now on sick leave. Yet the Treasurer's Office was a mess, and Davis had to send his private secretary, Mr. Mercer, to assist.[42] The state of crisis continued until April 1845, when Shelley, now recovered and in his customary role as auditor, provided Davis with some much-needed ammunition against Martin. Martin had demanded to be consulted in every minute aspect of expenditure during his periods of convalescence. Yet he failed to approve valid claimants' vouchers, while debts to the Treasury mounted. Accounts had fallen in arrears, so Davis instructed Bruce to suspend all government salaries and payments, with the important exception of wages to Chinese labourers in the public works.[43] If Martin had not yet alienated himself from every branch of the civil service, this now assured him of it. 'I am happy to say,' concluded Davis to Stanley, 'that, with one exception, the greatest harmony and desire to assist each other has prevailed in the different departments of this Government since my arrival.'[44]

Davis's eventual rebuttal of Martin's 1844 report to Lord Stanley was completed nine months later, in late April 1845. 'I will endeavour to show that the great mortality among the military, and (at the very first) among civilians, must be attributed to circumstances and causes sufficiently obvious to save the character of the climate.'[45] Poor architecture was the culprit. Instead of blaming land and climate as Martin had done, Davis blamed the failure in poor house construction, especially for the troops, arguing that this was the chief cause of the fatalities. He made three sequential points: The lack of good workmen in Hong Kong led to shoddy housing, with 'persons of all ranks being housed in dwellings progressing gradually from mere mat sheds to wooden and brick hovels of a somewhat better description'.[46] In consequence, most residents had, through speed and economy, to endure a 'pernicious system of ground floor apartments' many of which, he noted, remained. Therefore, it was hardly surprising that living conditions created the risk of sickness in a wet and windy climate like Hong Kong's.[47] Always eager to score points at the expense of his predecessor, Davis continued, 'the deplorable condition of things which I found on my arrival led me immediately to acquiesce in the request of Major General D'Aguilar that he should appropriate the ground on the side of the road opposite to the

"North Barrack" to the construction of permanent and proper accommodations for the troops'.[48] This was the site Pottinger had vehemently protested against giving up. Davis had thereby sealed the Ordnance District's fate and Pottinger's vision of Hong Kong as a coastal-edge, linear city, by now allowing the city's length to be breached by inserting a military enclave at its centre point.

Davis noted that 1844 was a year of significant improvement in health for all but military and police officers. Many of the latter had been seconded from the army, and either suffered from past fever or were now exposed for long periods outdoors. Colonial Surgeon Dr. Dill's enclosed report showed that from 1 July to 31 December 1844, a total of 97 government officers reported sick but with no fatalities, whereas 249 policemen had been taken ill and seven had died. Various other factors explained sickness among the troops. The Indian soldiers of the 4th Madras Native Infantry (MNI) were among the worst afflicted. They had arrived in Hong Kong sick from Singapore, having travelled 'in the condition of a flock of rotten sheep'.[49] The custom of saving almost their entire salaries for the benefit of their families by withholding sustenance for themselves caused them to faint with fatigue during their military exercises. As for the worst affected European regiment, the 98th, most were 'raw recruits from England, at the boiling age of 18 to 20, stimulated in a hot climate by continued drunkenness'.[50] One wonders if Davis's counterpart, Lieutenant-Governor Major-General D'Aguilar, concurred with his sharp commentary. Yet, for Major Edward Aldrich, superintending engineer and de-facto military architect for Hong Kong, Davis extended the warmest of praise. 'My chief hopes for the military are founded in the near completion of the excellent and ample quarters for both officers and men, under Major Aldrich's supervision, and when these are occupied I have little doubt of this Climate being found superior to that of most other countries.'[51] Though unintended by Aldrich, his military barracks, these Grecian forms so admired by Collinson and Cree, were to be held by their very public quality, as a vital experimental proof before the Davis administration. If poor architecture was central to the governor's rebuttal of Martin's thesis, then good architecture's remedial effects had to be shown to dispel any further doubts by the Colonial Office.

Davis's refutation had helped calm Stanley's permanent under-secretary. 'It seems to me,' said a relieved James Stephen, 'to have been fortunate that the enquiry was proposed; as the answer tends much to dispel Mr Martin's gloomy anticipations.'[52] Unfortunately, the British could not as quickly dispel a poor comparison of Hong Kong against Chusan within colonial debates. 'What is to be done about Chusan?' asked the *Friend of India* in late July 1845. 'The climate vies with that of the most favoured regions in the world. It is the Montpelier of China.'[53] The deaths of troops there in 1840, according to the Indian newspaper, were owing to mismanagement rather than any inherent unhealthiness.[54] Another Calcutta-based broadsheet, the *Englishman*, picked up the debate. 'Sir Henry Pottinger said in his speech at Liverpool, that he had given up Chusan, because it is too large. This we think is a mere excuse. It would require scarcely more means of defence than Hongkong, because there is no occasion to garrison more than the city of Tinghae [Dinghai].'[55] But the newspaper did agree that it was a political impracticality to retain Chusan. The *Bombay Times* lamented that it was 'a great misfortune that at the time of settling our dispute with China, the retention of Tinghae was not preferred to establishing ourselves at Amoy or Foo-chow-foo [Fuzhou], where so little trade and so few commercial facilities are now unhappily found to exist'.[56] Among the Indian press, Martin was seen to have brought to light 'the whole Davisian system of government', whereby '. . . if a secret plan has been preparing for removing from the barren reeks and feverish rice swamps of Hongkong to the more fertile and salubrious northern island, we can understand the policy of preventing people from spending their money in building'.[57]

Now back in Britain and a willing hostage of the evening banquet circuit, Sir Henry Pottinger was shocked to encounter a public mood volubly favouring Chusan over Hong Kong. On 11 December 1844, in his speech at the Merchant Taylors' Hall, London, he argued, 'I feel it right, on this most public occasion, to say that I look upon Hongkong still as the best position for British enterprise. Unfortunately it has been unhealthy; but there is nothing in its appearance or situation that should render it so, and those who would substitute Chusan for it are, in my humble opinion, in error.'[58] The local Hong Kong press agreed and were understandably incensed at their Indian colleagues. The *Friend of China* thought it absurd that the Chusan debate continued. 'The Chinese . . . would not even exchange it for Hongkong with all the houses, barracks, roads, drains, &c. upon which so much money has been expended.'[59] This, from an anti-government newspaper, was a sign that the Hong Kong community had turned. Now, at the end of 1845, residents were no longer interested in discussing the tired news about fever and ill health. Poor governance, crime, excessive costs, and draconian laws that stifled commerce were the real concerns. The editor demanded that Martin stick to his facts.

> Let him represent the *true* state of affairs to Her Majesty's advisers. Tell them that this petty island has a civil establishment which costs the country more than double what it ought to do—that for a Governor and a Lieut. Governor alone, there is an item of £10,000—that our police and our Magistracy cost more than that of colonies with double the number of inhabitants, scattered over a territory with a frontier of a hundred miles, which has to be protected against the savages by a mounted police—that trade has been driven from the colony—and that laws, the most arbitrary and unjust, have been attempted to be forced upon the colonists by a government that they cannot respect.[60]

In an apparent and cutting reference to Martin's first, anonymous contribution in the Hong Kong press as 'No Geologist', a local writer using the pseudonym 'An Amateur Geologist' dug the knife in. He reprimanded Martin for his misleading usage of language in describing the geology of Hong Kong.

> The mere circumstance of disintegration however will make no change on the materials as Mr. MARTIN would have us believe, misled apparently by the terms *decayed* granite, *rotten* rock and other such names applied to it, and drawing his conclusions from the same terms as applied to animal and vegetable substances . . . no such thing is the result of decay in granite, and to whatever cause the sickness of Hongkong may be attributed, some other source must be looked for than the gas proceeding from *rotten* rock.[61]

All of this had followed the final departure of Martin from Hong Kong. In mid-June 1845, he provided a perfect 'suicide' note to Davis, writing to him requesting a leave of absence of six months and curtailment of his salary to enable him to convey specific information he was not at liberty to disclose back to Whitehall. With characteristic melodrama, he wrote:

> I ask permission to forego all my salary,—to incur considerable expense,—to destroy perhaps my remaining strength by travelling during this hot and adverse season,—and further I propose to risk my commission in H.M. Service in order that I may have an opportunity of communicating personally to the Authorities at home, the result of my enquiries in this Country.[62]

Davis refused the application because he lacked the authority to grant such an unusual request.[63] 'Life or death,' protested Martin theatrically, 'is of little moment compared with the great interests which England has at stake in China.'[64] Martin tendered his resignation on 8 July 1845, and so departed one of the most controversial, peculiar, and yet peculiarly selfless members of the early government of Hong Kong.[65] He would continue to claim that he had merely surrendered his post temporarily. Still, neither Davis nor Stanley were unhappy to see the back of him.

Timing was everything. Had Martin written his July 1844 report a year earlier, the community's opinions of his views would have been different. London had taken his report seriously enough to require Davis to counter the detailed points made against Hong Kong's future viability. But the delay in despatches and continued improvements to the city's health provided a growing defence against his attacks. As early as mid-March 1844, two months before his arrival, local newspapers began to develop a hope that the epidemic of 1843 had been an aberration. The *Canton Press*, soon to wind up its operations, and writing wistfully from Macau, noted that most of the British were now determinedly pulling out of the Portuguese enclave.

> After a residence of nearly five years in Macao . . . many of the British merchants have either left or intend leaving for Hongkong shortly, so that after another month or two shall have elapsed, very few will remain domiciled here. We sincerely hope that the many cases of sickness we had to deplore last year, will be found by experience to have been produced by local causes, such as the free exposure to the sun, living in houses but ill protected against the weather, and others, rather than to any inherent unhealthiness of the climate of Hong Kong. The experiment, from the painful experience of last year is however a hazardous one; most of the new residents of Hongkong have now substantial houses to reside in and may therefore avoid many causes of sickness.[66]

In Christopher Munn's essay on Britain's short, volatile history with Chusan, he argues that before the restoration of the island to China there had been a 'certain symmetry' in the positive and negative views expressed by propagandists on Britain's future relations with China. Martin had represented the forces of optimism. That 'symmetry' was destroyed when Chusan was returned to China. While it had remained on the table, hopes had been maintained.

> Only Chusan, which paradoxically was under military rule and had only the most superficial experience of liberal British institutions, remained as a beacon of hope: the ambitious plans for its acquisition and development became almost the only slender link with the inflated dreams that had arisen out of the first 'collision' with China. When that connection was severed in 1846, the shift towards disillusionment gathered pace.[67]

Chusan held its final party, its equestrian 'Spring Meeting', on 29 May 1846. It was to have been held in March but was deferred 'on account of the weather'.[68] The departure of British troops from Chusan commenced a few days later, on 5 June, with the arrival of the steamer *Nemesis* from Ningbo, carrying on board four mandarins sent to take possession of the island.[69] The restoration was sealed by a proclamation on 16 July by Davis, who had travelled up in the steamer *Vulture* to officiate at the lengthy handover ceremony.[70] Thus ended the hopes of a British Chusan and, with it, a compulsion by observers to denounce an innate, physical unsustainability of life on the island of Hong Kong.

The task of building Hong Kong's colony could continue without apprehension in London. Health concerns would remain, and Martin's predictions of climatic retribution would linger in the minds of the European population. However, the mood had decisively swung. The focus now was on local spaces of viability within the city and not the city's viability in its entirety. As will be seen, localities of health and the properties built upon them would become pervasive markers in the town, denoting class and status—catalysts of desire in guiding subsequent urban expansion.

From Mat-Sheds to Mansions

By the beginning of 1844, the ubiquitous mat-shed form of architecture that dotted the city had begun to concentrate and embody within itself all that was thought bad about life in Hong Kong. It had become a prototype of paranoia, a progenitor of disease, criminality, and conflagration. This poor perception of such temporary structures benefited the commanding Royal Engineer, Major Edward Aldrich, as he pushed for an ambitious construction programme. With the arrival of his military superior, Major-General George Charles D'Aguilar, in December 1843, and reinforced by the transfer of governorship from Sir Henry Pottinger to John Davis (later 'Sir') in May 1844, there was to be a fortunate convergence of aims between these three individuals. The mat-shed was ideal fear fodder, serving as an *anti-model* for developing European residences across the city. All its essential detriments of dampness, poor ventilation, and ground-hugging cramped-ness—as experienced by the guinea pigs that were the military forces—could be reversed in a construction language that spoke of the attributes of the opposite. These opposing model exemplars were the buildings constructed by the wealthiest mercantile establishments, such as Dent & Co. or Jardine, Matheson & Co.

One of the most significant causes for the growing association of the mat-shed with ill fortune occurred in late 1843. In the early morning hours of Saturday, 28 October, a fire broke out in a building appropriated for the destitute wives and families of the soldiers of the 55th Regiment. Many of these soldiers had perished from malarial fever months earlier at the West Point Barracks.[71] Adding to their grief, these families now lost their entire possessions. The following Wednesday morning, on 1 November, another fire broke out in one of the outhouses attached to the premises of Chinam's Hong on the Queen's Road.[72] Both structures were 'mat-sheds', buildings of a temporary, and now, too recognisably flammable nature. 'There are not in all Hong Kong,' reflected the editor of the *Friend of China* in the same edition, 'more dangerous, unseemly and unhealthy buildings than those mat outhouses attached to the godowns [warehouses] in Queen's Road: surely the Government:—the Committee of public health, or some other department has the power of abating the nuisance and preventing a fire on a large scale, which assuredly those mat houses are well prepared to engender.'[73]

By 1844, many in Hong Kong felt that the mat-shed had served its purpose. It had started life as an infinitely adaptable construction kit suited to the practical needs of both the military and merchants. Rapidly deployable, it transformed into almost every building typology imaginable: from the storage of troops (the barracks) to the storage of cotton (the godown), and from the site of mammon (the market bazaar) to the place of worship (the colonial 'mat church'). However, following the Hongkong Fever of 1843, more solidly constructed buildings were demanded as safer and more morally respectable. And so, the mat-shed began to take on a dubious nature. Its very materials were considered a cause of sickness and a potential tinderbox. It also developed a reputation as a concealer of immorality, a dwelling place of crime and debauchery.

In addition, the existence of the mat-shed had become somewhat of an anachronism, a dated component of the city's founding mythology. Newer residents listened in disbelief at recollections of the physical state of the settlement just a mere three years before. For instance, the original hardship of William Caine—Hong Kong's elder statesman and its chief magistrate—was romantically recollected. He had, it was told, been 'cast, as it were, on the side of a barren mountain, with literally nothing but a mat hut to shield him from the weather . . . without Architect or Engineer, a suitable Jail, Court-house, &c., rose under his indefatigable industry and auspices'.[74] The mat-shed was considered best relegated to such stories. For the British, the era of this despised building type as a domestic necessity was thought to be over. Nevertheless, its use would persist.

When D'Aguilar and his party arrived in late December 1843, finding suitable accommodation for the major-general, his military sons Charles and Henry, and his small retinue of staff proved challenging.[75] Major-General Saltoun's house, rented from Jardine Matheson, was, as Pottinger noted, 'one of the very earliest in the Colony at a moment that even the retention of this Island by Her Majesty was a matter of doubt'.[76] Understandably small, the house was ill-adapted to an officer of D'Aguilar's rank and with his considerable entourage. He was, after all, the new lieutenant-governor. Pottinger had thought the house unalterable apart from tearing it down.[77] In any case, the hill upon which it stood, Cantonment Hill, had been offered up to the military, pending London approval, after which it was intended to be shaved down.[78]

While he waited, D'Agular rented a private house belonging to a Mr. Scott.[79] Finding it confining he decided to move to a larger house, in fact a hotel on a lot between the Queen's Road and Stanley Street called the *Victoria Hotel* belonging to William Lane[80] since it was, as Pottinger explained to Lord Stanley, 'the only one in this Colony that could be procured on any terms'.[81] That left the 'only hotel' available in the city, the *Waterloo Hotel*, as a source of much complaint, causing one visitor to bc 'perfectly disgusted with the cool assurance and extraordinary impudence' of the owner, Mr. Lopez, in allowing 'orgies, which the proprietor permits to be carried on nocturnally'.[82] Lopez kept his dubious monopoly until March 1845 when the new *British Hotel* announced itself to the visiting public as 'a commodious house' at the corner of Graham Street up the hill and to the south of the Queen's Road.[83] Meanwhile, seemingly oblivious to the scandals, D'Aguilar moved into Lane's nearby property on 10 February.[84] The street adjacent to where he resided would later be given his name.

After much wrangling as to his terms of compensation, Pottinger agreed that D'Aguilar should draw a tent allowance, known in India as 'batta', as if he were an Indian officer on field service in China.[85] The rent was a hefty 300 rupees, of which the major-general agreed to temporarily cover 200, the remaining 100 rupees coming from the Civil Treasury 'until public quarters can be built'.[86] In light of the burden he was making, D'Aguilar was anxious to commence Aldrich's plans for constructing the barracks and particularly that of his future home, Headquarter House (the site of Saltoun's residence), and to see it completed as speedily as possible. Headquarter House would later be known as Flagstaff House, and is now home to the Museum of Tea Ware in Hong Kong Park. Throughout 1844, the new major-general would also become increasingly familiar with the historic vices of the dreaded mat-shed and initiate a more aggressive and expensive programme of military billeting for his officers and troops across the city (**fig. 5.3**).

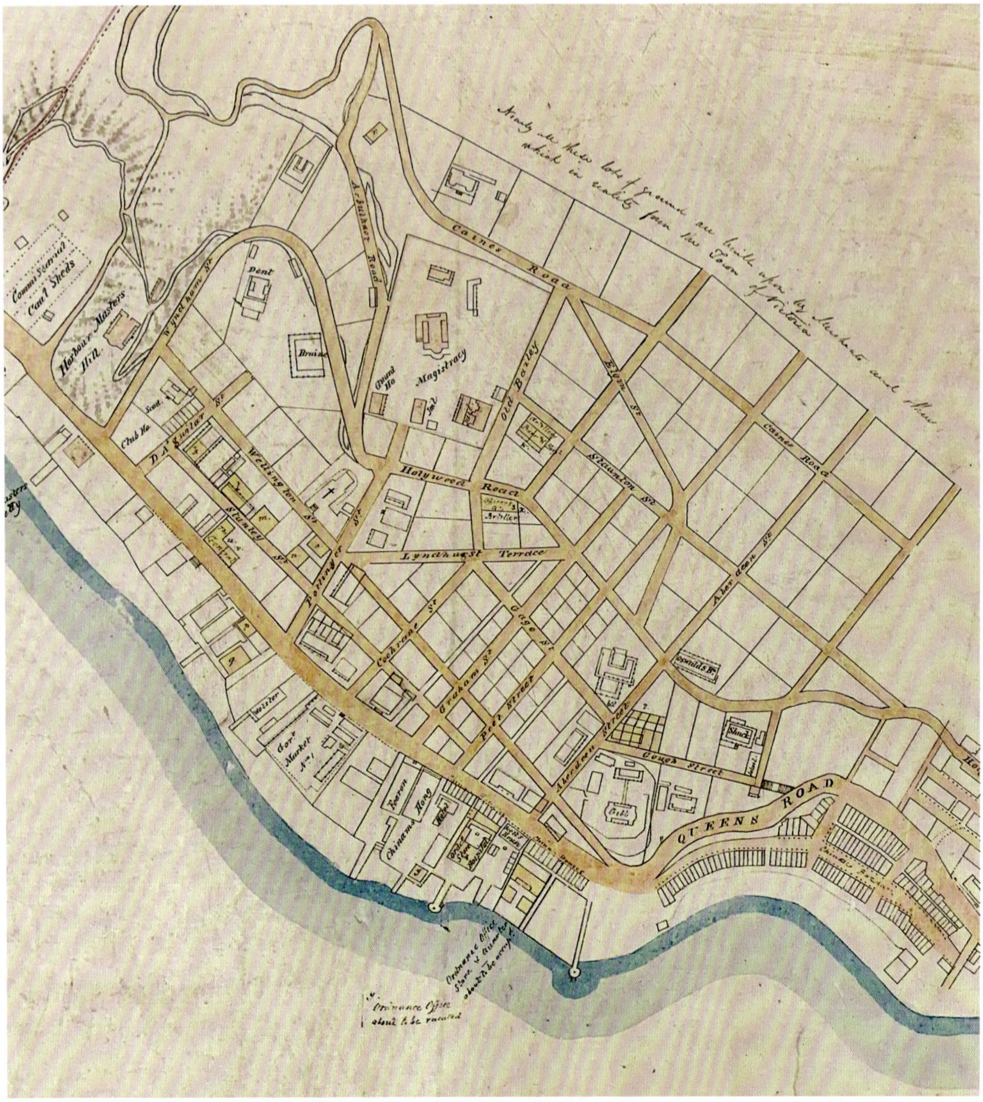

Fig. 5.3. Surveyor General's Dept., 'Plan of Victoria, Hong Kong', Billeting of Troops Shown in Yellow (detail), 12 May 1845. Ink and watercolour on paper. © The National Archives, Kew (WO 78/479).

By mid-1844, many residents believed there was a tangible connection between poor accommodation and sickness. The recent suffering of the temporary police force, a unit quickly established by D'Aguilar, merely amplified this opinion. From the beginning, the major-general had proved to be a more civically proactive commanding officer than his predecessor. For example, he had taken the role of lieutenant-governor seriously enough to immediately offer the assistance of his 55th Regiment as a gendarmerie for the colony until the civil government could establish a permanent unit.[87] The men who had suffered at West Point were given these duties as a relief measure. However, D'Aguilar did not realise that in the new course of their duties, their exposure at night to mosquitoes, including a number recently immunocompromised having recovered from malaria, would lead to further casualties.

This makeshift police force was distributed broadly across the island, with some, as in the case of the 98th Regiment, put in temporary accommodation in the south-eastern fishing village of Chek Chue—a place notorious for pirate attacks and robbery.[88] In Victoria proper, police were given a few rooms of the Seaman's Hospital on Hospital Hill in Ha Wan (Wan Chai); in a house provided in the soon-to-be-demolished Upper Bazaar near the Mess Room of the 41st Madras Native Infrantry; and in outhouses attached to the seaward residence of Mr. Edgar in the Sai Ying Pun area along the west side of the city.[89] These strategic posts were necessary for police on night guard duty.[90] Most of the day patrol were accommodated centrally within their various barracks.

Perhaps sensing the stretched and weak police security on the island by opportunists, a spate of audacious domestic robberies took place over this period. 'These affairs,' wrote Edward Cree, 'are constantly occurring at Hong Kong where the Chinese are most expert and daring robbers.' As an example, Cree records in his diary for early March a meeting he had with his friend Mrs. Alderman White and her distressed ward, Miss Mary Ann Le Foy. 'Monday 4 March 1844: Called on Mrs Alderman White, whose house has been broken into by a party of Chinese robbers. She gave a graphic description of the affair, and Miss Le Foy added she had 50 Chinamen in her bed room, that she jumped out of bed and, without dressing, ran down to the 41st Quarters to fetch up the guard, but before she got back the robbers had decamped.' So apparently graphic was the scene described by the woman that for the young naval surgeon, it seemed to excitedly paint itself in his diary, the room hurriedly drawn in confused perspective. For him, it is a scene full of racialised and sexualised theatricality, set as if on stage (**fig. 5.4**). Brown, shirtless, snarling men are packed into the foreground. The pale ward clutches her diaphanous nightdress to her bosom as she leaps

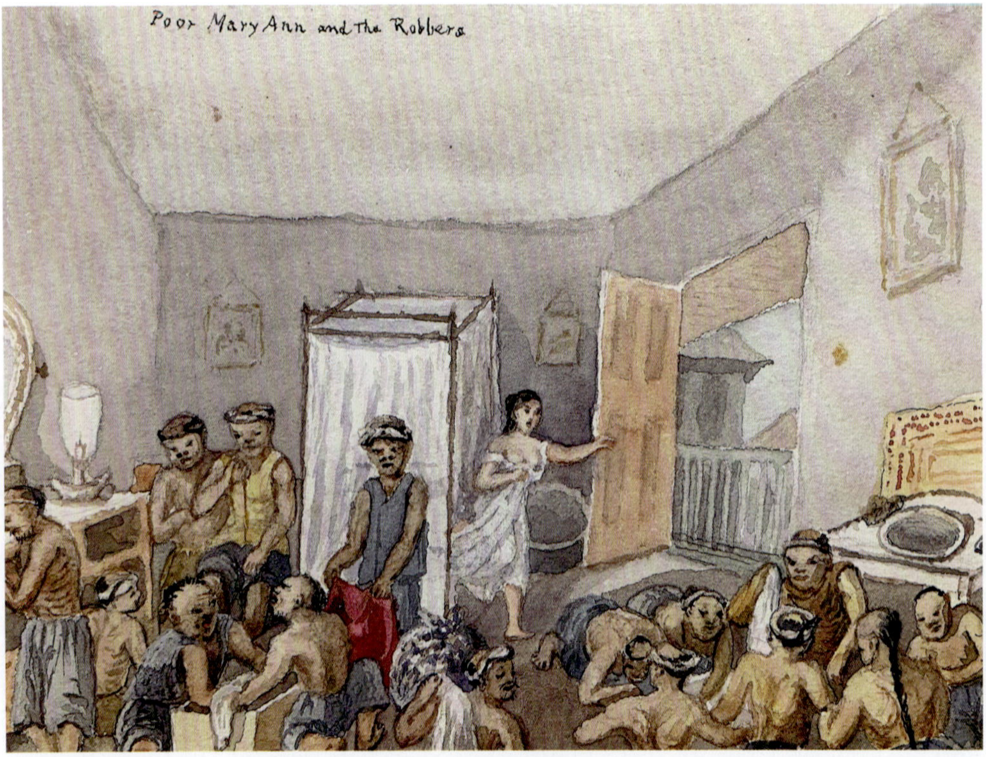

Fig. 5.4. Dr. E. Cree, 'Poor Mary Ann and the Robbers', 4 March 1844. Watercolour on paper. © National Maritime Museum, Greenwich, London (CRJ/8).

from the four-poster bed and through its netting towards the door, stage left. Evidently, Cree knew the house's layout sufficient to show that Miss Le Foy lived on the upper floor, her room facing a balcony. His illustration of the furniture and accoutrements within the room may or may not have been fantasised, but they are a convincing depiction of the interior of a mid-1840s European's bedroom on the island. The '50 Chinamen' is an evident exaggeration even Cree could not accommodate to fit within the reimagined drama. 'Mrs White did not lose much by the Chinese plunderers, some clothes and nothing of much value. Poor Mary Ann lost the clothes she was going to put on—but they had a great fright.'[91]

By late April, malaria had decimated the police force. Colonial Surgeon Dr. Alexander Anderson had few doubts about the cause. Pottinger quickly wrote to Chief Magistrate William Caine, telling him that Anderson blamed 'the Mat Barracks within the Cantonment and which he mainly attributes to the nature of those buildings'.[92] This was merely the first reappearance of the fever. 'The constant exposure both night and day to which the policemen are necessarily subjected, must always make them liable to much sickness,' Anderson later wrote to the new governor, John Davis.[93] 'The majority of men,' he observed, 'have served long in warm climates, India principally—and have had their constitutions previously much injured. . . . the men are badly housed; no stations have yet been built for them, and the houses in which they are located, have neither sufficient accommodation for this climate, not the comforts necessary for men so much exposed out of doors.'[94] Anderson also noticed that as with the previous year, 1843, most members of the civil government had enjoyed relatively robust health, arguing that 'the comparative exemption of those among the civil community last year, who had good and well-seasoned houses, from severe sickness, would point out this as a powerful means for the preservation of health'.[95]

Using a table to back his claim, Anderson showed that from the five months 1 January to 31 May 1844, a total of 46 civil servants and clerks (mainly those poorly-housed) had been admitted for medical treatment, 59 prisoners, and 73 wives and children of policemen, while a total of 130 policemen were treated.[96] Many of these patients were sent to the Seaman's Hospital, while others were placed in the hospital of the 98th Regiment at Chek Chue. Though fatalities were low—a total of seven—the disproportion of afflicted police and their families compared with more numerous classes of clerks and civil servants was alarming.

Davis eventually replaced the European police with 'native' officers, Hindustani and Malay. As he justified to Stanley in November 1844, their constitution could better deal with the climate, while they had one extra advantage: 'The difficulty of maintaining an European force in health and efficiency in this climate, will I have no doubt render it necessary to adopt a Malay or Native Police for the performance of the bulk of the duties. This class of persons possess an additional recommendation from their superior habits of sobriety, and, with European superintendence, are fully equal to the due restraint of the Chinese population.'[97] Davis's admiration for Asian temperance was matched by a shocking, wilful ignorance of the rampant sicknesses of Indian and Malay troops—the native infantry—in the summer of 1844. In this light, why were their constitutions thought any different from the European infantry?

D'Aguilar, too, had initially ignored their plight. In anticipation, he had placed all the European troops in more comfortable and expensive private accommodation (billeting) across the city during the spring months of 1844, while leaving those non-Europeans such as the 4th MNI in the now dreaded old style of mat-shed barracks. 'We would declaim all intention of wishing in the most remote manner to censure the Commander of the Forces in China,' the *Friend of China* censured. 'The fact however that much of the sickness which prevails in the 4th MNI is to be ascribed to the barracks which they inhabit,—if they can be dignified with the name of barracks—and the locality in which they are built is undeniable' (**fig. 5.5**).[98] In the same article, the editor described the mat-shed site as 'wet and spongy' and 'placed in a low flat between two ridges, with a gulley on the one side and a stagnant ditch on the other'.[99] It seemed that site-lore had evolved into a fine science for Hong Kong observers. These native barracks were trapped in a cleft, lacking contact with breezes except from the north. Their internal air was subsequently considered 'poisoned' by malaria, which spread through the barracks, striking down two hundred of the approximately five hundred troops in residence.[100] The newspaper surmised:

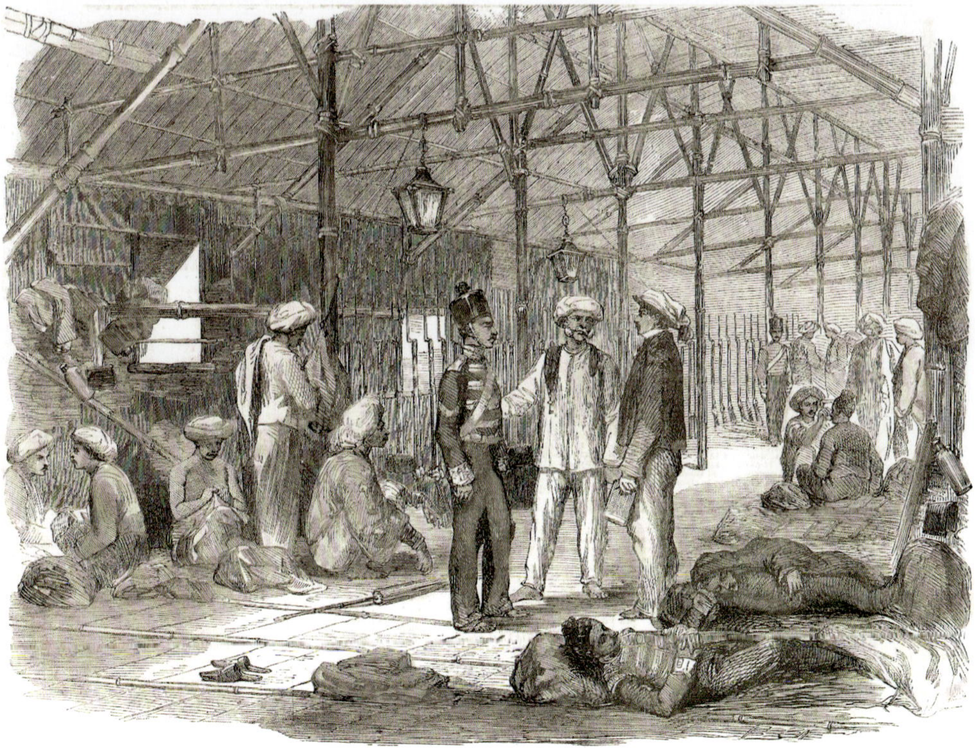

Fig. 5.5. Anon., 'Interior of a Mat Shed in Hong-Kong.' Engraving. *Illustrated London News*, 15 August 1857.

> It is the opinion of the most intelligent of the colonists, that last season one cause of sickness was the insufficient way in which many of the inhabitants were housed; and this summer it is confidently anticipated will prove less fatal, from the very circumstance of most of the inhabitants, *and all European troops*, being provided with better accommodation. The condition of the Indian soldier in this respect is not one whit better that it was a year ago. The same damp situation, the same mat hovels for barracks, and we regret to say, the same alarming degree of sickness and death which cut up the 41st, is now committing equal, if not greater havoc among the 4th.[101]

D'Aguilar, stung by similarly bad publicity as Saltoun had been with West Point a year earlier, applied to Davis for assistance. 'Major General D'Aguilar,' wrote Davis to Lord Stanley, 'applied to me for a site on which he might at once commence the erection of Barracks in lieu of the wretched mat-sheds in which the Sepoy troops have been hitherto housed, and to which the sickness and mortality among them had been principally owing.'[102] The site offered by the governor was south of the Victoria Road (the new name for this stretch of the Queen's Road and later renamed 'Queensway'), within the Ordinance District and opposite the North Barracks.[103] In the meantime, as a stopgap, an advertisement appeared in the local press from the Office of Ordnance.

> LARGE BUILDINGS REQUIRED FOR MILITARY PURPOSES.
>
> Merchants or others having large Buildings in Victoria, which they may be disposed to Let for Military purposes, with immediate possession, are requested to forward Tenders, Specifying the situation and description of the Buildings and the terms of letting . . .[104]

The military began to commandeer godowns since they were considered the most substantial building type in the city suited for conversion into barrack housing. One such building that the army rented was Gillespie's old warehouses, renamed 'Gillespie's Barrack'.[105]

Mat-sheds had been thought of as a source of sickliness, but they were also overtly vulnerable to fire. One of the most significant fires occurred at about ten in the evening during Queen Victoria's birthday celebrations on Saturday, 24 May 1845.[106] According to the *Hongkong Register*, 'the flames spread with the greatest rapidity and at one time extended over a space of fully 250 yards, including the Eastern bazaar and a long range of matsheds occupied by the Carpenters engaged on the government buildings'.[107]

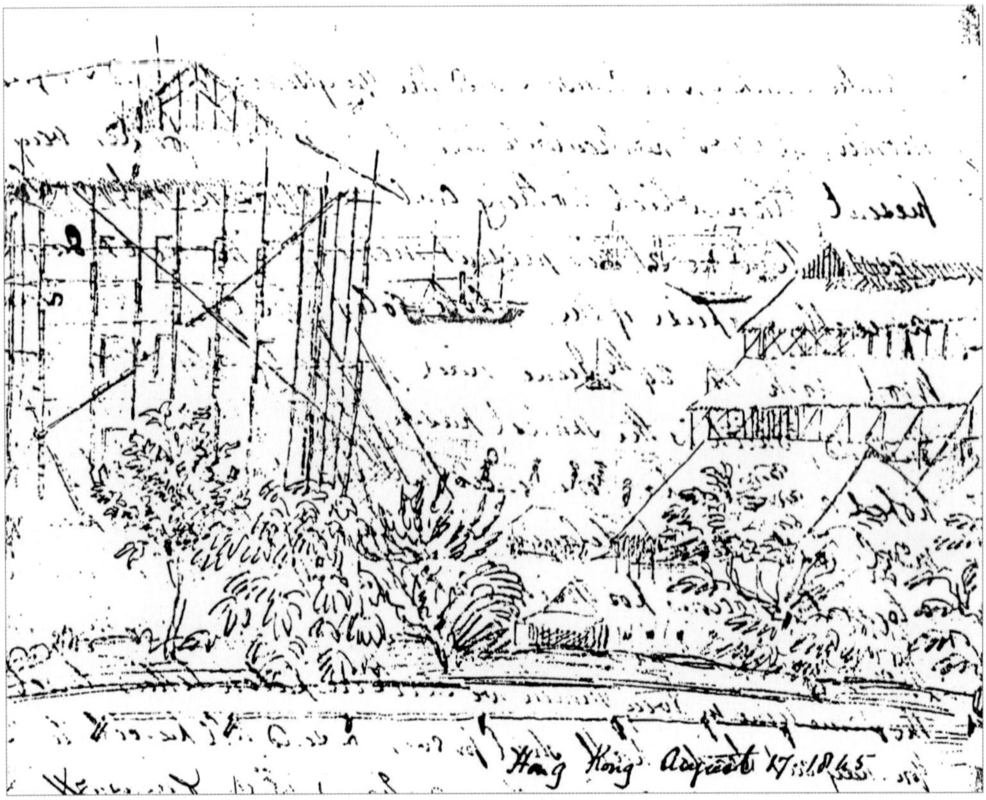

Fig. 5.6. Lt. T. B. Collinson, Sketch of Ordnance District Mat-Sheds, 17 August 1845. Ink on paper. © Hong Kong Public Records Office (*Transcripts*, HKMS 140-1-1).

The *Friend of China*, with typical mordancy, remarked, 'In the evening there was a ball at Government House which passed off tolerably well as the first government ball at Hongkong. Causes, unexpected, had the effect of brilliantly illuminating the town and harbour in the evening, though at the expense of a destruction of property which will fall heavily upon many poor people.'[108] These were the large mat-sheds along the waterside within the Ordnance District and below Cantonment Hill, protecting the carcass of the Military Hospital and other public buildings under construction.

Somewhat poignantly, Lieutenant Collinson had had these exact structures on his mind, having been asked by his superior, Major Aldrich, to draw them for the article he was preparing for the Royal Engineer's 'Professional Papers' (see **fig. 4.10**). He drew the reconstructed mat coverings in a letter to his father that August (**fig. 5.6**), adding:

> Those large buildings in the picture are specimens of Chinese ingenuity in scaffolding. When they are about to build a house in Hong Kong, they put up a shed of the length, breadth & height of the house before they do anything else—There is one over the new hospital like those, 240 ft. long 60 feet broad & 60 feet high, all of bamboos about as thick as your arm. . . . It was the hospital shed that caught fire on the Queen's birthday, when Dick climbed up one of the poles in his coat & epaulettes & cut away the lashing with his sword.[109]

Bernard's brother, Captain Richard Collinson, was among those brave officers who had run out of the ball, dressed in their dinner uniforms, pitching down Government Hill towards the inferno. With the favourable circumstances of a calm, windless night, Richard's actions had saved the Commissariat stores and two large houses, together with connecting godowns.[110] Unfortunately, all the timberwork for the doors and windows to the hospital had been added that day and was destroyed. So too were much of the contractors' on-site materials.[111] This disaster would contribute to the eventual suicide of the main contractor, Achou.

Though many domestic and commercial fires had broken out frequently across the city, it was a fire of this magnitude, and on government property, that brought about a change in the law. C. B. Hillier, the 'officiating' chief magistrate, issued a notice to the public that September.

> In consequence of the frequent and dangerous FIRES of last Dry Season, Notice is hereby given, that no MAT SHEDS, or GRASS BUILDINGS of any description, will be permitted after the 1st day of October; and the Public are hereby informed, that the Police will remove all such after the above mentioned day.[112]

The notice claimed to target and remove mat-sheds to prevent fires, but the truth, as ever, was more complex. The government itself continued to use mat-sheds both for housing 'native' troops and in surrounding and protecting the construction of buildings, though as the *Friend of China* conceded, 'in this climate it is impossible for men to work in the sun, and therefore an awning of some kind is necessary'.[113]

After the notice was released, the police raided several mat-sheds within Chinese districts, suspected of harbouring criminals conducting illegal activities. Since Hillier's notice, it had become easier to doubt and target the purposes of mat-sheds that remained standing in non-European areas. Under the command of the new superintendent of police, Charles May, officers raided a gambling establishment near East Point 'in the neighbourhood of a sing song mat-house. . . . A mat-house with eight tables was found and a goodly number around each'.[114] May estimated a significant crowd of between two and three hundred assembled inside, of which he had five arrested. The following month, the murder of Mrs. Clarke, an English blacksmith's wife, at her home, provided a pretext for police to raid 'a mat shed in the vicinity of Mr. Clarke's house on the morning after her murder'. Though, as the pro-government *China Mail* baldly recorded, the 'inmates had absconded but shortly before, leaving behind them some books and papers and other small articles'.[115]

One writer, *Vindex*, decried the double standard. 'I have this moment returned from an early walk and perceive among other matters that His Excellency's Mat Sheds, with those attached to the Post Office, Sepoy Barracks, and the General's new House are yet standing.'[116] Those mat-sheds around the military works would only be abandoned once they had served their purpose and the buildings were complete. Appallingly, these included new mat-shed barracks for the 42nd Madras Native Infantry, built for them while they waited for their adjacent permanent accommodation to be completed. D'Aguilar's and Davis's racially discriminatory policies—billeting for Europeans, mat-sheds for non-Europeans—were still firmly in place. Fortunately, the Indian troops were able to move into their finer barracks just before their older premises, now empty mat-sheds, were engulfed in fire in May 1846, almost a full year after the great Ordnance District fire. In recording the burning of these, the *Hongkong Register* observed, 'But such should bear in mind that we still retain in Hongkong, "the good old plain," of having one law for the governed, and another for the Governors. . . . The loss can only be trifling, and probably might have been a blessing to the poor Sepoys had it occurred long ago, and saved them from living in hovels compared to which many a kennel would have been a luxury.'[117]

1846 would be the first year that D'Aguilar could objectively test the health of his military forces in Hong Kong. 'The hot season has already set in,' he wrote as lieutenant-governor to the new British colonial secretary, William Gladstone, in mid-April. 'And for the first time since the occupation of the Island, the Troops are properly housed in substantial barracks. . . . It is moreover of the last importance to our commercial interests and to the revenue connected with them, to test this climate fairly, and this is the first year that any reasonable means have been afforded me for this essential object.'[118] By mid-July, D'Aguilar was able to write again to Gladstone, confirming that the troops had experienced the healthiest year to date and that they had suffered 'no mortality'.[119]

Aldrich's magnificent barracks complex, the Officers' Quarters below, and rising above and behind it, the parallel ranges 'B' and 'C' of the soldiers' barracks, was now almost complete. (B and C would take a little longer to finish.) Nevertheless, by now, the entire cantonment could comfortably house nine-hundred soldiers, approximately three-quarters of the whole island's forces. The remainder were housed on the north-eastern and south-eastern sides of the island in older, refurbished accommodation at Sai Wan (now Chai Wan) and Chek Chue (renamed in English as 'Stanley').[120] As officers and troops transferred to their new, permanent accommodation, they created an acute rental crisis, causing a surplus of private housing to become vacant. Adjacent, competing advertisements appeared in the newspapers that late summer with homes to let, such as C. W. Bowra offering 'TWO [houses] in *Stanley Street*, formerly occupied by the 18th ROYAL IRISH', and Smith & Brimelow with 'a convenient suit of ROOMS above the premises . . . at present occupied by Col. FARQUHARSON'.[121]

Since 1844, there had been a steadily growing stock of buildings offered either for let or sale, particularly around the area of the new Hollywood Road within the eastern edge of the Western District (now part of the Central District), as the government released extensive, smaller plots of land. To meet the supply, advertisers evolved an increasingly sophisticated language of enticement that reflected purchasers' needs and desires. Tracing this may be of considerable value in understanding the development of early Hong Kong.

On 9 October 1843, Gibb, Livingston & Co. decided to sell their estate. This was that remarkable enclave that the Rev. James Legge would describe in his recollections of 1843.[122] Selling it towards the closing stages of the Hongkong Fever they advertised it as 'A desirable detached two Storied Residence, situate within a Ring Fence and situate in the Healthiest part of the Island'.[123] It was one of the first private attempts to commercially promote a specific locale in Hong Kong based on health claims. But it was commercial storage that led the way in catering to the population's desires for greater space and good ventilation. It seemed that placing objects of value above personal comfort was the first instinct of Hong Kongers. For instance, the *Friend of China* could advertise in early June 1844 of 'Goods and merchandize of all descriptions received and carefully stored in spacious, airy and secure Brick Godowns situated 18, and 56 Queens Road upon moderate terms'.[124] By late 1844, however, advertisers had fully appropriated the language of storage, those 'spacious' and 'airy' godowns and, combined with Gibb, Livingston & Co.'s clever marketing of location, produced a reusable template for selling domestic properties.

Parsee merchant Framjee Jamsetjee's bungalow, for sale that October, was described as 'commodious' and in 'a perfect state of repair'. It commanded 'a fine view of the harbour and shipping' and, in terms of location, 'the situation is healthy'.[125] A few months earlier, Fletcher & Co. offered to let 'The spacious and airy Bungalow, situated on Oswald's Hill, behind the house occupied by Messrs. Murrow & Co., having a very commodious Office, with a Treasury, and a commanding view of the Harbour'.[126] Of all buzzwords, 'commodious' was the most abused, invariably appearing in housing advertisements from 1844 to 1846. It was, after all, in tiny and cramped Hong Kong that the desire for space was at its most obsessive.

One of the peculiar statistics to emerge from the grim headcount of sick and dying between 1841 to 1843 was the surprising healthiness of prisoners lodged in William Caine's prison complex, situated a little above and to the east of the Upper Bazaar (and where it has remained, locally called *tai kwun* or 'big station'). The bluff it perched upon was known as Magistracy Hill. Writing in October 1843, the *Chinese Repository* commented that there were an average of sixty inmates at any one time. Yet, of those, only nine had died throughout the entire three years of occupation. 'Of those nine, some were debauched opium smokers—who died for want of that which caused their death. Two or three only died of fever.'[127] It continued,

> It might indeed be worthwhile to inquire, and to ascertain if possible, why there has been so much less sickness in the prisons than in the barracks at Hongkong, during the last twenty-six months. When of seventy men in the artillery lines, not more than fifty were reported *fit* for duty; not more than three, of nearly an equal number in the jails, were *unfitted* by sickness to perform 'hard labor'. In not a few cases, men have gone in sick, and come out well.[128]

Of course, this sense of injustice prompted an expected response from the administration, increasing the number of prisoners used in civil construction for such public works like roads and drainage. But also, from 1844, the area around Caine's house, his prison and magistracy, acquired heightened kudos for the private-property speculator as one of the healthiest and therefore desirable parts of the city. The area gained a new aura, helped immensely by the 1844 and 1845 reorganisation and expansion of streets across the district under Davis. And so was born the lower portion of an area later to be named the 'Mid Levels'.[129]

By the beginning of 1845, the explicit nearness of a property to William Caine and Magistracy Hill had become a strong selling point. A carpenter, John White, for instance, advertised 'A Verandah Cottage, containing two Rooms, situated at the west-end of Major Caine's premises and commanding a delightful view of Victoria Harbour'.[130] The auctioneer C. Marwick, one month later advertised 'That beautiful Cottage situated "South East" of the Hon. Major William Caine's Residence, and lately occupied by the Hon. P. J. Sterling "Attorney General". . . . The above House is situated in a most healthy Part of the Island, and has a beautiful commanding view of Victoria Harbour.'[131] By April 1845, the road to the south adjoining the rear of the prison site had become known as Caine's Road, and all that was now required was to advertise the fact as often as possible. 'An elegant and well-built house in Caine's Road, contains ten rooms and a spacious Hall 45 feet long by 23 feet wide.'[132]

Advertisements soon grew in detail, the selling points had become more varied, and the lifestyle options more flexible. Jamieson How & Co., unable to proffer the health of their location (the premises for sale was 'situated on the ridge at West-point'), compensated for the unfortunate locale by way of the property's size, luxurious facilities, and in its capacity to expand. Advertising in mid-July 1845, they offered

> A substantial House, consisting of two Sitting rooms, each 30 feet by 20, and in height 17 feet, separated by folding doors; five good sized bed rooms, with Dressing and bath room each; two Servant's rooms; a front and a back Verandah, closed with Venetians, each 100 feet long, 12 feet wide; flat roof, convenient for exercise, and affording a fine view of the harbour and its entrances. The Halls and foundation constructed purposely to admit of the addition of an upper Story.[133]

A fascinating advertisement appeared that same day for one of the stately harbour-front merchant houses in the city's centre. Gibb, Livingston & Co. offered to let their 'large House on the Queen's Road, next to Messrs. DENT & Co's. premises'.[134] The rooms on every floor were listed and dimensioned. They provide an insight into the spatial sequence of rooms within a marine-lot merchant's house. Here was an A–B–A (room–hall–room) arrangement across a floorplan not unlike a Venetian palazzo. The three-storey structure consisted of storage and offices on the ground floor; a central hall or salon stretching north to south (or from harbour-side to mountain-side) on the upper two levels; with an inset, covered balcony or veranda, harbour-side, along the upper hall; and with more minor, ancillary rooms placed upon either side of the halls, east and west.

Containing on the ground floor:—

	5 Rooms or Godowns		35 feet + 21 feet.
	2 Do.	do.	35 feet + 16 feet.
First Floor	5 Rooms	-	35 feet + 21 feet.
	1 Do. -	-	21 feet + 15 feet.
	1 Do. (large)	-	80 feet + 16 feet.
Second Floor	1 Large Hall in centre		85 feet + 45 feet.
	2 Rooms	-	20 feet + 20 feet.
	1 Do. -	-	16 feet + 10 feet.
With a Verandah to Sea frontage			85 feet + 16 feet;
	a Compound		40 feet + 40 feet.

And out houses, containing 15 Rooms, each 15 feet + 10.[135]

Three-storey buildings were still a relative rarity since the first example on the island, Jardine Matheson's East Point offices, had been built to then soon collapse, in 1843. But the broadest cluster of these titans could now be found vying for attention along that same stretch of the Queen's Road as Gibb, Livingston and Co.'s merchant house. We are fortunate to have two drawn views along this stretch, showing temporally close but distinct stages of urban development. One is the familiar view by the Scottish architect and road-construction overseer Murdoch Bruce, published as a print in 1846, drawn above from the edge of Murray's Battery (**fig. 5.7a**). The other, is by the English architect Edward Ashworth, and is a recently discovered line drawing predating Bruce by at least a year (**fig. 5.7b**). Here, by way of a better angle, the southern façades and their relative heights are visible. Beyond Dent & Co.'s merchant house (on the site of The Landmark complex)—one part of its property having a proprietary flat roof and an out-slung and extended grilled balcony—can be seen the Gibb, Livingston & Co. building. Behind this rise many more three-storey properties, including to the left what would become the premises to the first Hong Kong Club. It is possible that Bruce borrowed the idea for this view after seeing Ashworth's work (they also produced matching views along the Ordnance District), though the promontory would have been an obvious perch from which any urbanist might be inspired to produce a sketch.

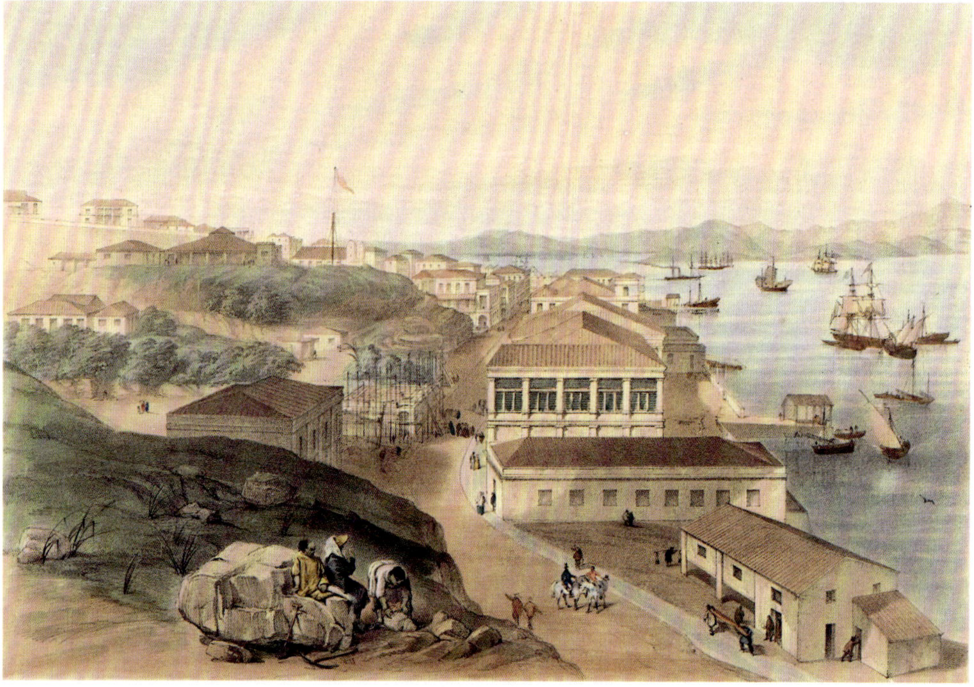

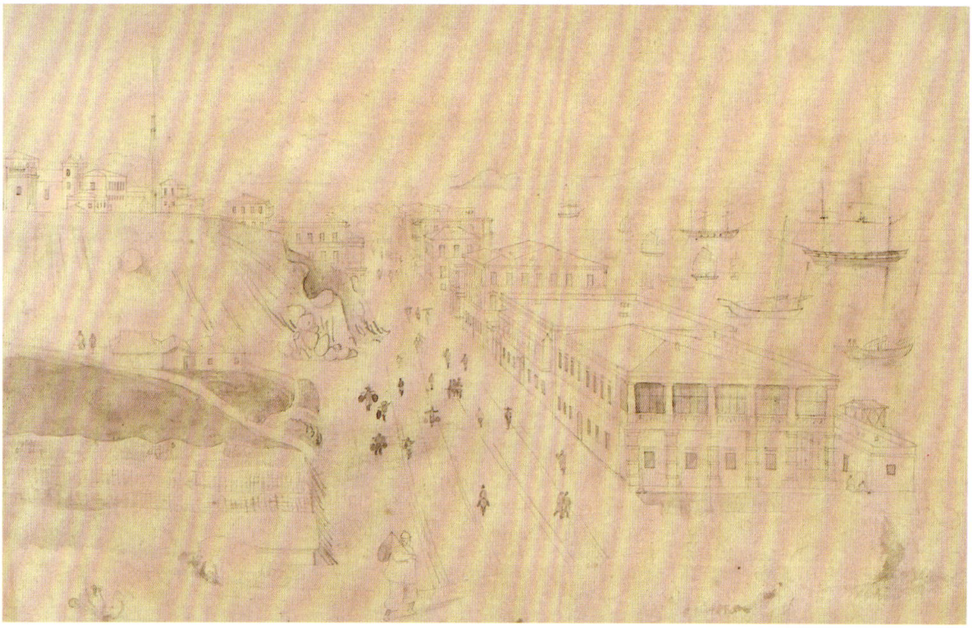

▲ **Fig. 5.7a.** M. Bruce, *View of Hong Kong and the Harbour Looking West from Murray's Battery*, ca. 1845–1846. Coloured lithograph. © Hong Kong Museum of Art Collection (AH1964.0389.001).

▼ **Fig. 5.7b.** E. Ashworth, 'Part of Queen's Road looking to the Principal Street of the Town of Victoria, Hong Kong, China', ca. 1844–1845. Graphite with sepia wash. © Hong Kong Museum of Art Collection (AH2015.0010).

For properties lacking contact with the waterfront, a property's raised situation above the city's old datum, the coastal Queen's Road, was becoming increasingly desirable as a means of gaining visual access to the harbour. More than seeking a good view, this also implied privileged access to guaranteed, health-giving flows of air. *Height*, that is, either in terms of prospect or a building's actual tallness, was emerging as an emblem of need. Houses of note had begun by selling their convenience, healthy location, and vantage. For example, R. Oswald described his properties as 'Two small convenient Houses situate[d] in a central and healthy part of the town, commanding a fine view of the bay'.[136] Some sellers promised that their location offered the security of such a view for the foreseeable future. 'DESIRABLE PROPERTY FOR SALE—INLAND lot No. 5 . . . in a central and business part of the town, and commanding a fine view of the harbour which cannot be cut off by any buildings to be erected.'[137] Yet, if one did not possess a marine lot, the only way of ensuring an uninterrupted enjoyment of the harbour was to build upon a higher location. So desperate was the desire to climb that this new style of high-altitude living was caricatured by visiting Chinese artists, such as Piqua (**fig. 5.8**).

By late 1845, undoubtedly influenced by the glamour of the tall merchant palaces along the Queen's Road strip, and to escape the perceived miasmas that hung upon the lower reaches of the city, three-storey residences began to rise within the elevated district west of the prison and newly reconfigured upon the bones of the Upper Bazaar, this new 'Mid Levels'.

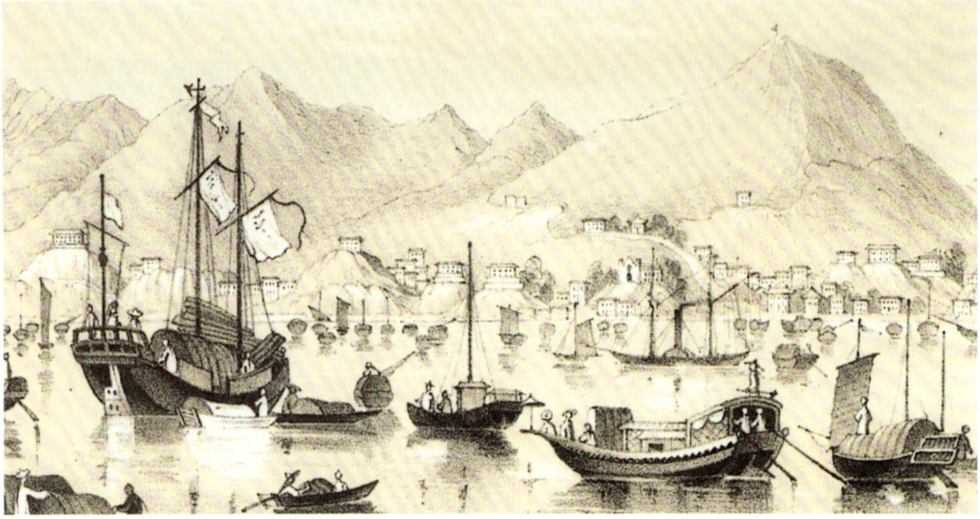

Fig. 5.8. B. Clayton, 'View of Victoria Town—Island of Hong Kong' (detail), ca. 1845, after a painting by Piqua. Lithograph. Miss (Julia) Corner, *The History of China and India, Pictorial & Descriptive*, London, 1846.

> TO LET AT A MODERATE RENT
>
> THAT fine commodious and airy block of building containing two houses in Hollywood Road directly at the back of Gough Street. Those houses are of three stories with verandahs, godowns, stables, bathrooms, &c., &c.
>
> They command a fine and uninterrupted view of the bay, and being situated in the most respectable part of the west end of the town are a most eligible residence.[138]

John Carr, the editor of the *Friend of China*, placed a personal advertisement of his own in the newspaper to let out 'A three-story veranda house in the west end of Gough Street. In building, every attention has been paid to the tropical climate, and the house will be found replete with conveniences.'[139] 'Every attention' meant moving from outside concerns of a building towards its interior life, the mark of a house of healthfulness and quality. The 'conveniences' of this interior referred to self-contained bathing and toilet facilities, to 'every description of PUMPS, PIPES, and WATER CLOSETS, BATHS (Warm and Shower)'.[140] These, together with rooms of spaciousness and dryness upon a site that was well-drained, offered a highly attractive rental proposition for a Hong Kong resident of the mid-1840s.

In the most detailed property advertisement yet provided, taking up almost half a column of newsprint, the auctioneer W. H. Franklyn announced several sets of houses soon to be put under the gavel. Occupying the Aberdeen and Wellington Street areas, 'The above Houses were carefully built, regardless of Expense, under the Superintendence of Europeans, they are well-drained, in excellent repair, and situated in one of the most healthy and respectable parts of the Town, being in and adjoining one of the most fashionable Streets. They are formed for a refreshing coolness, not to be found in less elevated and more crowded localities.'[141] In addition, Franklyn added a special note to the speculator.

> TO THE CAPITALIST
>
> This presents a safe and rare opportunity for investing Money, which will continue to yield a high rate of Interest, as the situation will always insure Tenants, and become more valuable from year to year. To those requiring a Residence an opportunity now offers itself of procuring one delightfully situated, dry, and well aired—no small consideration in this Climate.[142]

Informed by their Hong Kong 'correspondent', the *London Evening Mail* found this hyperbole incredibly amusing.

> If we turn to the columns of the colonial newspapers, especially those occupied by advertisements, much instruction may be gleaned. There we may read a whole list of houses to let, from the 'spacious and airy bungalow', to the 'large houses of business with a sea frontage and godowns, &c.'; while so many valuable 'waterside properties', are advertised 'at a moderate rent', that a stranger might be disposed to think some good-natured capitalist has been building these commodious properties upon the most purely disinterested motives, 'moderate rent', having been a condition hitherto unknown in Hongkong.[143]

However, by now, a large class of gentlemen could only entertain a 'moderate rent'. For those of lesser means, lodging within a household was one of the few options available. One room to let as bed and board was 'offered in a quiet, genteel family the situation particularly healthy, good airy Bed Room, and cheerful society'.[144]

Dry, airy rooms, it seemed, mattered a great deal. In addition to constructing a building upon an appropriate, that is, a dry, well-drained and ventilated site, there was also a consensus by Europeans in Hong Kong that new buildings had first to be 'cured'. The plastered walls had to have adequately dried out before inhabitation. One medical article appeared in the *Friend of China* in February 1846, reminding purchasers of the fact. In a paper entitled 'Influence of Newly-Built Houses on Health', a German physician, Dr. Reidel of Berlin, wrote of three issues arising from a newly constructed dwelling that was dangerous to the occupant. First, he argued, new buildings held increased amounts of water vapour in the air, affecting breathing. Wood could remain damp. Stonework needed a long exposure time to sufficiently dry, while 'the walls of those houses remain damp longest which have been plastered immediately after their completion'.[145] Second, the spent air from our breathing, that is, 'the proportion of carbonic acid [what we now consider as CO_2] is diminished by the mortar which attracts it from the air; it may also be attracted to certain colours such as those containing acetate of copper'. Third, 'deleterious ingredients' such as lime particles, oils and 'metallic colours', and 'combinations of lead, copper, and arsenic' used to prepare paints, had been proved, he argued, to sit in the atmosphere, released by the evaporation process.[146] He called for careful examinations of any materials used before their incorporation into the structure of a building, and he suggested a sufficient drying-out period of half a year for houses built in the countryside, but one year within a town setting, due to surrounding buildings cutting off air exposure. He also recommended, in the case of remedying a damp room, that drying and ventilation should not be confined to the one space but all adjoining rooms and that 'drawers and other furniture should not be placed too near the damp walls'.[147]

Light, movable furniture were items in greatest demand in Hong Kong, a trend acquired from bungalow life in India. We saw such items drawn in T. B. Collinson's letter to his mother from his Royal Engineer's bungalow 'Letter G' built on Cantonment Hill and sketched in late 1845 (see **fig. 2.16**). These items with their airy quality were considered more conducive to maintaining good health, as they allowed dryness and aeration with the added advantage of minimal size and weight in shipping. For instance, the cabinet makers Currie & Co.—'the oldest establishment in the Presidency' of Calcutta—offered residents of Hong Kong 'every requisite in Furniture of a novel and portable description by which more than half the expense hitherto will be saved'.[148] They assured customers that their flat-pack approach would not compromise on the finished appearance and that 'the arrangement of the different parts will be so clear and distinct that the most inexperienced will be enabled to put them together'.[149] For those determined upon a life of reclining and snoozing in the tropical heat of the colony, W. H. Franklyn offered 'RECLINING CHAIRS, the most luxurious, in Crimson and Purple Morocco, adjusting themselves to the posture, and in which to sit and repose, and, 'Unrivalled COUCHES, SOFAS, and OTTOMANS, with spring Horse-hair Cushions, wooing balmy sleep to the fortunate possessor'.[150] Finally, if breathability and portability of furniture was a concern, particularly for the military and the club member, shipments of cane-bottom furniture, familiar designs adapted for the hot and humid climate, would frequently find their way via the occasional merchant's ship. 'TO THE CLUB HOUSE, ARMY AND NAVY MESSES &c. Just arrived ex *Alfred*, seven dozen Cane bottom Chairs, best London make, remarkably strong and a mere feather weight for lifting; imitation Rosewood, Mahogany and Satinwood.'[151]

For the wealthy merchant classes, that is, those in possession of a substantial garden, the importation of good trees and plants was equally important to a comfortable home. As far back as early 1843, preparing for his imminent move from Macau to Hong Kong, Alexander Matheson wrote to Manila and his relation and agent there, James Adam Smith. 'We propose moving in about a month to Hongkong which will soon be, next to Calcutta, the most important commercial town this side the Cape. We shall be much more comfortable there than we have ever been in China. If you have an opportunity, I wish you would send me a dozen of young mango trees for my Black-Mount garden.'[152] Framjee Jamsetjee, still apparently unable to sell the bungalow he had put up for purchase a year before, found that he was now able to advertise it as a 'property beautifully situated by the water side, with a fine view of the Bay, surrounded by a Garden stocked with the choicest plants which have been imported at great expense and now in a flourishing condition'.[153]

However, of all the successful planting schemes in Hong Kong, none were more impressive than that of Dent & Co.'s magnificent garden at 'Green Bank', a large house built in an elevated position by Wyndham Street and close to the Magistracy (on the site of Lan Kwai Fong). Significantly, the garden sat in a valley declivity—a feared site of sickness—as if to tauntingly boast by its presence that this botanical experiment would banish past fears. A winding path climbed out of its bowl to the house and its terrace. Green Bank's collection was enriched immeasurably in 1845 by the transplantation and incorporation of most of the plants that had once belonged within the famed Macau garden of the late Thomas Beale (**fig. 5.9**).[154]

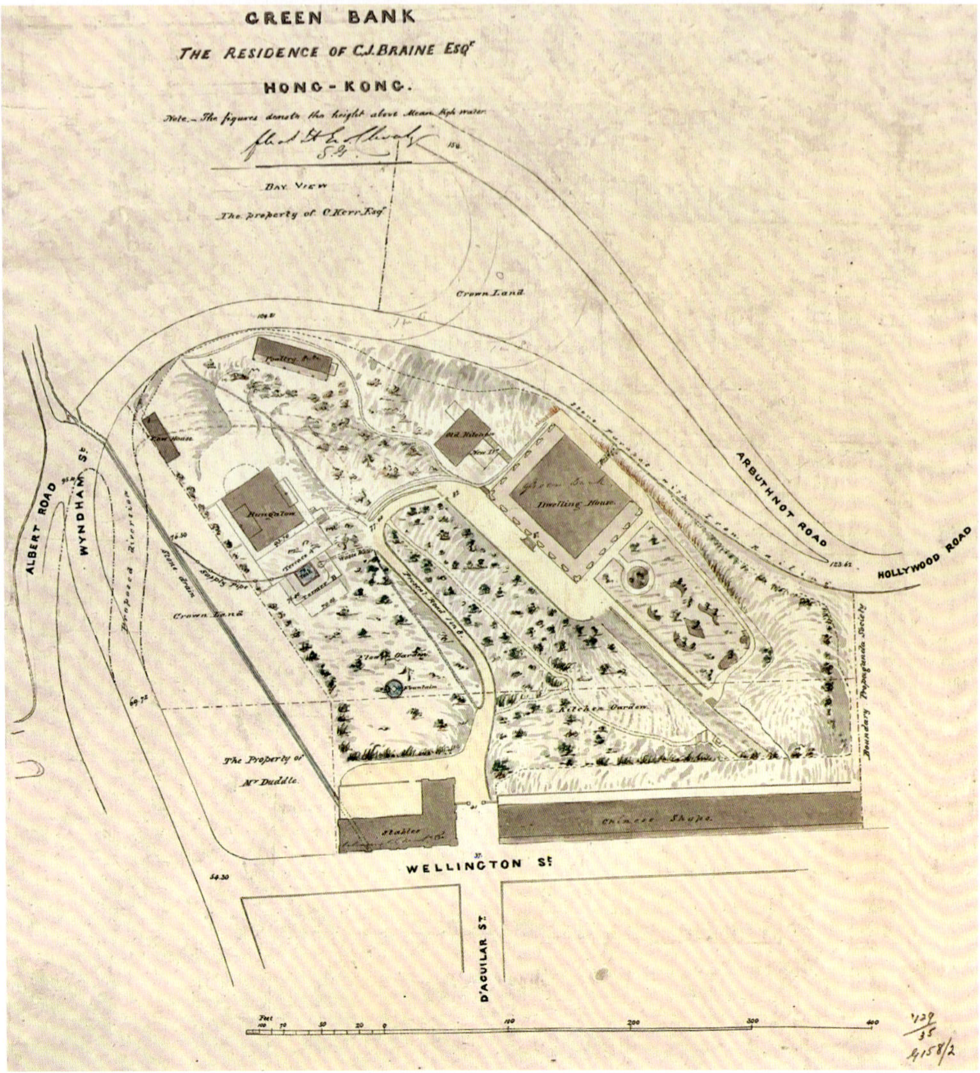

Fig. 5.9. C. Cleverly, Plan of 'Green Bank', ca. 1850. Ink and watercolour.
© The National Archives, Kew (MPG 1/158).

Under the custodianship of Charles Joseph Braine, a partner at Dent's, the garden at Green Bank appropriated the plot of the first colonial house built on Hong Kong Island. This peculiar home had originally belonged to William Caine and was built in a local vernacular style in the form of a surprisingly elaborate Chinese bungalow. There it remained, an architectural seed around which the lush garden was laid out (see **figs. 2.19** and **5.10**). Even the renowned botanist, Robert Fortune, during his visit to the island, noted that 'the barren soil, the burning sun, and the dry air, are all much against success; but on the other hand, you have only to look to the healthy and flourishing trees and shrubs on Messr. Dent & Co.'s property, to prove that all these disadvantages can be overcome with a little attention and skill'.[155] Merchants such as Dent, by introducing a wide variety of botanical species to the island, were leading the way in experiments that would influence the afforestation of Hong Kong a few decades later.

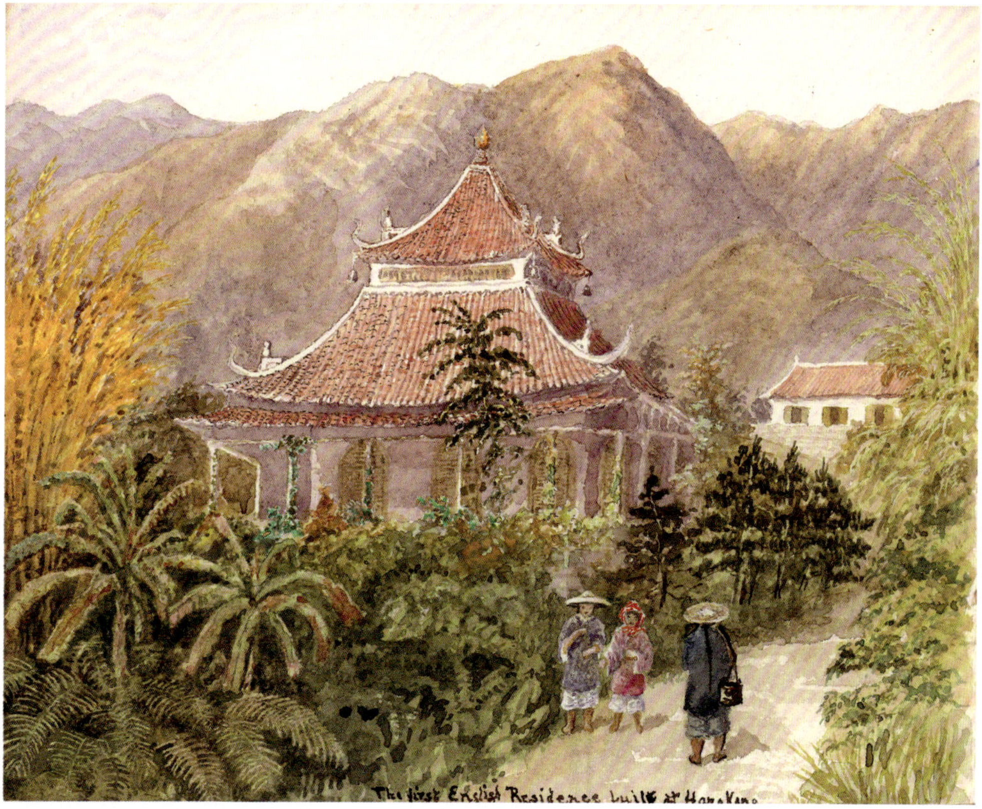

Fig. 5.10. Dr. E. Cree, 'The First English Residence Built at Hong Kong' (Dent's bungalow within Green Bank), 1 January 1844. Watercolour on paper. © National Maritime Museum, Greenwich, London (CRJ/8).

Robert Fortune made a brief stop in Hong Kong in late 1844 before embarking on his arduous, year-long voyage into China to identify and collect specimens unknown to the European collector. These fragile samples were sent back to the Horticultural Society of London in custom-built glass containers (terraria) known as Wardian cases designed by Dr. Nathaniel Bagshaw Ward, an East-London physician and fern enthusiast.[156] During his stay, Davis asked Fortune his opinion on which species of trees and large shrubs were the most suitable for successful integration into the soil and climate of Hong Kong. Fortune enthusiastically provided a list of twenty-three plants. At the top of his list was the banyan *Fictus Nitido*, a native China pine called *Pinus Sinensis*, and the coniferous cypress *Cunninghamia Lanceolata*. He also shared the thoughts of Matheson, recommending numerous fruit trees, including mango, guava, lychee, loquat, and orange trees. However, his principle was simple. 'You cannot do wrong in planting anything found growing wild on the Island.'[157] It was claimed that long-time Chinese settlers had stripped the island of grasses and young saplings before they had time to grow. Fortune recommended that the government ought to inflict the 'severest penalties' upon those who persisted in this damage. He explained that the *Fictus Nitido* grew well in barren soil and felt confident that it would be ideal for planting along the sides of the Queen's Road and other roads that were now under construction. Fruit trees and willows could likewise flourish along roadsides, ensuring, that is, that fruit trees were planted in richer soil while willows were placed in damper locations. Bamboo would serve as cover within ravines, and the *Pinus Sinensis*, as with other coniferous trees, 'would succeed well in almost any situation, from the tops of the hills down to the level of the sea'. 'I have no doubt,' he concluded, 'that trees and shrubs would exert a powerful *Mechanical* and *Chemical* influence on the *air* of the Island, preventing in a great degree that *reflection* which is so disagreeable and injurious to health, and rendering it more fit for the purpose of respiration.'[158]

Despite Davis's willing ear, Fortune would repeatedly appeal to the colony's government over the following years, imploring them to adopt his arboreal programme of reafforesting the island. But it would take some time before the natural environment reached a level of growth that could provide a degree of coolness and shade that Hong Kong Island would eventually become accustomed to. Nearly five years later, William Morrison, Hong Kong's new colonial surgeon, would strongly defend Fortune's neglected vision in his 1849 Blue Book report.

> Every man who plants and nurtures a tree or shrub, nurtures his own existence; he is unconsciously acting in obedience to the sanitary laws of nature: he is, in the exercise of a simple and refined pleasure, creating a safe vent for the noxious residue of his own respiration, and the source of a life-invigorating gas. It is much to be regretted that the Government, in apportioning the building sites in Victoria, did not encourage and enforce the formation of gardens.[159]

Morrison would put this belief into practice by planting a grove of bamboo along the ground south of the Murray Barracks, whose military inhabitants (as will be recounted in the next chapter) suffered terribly from malaria during a contained outbreak in 1848. The waving fronds of this fast-growing grass were believed by many to directly improve the health of the resident soldiers, if it was to be believed, by the action of disturbing the surrounding air.[160]

Nevertheless, even by late 1845, Victoria had transformed itself into a settlement that caused many arrivals to marvel. When Imperial Commissioner Qiying made his second and final trip to the colony on 20 November that year, there was sufficient confidence among residents that the altered state of the city since his last visit would both surprise and delight the old official, as indeed it did.[161] The *Friend of China* purred, 'what with the increased observation of British character he will thus obtain—together with the greatly altered and improved appearance of the Island, since his last visit . . . a large and handsome Town has risen'.[162]

The *Hongkong Register* was one of a few critics to point out that Hong Kong had indeed improved dramatically since Qiying's last visit, especially the architecture of commerce. 'But while such displays of private enterprise cannot fail to attract his attention, what must be the opinion of the proceedings of our government . . . what a contrast to this is exhibited by the Civil department. . . . The public buildings for them are in a worse state than at his last visit.'[163] So too, it complained, were the state of the roads. 'The portion of the Queen's Road opposite the new buildings intended for Officers Quarters is the most rugged on the whole line.'[164] Murdoch Bruce, responsible for the highway, honestly captured this embarrassing stretch in front of the Officers' Quarters in one of his lithographs, compelled to seek the gritty to meet his picturesque objectives (**fig. 5.11**).

Qiying, carried aloft in his sedan chair, was perhaps less observant of the potholes. But there was another, a minor Chinese official in his retinue, who marvelled at the sight of the city. A man named Tung, a poet and scholar, was moved to write a 'sonnet' on board

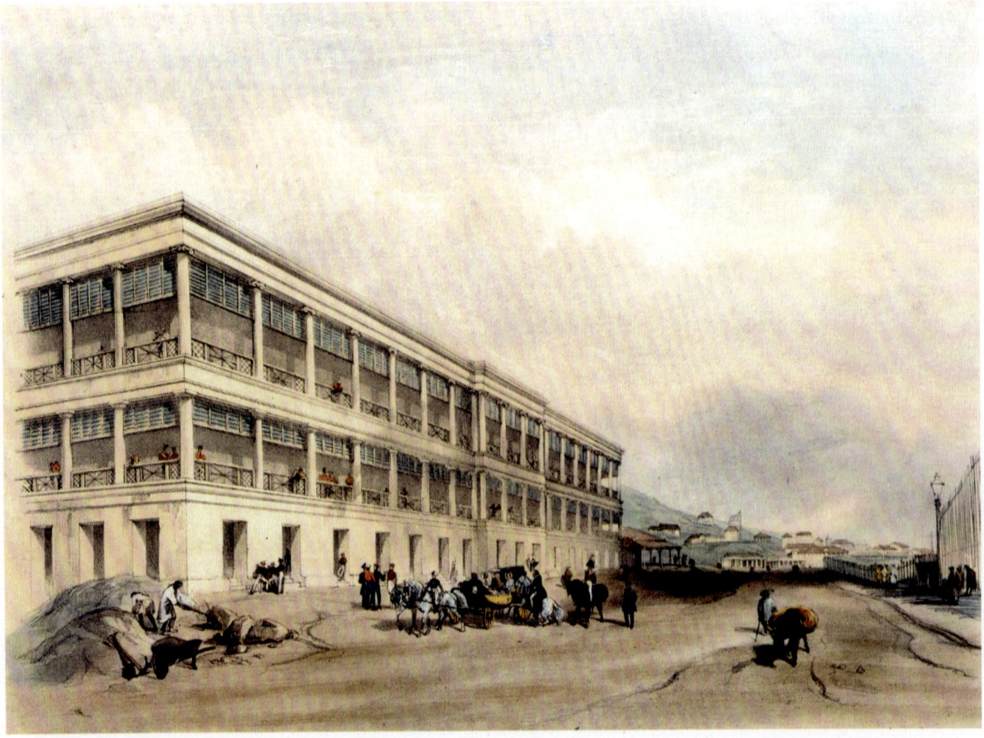

Fig. 5.11. M. Bruce, *The Officer's Quarters Looking Towards Victoria*, 1846. Coloured lithograph. © Hong Kong Museum of Art Collection (AH1964.0389.006).

the steamer *Vixen* as he travelled back to Canton (Guangzhou), his eyes transfixed upon the fading palaces tumbling down the hillsides. It was translated on the spot, most likely, by the Hong Kong Chinese Secretary, the Lutheran missionary Karl Gützlaff.

> I gaze upon yonder royal white city, on the high cliffs, while the shades of evening gather round it. There it stands, lonely as a palace built upon a rock.
>
> The sun has disappeared beneath the waves, but my lingering eyes still turn to it with straining fondness. The southern stars that gleam upon its snow-white walls look beautiful and bright as glittering flowers.
>
> And now I sleep with bitterness, and as I sink upon my pillow, the splendid town is present to me still. I behold even in my sleep the fragrant incense urn dispensing its thousand gushing streams over the mountains, while the city's white abodes seem glittering in the morning sun.[165]

> . . . The scene is changed—The bright moon issues from the parting clouds, and spangles with her light the feathery bamboo and the shrubby jessarmine, that overarch the islet's thousand habitations; and soon the silent morning sun starts from her golden sleep, and sheds a liquid lustre on the rocky steeps that bear aloft a thousand glittering and spacious mansions.
>
> Yet on this spot ere-while were only to be seen the hovels of the roving fishermen. Where are they?—gone like the swallows of departed autumn![166]

Hong Kong had survived repeated onslaughts of malaria. Indeed, the supposed miasma was thought to hang along its lower reaches, causing newer properties to climb ever upwards. The settlement had also survived subsequent attacks by government officials, foreign observers, exploitative practices, arson and other fires, unhygienic sewers, insubstantial roads and drains, and poor buildings. During these three years, from the last months of Pottinger's administration to the first years of Davis's, the city gained a form and dignity hitherto unimaginable. It was undoubtedly true that below this surface remained a rough, unresolved set of severe municipal and economic problems, particularly an inequitable relationship between the commercial and governmental forces of the island colony that would only be resolved in 1847 and 1848 by a parliamentary inquiry and the replacement of a governor. Trade remained stagnant, and the social neglect of the principal constituents of Hong Kong, the Chinese community, was deplorably apparent. But, through reasons always self-motivated, often unethical, and occasionally blinkered, various physical programmes merged to produce a settlement of now notable civic appearance and character. As a result, this new city began to imprint itself upon its ramshackle collection of citizens in a first attempt at an urban 'Hong Kong' identity.

Notes

1 National Library of Australia [hereafter NLA]; Mfm M602, Papers of Edward Ashworth (File 3), Notebook from 8 May 1844, entry undated (ca. July 1844).

2 Hong Kong Public Records Office [hereafter HKPRO]; file: HKMS 140-1-1, 'Transcripts of Correspondence of Lieut. Thomas Bernard Collinson R.E. Dec. 1838–29 Mar. 1846' [hereafter 'Transcripts'], T. B. Collinson, Hong Kong, to Rev. J. Collinson, Boldon Rectory, Gateshead, 22 Jan. 1846.

3 Edward Cree, *Naval Surgeon: The Voyages of Dr. Edward H. Cree, Royal Navy, as Related in His Private Journals, 1837–1856*, ed. Michael Levien (New York: E. P. Dutton, 1982), 142, 179.

4 *Canton Register*, 12 Jan. 1841.

5 *Canton Register*, 19 Jan. 1841.

6 *Canton Press*, 15 May 1841.

7 G. B. Endacott, *A Biographical Sketch-Book of Early Hong Kong* (Singapore: Eastern Universities Press, 1962), 72.

8 Ibid. See also Frank H. H. King, 'Martin, Robert Montgomery', *Oxford Dictionary of National Biography*, vol. 36 (Oxford: Oxford University Press, 2004), 974.

9 Ibid.

10 *Friend of China*, 8 May 1844. Included in the retinue were F. Bruce, Colonial Secretary; R. D. Cay, Registrar; Mr. Mercer, private Secretary to the Governor; and Mr. Shelly, Auditor.

11 *Friend of China*, 20 Apr. 1844.

12 As stated at the beginning of the article.

13 Ibid.

14 Ibid. My belief that this article was planted by Martin is further strengthened by his own inclusion of this same article in his printed collection to Parliament in 1846 entitled *Reports, Minutes and Despatches, on the British Position and Prospects in China*, whereby Heyne's account forms a footnote for his arguments on the 'rotten granite' of Hong Kong. See The National Archives, Kew [hereafter NA]; Colonial Office [hereafter CO] 129/18: 465–466.

15 *Friend of China*, 23 Aug. 1845; *China Mail*, 4 Sep. 1845 (Advertisement dated 21 Aug. 1845).

16 Ibid.

17 *Friend of China*, 25 May 1844. First part of Martin's essay.

18 *Friend of China*, 1 June 1844. Concluding part of Martin's essay.

19 Ibid.

20 CO 129/6: 302, Davis to Stanley, 29 June 1844.

21 CO 129/6: 306–306a, Martin to Davis, 17 June 1844.

22 Ibid., 307a.

23 Ibid., 309a.

24 Ibid., 311–311a.

25 Ibid., 313a.

26 Ibid., 313a–314.

27 *Friend of China*, 7 June 1844.

28 CO 129/6: 318a, Davis to Stanley, 2 July 1844.

29 CO 129/6: 375–376, Davis to Stanley, 2 July 1844.

30 Ibid., 376.

31 CO 129/7: 49–93. Included as part of the correspondence of Davis to Stanley.

32 CO 129/7: 50a, 'Physical Aspect', *Report on the Island of Hong Kong*.

33 Ibid., 51–51a, 'Geology'.

34 Ibid., 53a, 'Climate'.

35 Ibid., 55, 'Diseases and Mortality'.

36 Ibid., 55–55a.

37 Ibid., 55, 58a, 59–60.

38 CO 129/7: 44–44a, Davis to Stanley, 2 July 1844.

39 Ibid., 45a.

40 Ibid., 47.

41 CO 129/7: 102–102a, Davis to Stanley, 26 Aug. 1844.
42 CO 129/7: 239–240, Davis to Stanley, 25 Nov. 1844.
43 CO 129/11: 253–263, Davis to Stanley, 13 Apr. 1845.
44 Ibid., 253a.
45 CO 129/11: 277a, Davis to Stanley, 25 Apr. 1845.
46 Ibid., 278.
47 Ibid., 278–278a.
48 Ibid., 278a–279.
49 Ibid., 280a.
50 Ibid., 281.
51 Ibid., 281a.
52 Ibid., 287a.
53 *Friend of India*, 31 July 1845, as reprinted in the *Hongkong Register*, 9 Sep. 1845.
54 Ibid. The *Friend of India* referred to the 26th Regiment of the Cameronians, though it has its year confused, meaning to say 1840 rather than, as it stated, 1841.
55 *Englishman*, 2 Aug. 1845, as reprinted in the *Hongkong Register*, 7 Oct. 1845.
56 *Bombay Times*, 13 Aug. 1845, as reprinted in the *Hongkong Register*, 4 Nov. 1845.
57 *Englishman*, 17 Sep. 1845, as reprinted in the *Hongkong Register*, 4 Nov. 1845.
58 Extract from the *Monthly Times*, 7 Jan. 1845, as recorded in the *Friend of China 'Extra'*, 14 Apr. 1845.
59 *Friend of China*, 26 Nov. 1845.
60 Ibid.
61 *Hongkong Register*, 16 Dec. 1845.
62 CO 129/12: 221–221a, Martin to Davis, 18 June 1845.
63 Ibid., 222a–223.
64 Ibid., 226.
65 CO 129/12: 270–271, Martin to Davis, 8 July 1845.
66 *Canton Press*, 16 Mar. 1844.
67 Christopher Munn, 'The Chusan Episode: Britain's Occupation of a Chinese Island, 1840–46', *The Journal of Imperial and Commonwealth History*, vol. 25, no. 1 (Jan 1997): 105–106.
68 *Hongkong Register*, 30 June 1846.
69 Ibid.
70 *Hongkong Register*, 11 Aug. 1846.
71 *Friend of China*, 2 Nov. 1843, as recorded in the *Canton Press*, 4 Nov. 1843.
72 Ibid.
73 Ibid.
74 *Friend of China*, 27 July 1844.
75 D'Aguilar arrived with his personal staff on H.M.S. *Castor* on 27 Dec. 1843, as announced in the *Canton Press*, 30 Dec. 1843. For the date of his arrival see the *Canton Press*, 6 Jan. 1844.
76 CO 129/10: 621a–622, Minutes of Woosnam (Pottinger) at the Executive Council, 22 Jan. 1844.
77 Ibid., 622.
78 Ibid., 621–621a.
79 CO 129/5: 124a, Captain Henry D'Aguilar, Assistant Military Secretary (AMS) to D'Aguilar, to Woosnam (Pottinger), 9 Feb. 1844.

80 Colin Crisswell, *The Taipans: Hong Kong's Merchant Princes* (Hong Kong: Oxford University Press, 1981), 99. William Lane went on to join his brother Thomas Lane and Ninian Crawford's ship's chandlers on the Queen's Road, becoming a partner of 'Lane Crawford' in 1860. Ibid., 99–100.
81 CO 129/5: 116a, Pottinger to Stanley, 10 Feb. 1844.
82 'Antihumbug' writing in the *Friend of China*, 22 June 1844.
83 *Friend of China*, 29 Mar. 1845 (Advertisement dated 14 Mar. 1845).
84 CO 129/5: 124a, Captain D'Aguilar, AMS, to Woosnam (Pottinger), 9 Feb. 1844.
85 CO 129/10: 644a, Woosnam (Pottinger) to Captain D'Aguilar, AMS, 8 Feb. 1844.
86 Ibid., 645a.
87 CO 129/10: 623a, Minutes of Pottinger to the Executive Council, 24 Jan. 1844.
88 CO 129/10: 627a–628, Woosnam (Pottinger) to Captain D'Aguilar, AMS, 26 Jan. 1844.
89 CO 129/10: 674–674a, Woosnam (Pottinger) to Captain D'Aguilar, AMS, 26 Feb. 1844. See NA; MPH 1/867 (extracted from WO 44/68), for survey plans converting Mr. Edgar's House as barracks and a battery, Sai Ying Pun, dated 22 July 1854 and 14 Feb. 1855.
90 Ibid., 674a.
91 National Maritime Museum, Greenwich, London [hereafter NMM]; CRJ/8, Private Journal of E. H. Cree, 4 Mar. 1844.
92 CO 129/10: 772, Woosnam (Pottinger) to Caine, 1 May 1844.
93 CO 129/6: 149a, Anderson to Davis, 15 June 1844.
94 Ibid., 150.
95 Ibid., 150–150a.
96 Ibid., 155.
97 CO 129/7: 168–169, Davis to Stanley, 2 Nov. 1844.
98 *Friend of China*, 10 July 1844.
99 Ibid.
100 Ibid.
101 Ibid.
102 CO 129/7: 23a, Davis to Stanley, 16 Aug. 1844.
103 Ibid.
104 *Friend of China*, 31 Aug. 1844 (Advertisement dated 30 Aug. 1844).
105 As referred to in paragraph XV of D'Aguilar's 'Rules' to troops in the event of an outbreak of fire in the city. See *China Mail*, 20 Nov. 1845.
106 *Friend of China*, 28 May 1845.
107 *Hongkong Register*, 27 May 1845.
108 *Friend of China*, 28 May 1845.
109 HKPRO; 'Transcripts', T. B. Collinson, Hong Kong, to Rev. J. Collinson, Boldon Rectory, Gateshead, 17 Aug. 1845.
110 *Friend of China*, 28 May 1845.
111 Ibid.
112 *China Mail*, 11 Sep 1845. Notice dated 5 Sep. 1845.
113 *Friend of China*, 28 May 1845.
114 *Friend of China*, 24 Sep. 1845.
115 *China Mail*, 9 Oct. 1845.

116 *Friend of China*, 1 Nov. 1845.

117 *Hongkong Register*, 12 May 1846.

118 CO 129/16: 236a–237, D'Aguilar to Gladstone, 25 Apr. 1846.

119 CO 129/17: 38a, D'Aguilar to Gladstone, 25 Apr. 1846.

120 Ibid., 236.

121 *Friend of China*, 22 Sep. 1846. Advertisements dated 11 Aug. 1846 and 26 July 1846 respectively.

122 James Legge, 'The Colony of Hong Kong—From a Lecture by the Rev. James Legge, D.D., L.L.D., on Reminiscences of a Long Residence in the East, Delivered in the City Hall, November 5, 1872', *China Review*, vol. 3 (1874): 164.

123 *Friend of China*, 9 Jan. 1844.

124 *Friend of China*, 8 June 1844.

125 *Friend of China*, 30 Oct. 1844. Advertisement dated 22 Oct. 1844.

126 *Friend of China*, 21 June 1845. Advertisement undated.

127 'Art. IV. Record of criminals, European and Chinese, lodged in jails at Hongkong, from 9th of August, 1841, to the 18th of September 1843', *Chinese Repository*, vol. 12, no. 10 (Oct. 1843): 534–535.

128 Ibid.

129 'Mid Levels' is now more precisely thought of as the area above (south) of Caine Road, though it should be considered historically as an organic extension of an original settlement below, now known since recent years as the 'SoHo' district (meaning 'South of Hollywood Road').

130 *Friend of China*, 1 Jan. 1845.

131 *Friend of China*, 8 Feb. 1845.

132 *Friend of China*, 5 Apr. 1845. Advertisement by Hughesdon & Co., undated.

133 *Friend of China*, 19 July 1845. Advertisement dated 18 July 1845.

134 *Friend of China*, 23 July 1845. Advertisement dated 18 July 1845.

135 Ibid.

136 *Friend of China*, 13 Aug. 1845. Advertisement dated 1 July 1845.

137 *Friend of China*, 20 Aug. 1845. As advertised by N. Duus and dated 19 Aug. 1845.

138 *Friend of China*, 20 Sep. 1845. As advertised by W. H. Franklyn and dated 2 Sep. 1845.

139 *Friend of China*, 26 Nov. 1845. Advertisement dated 18 Oct. 1845.

140 *China Mail*, 18 Dec. 1845. As advertised by Arthur Carlin and dated 5 Nov. 1845.

141 *China Mail*, 5 Feb. 1846. Advertisement dated 29 Jan. 1846.

142 Ibid.

143 *London Evening Mail*, 29 Sep. 1845. As reprinted in the *Hongkong Register*, 12 May 1846.

144 *Hongkong Register*, 21 Jan. 1845. Advertisement dated 29 Nov. 1844.

145 *Englishman*, 2 Dec. 1845. As reprinted in the *Hongkong Register*, 10 Feb. 1846.

146 Ibid.

147 Ibid.

148 *Hongkong Register*, 3 Sep. 1844.

149 Ibid.

150 *China Mail*, 5 Feb. 1846. Advertisement dated 24 Jan. 1846.

151 *Friend of China*, 13 June 1846. Advertisement dated 11 June 1846.

152 Cambridge University Library, Jardine Matheson Archives [hereafter JMA]; C6/3, A. Matheson to James Adam Smith, Manila (Macau, 13 Feb. 1843).

153 *Friend of China*, 7 June 1845. As advertised by W. H. Franklyn, undated.

154 Robert Fortune, *A Journey to the Tea Districts of China* (London: John Murray, 1852), 6.

155 Robert Fortune to Frederick Bruce, Colonial Secretary, Hong Kong, 9 Dec. 1844, as reprinted in the *China Mail*, 8 May 1845.

156 'We believe that during the last two years and a half he [Fortune] has sent to the Horticultural Society of London about seventy glazed cases full of living plants, besides a large collection of dried specimens both of plants and animals. . . . He has had the gratification before leaving China to learn that a good many of the cases have arrived safely, and that comparatively few plants have perished on the long voyage.' *Hongkong Register*, undated, as reprinted in the *China Mail*, 1 Jan. 1846.

157 Ibid.

158 Ibid.

159 CO 133/6: 99a, William Morrison, 'REPORT of the COLONIAL SURGEON on the Diseases and Climate of Hong Kong, 1849', *Hong Kong Blue Book: 1849*, 25 Mar. 1850.

160 James Legge, 'The Colony of Hong Kong', 166.

161 'As the *Vixen* approached Hongkong, the changed appearance of the place since he last saw it, struck Keying with surprise', *China Mail*, 4 Dec. 1845.

162 *Friend of China*, 22 Nov. 1843.

163 *Hongkong Register*, 7 Oct. 1845.

164 *Hongkong Register*, 18 Nov. 1845.

165 The translator notes that 'Hongkong in Chinese signifies the *Urn of fragrant streams*'.

166 Tung's 'Sonnet', *China Mail*, 11 Dec. 1845.

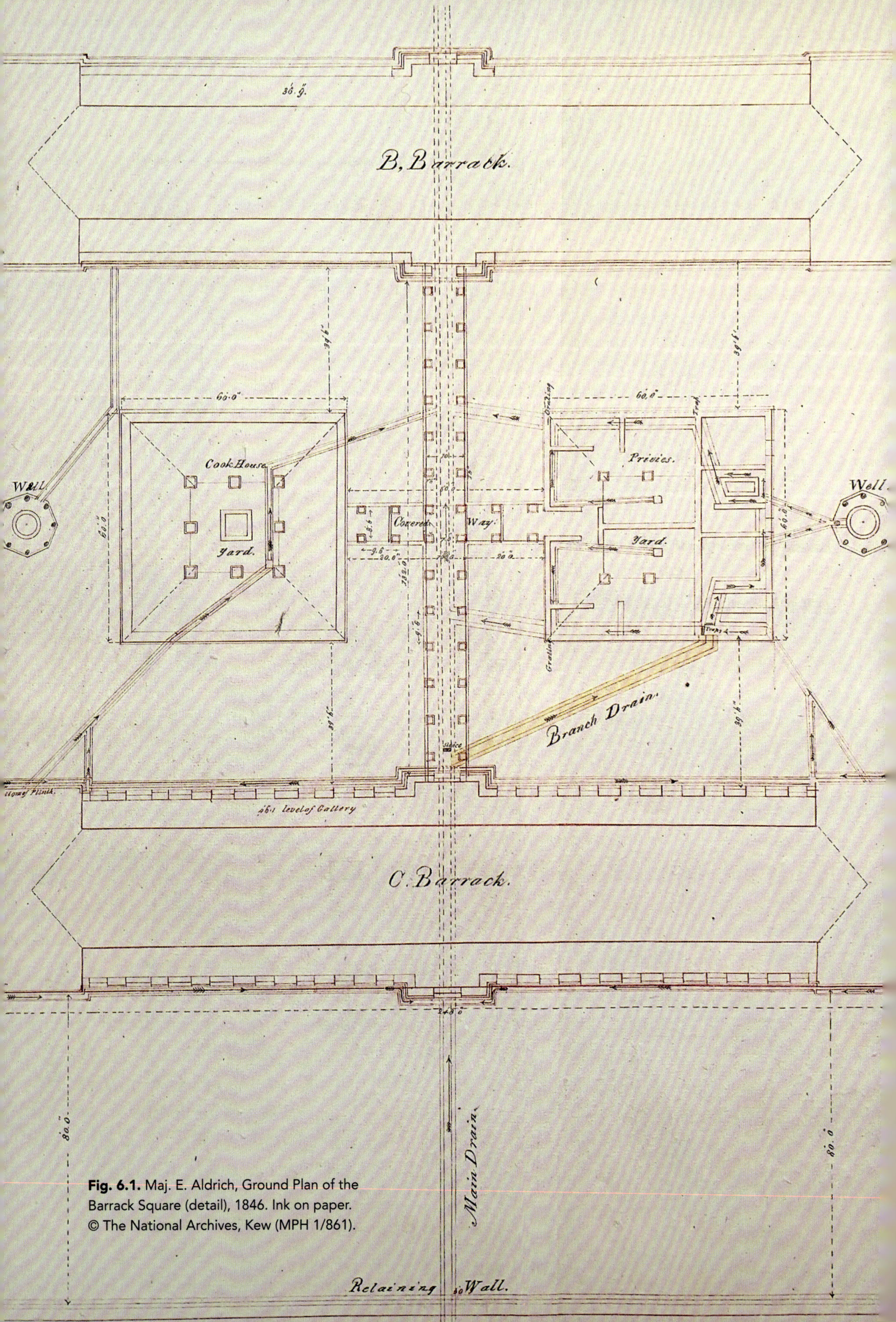

Fig. 6.1. Maj. E. Aldrich, Ground Plan of the Barrack Square (detail), 1846. Ink on paper. © The National Archives, Kew (MPH 1/861).

CHAPTER 6

An Outbreak in Miniature, 1847–1849

In March 1847, 195 troops from the 95th or Derbyshire Regiment of Foot journeyed to Hong Kong from Ceylon (Sri Lanka). They were being sent to the colony to replace the long-serving 18th Regiment.[1] The two ships conveying them were small and typically overcrowded. One ship, the *Minerva*, carried a complement of 13 officers, 20 sergeants, 10 drummers, 16 corporals, and 330 privates, together with 18 wives and 29 children.[2] Part of Major Edward Aldrich's Murray Barracks remained incomplete. Soldiers were scattered and billeted, including many put within a makeshift barracks at Central that used to be Gillespie's famous set of warehouses. Conversions for military use were commonplace. So, on arrival, the military passengers of the other ship, the *Castle Eden*, were placed in the Albany Barracks, a long row of four houses initially intended for civil government officials built high up behind Government Hill. Some were also put in Keying House, a new building by the public landing place that Imperial Commissioner Qiying occupied during his 1845 visit.[3]

Aldrich's project took nearly one more year to complete. But by January 1848, the 95th could, at last, be housed in the completed Murray Barracks 'ranges' (or blocks) 'B' and 'C': two parallel, long rectangular buildings that marched up the hill above the Officers' Quarters and the military hospital below, with Range 'C' placed above 'B' and against the mountainside. Aldrich conceived of the Murray Barracks—the Officers' Quarters and Ranges B and C—as a united complex, threaded together by the umbilical chord of a descending, central covered link placed above the main drain. This sheltered passage–drain connected the kitchens (cookhouse) and toilets (privies) to the barracks, providing continuous cover in order to prevent a soldier's exposure to the sun or rain (**figs. 6.1** and **6.2**). The final relocation of troops into the Murray Barracks coincided with the arrival of

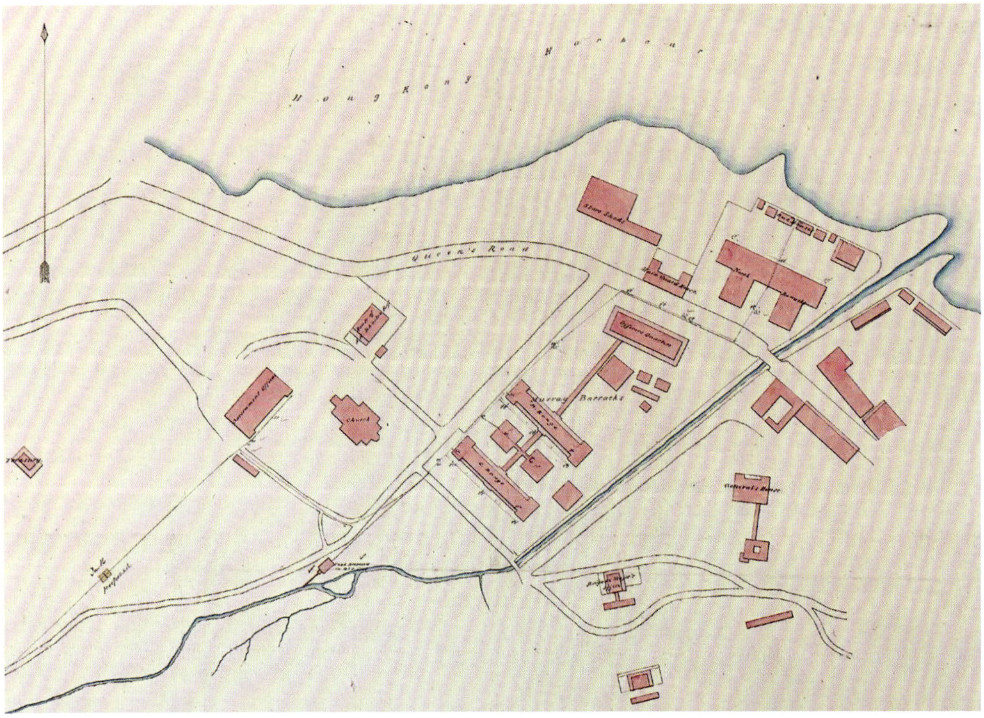

Fig. 6.2. Lt. J. J. Wilson, 'Plan of Part of the Cantonments at Victoria, Hong Kong', 1850. Pen and wash on paper. © The National Archives, Kew (MFQ 1/962).

the new major-general-cum-lieutenant-governor, William Staveley, in late January 1848. He replaced Major-General D'Aguilar, whose departure was marked by a ball held at the Officers' Mess (the principal dining and social space) within the lowest block of the Murray Barracks. This was the earliest to be completed and the grandest of the set, the Officers' Quarters.[4]

For the unfortunate 95th Regiment, the relative comfort of their new accommodation was to be short-lived. By May 1848, 44 men from the regiment had died of malarial fever, with a further 37 invalided. This outbreak started an all-too-familiar pattern that would imitate a similar curve of mortality experienced across the same months during 1842 and 1843. In June, a further eight men succumbed. Then, in July, the mortality rate shot up to 37; and by August, the regiment lost another 47 soldiers. Four women and four children also died.[5] August was the worst month, with subsequent numbers of cases sharply dropping as the days began to cool.

When the *China Mail* eventually published these findings, an odd thing became apparent. Despite several different regiments present in the barracks, the majority of cases comprised members of the 95th Regiment.[6] Many of these patients would later die in hospital beds.[7] However, when military investigators attempted to trace back the cases to their barrack locations, there was a considerable shock. Instead of a general spread, precise spatial positions within the brand-new and substantially built complex, those 'excellent and ample quarters' lauded by Davis in mid-1845 could be pinpointed as containing the highest mortality rates. It was as if an island-wide terrain of fear that had gripped the Hong Kong population from 1841 to 1844 had shrunk into a peculiarly minute world of rooms within a single pair of barrack blocks—an outbreak in miniature.

This short, concluding study is an account of the remedial measures prescribed and debated over, centred on this outbreak, and is used to illustrate just how far discourses, views, and scepticisms had evolved within and without the Hong Kong military community since the Fever of 1843. It will also serve as an epilogue to this journey, the medical education of Hong Kong residents manifested in the first crafting of their city.

The 1848 Barrack Fever

The position and orientation of the Murray Barracks was not a new controversy; it had been debated once before. In a strangely prescient article written in late 1845, months before the first phase of the barracks—the Officers' Quarters—was completed, the *Friend of China* made a prediction.

> The site chosen for the military buildings with the exception of the Hospital and the General's house—is in our opinion a bad one. Standing on a low, and formerly a swampy piece of ground, in front of an amphitheatre of hills, the water from which finds an escape through the hollow in which they are placed, it appears to us that the position is not one favourable to health, as the buildings with every precaution to draining, will be damp at the very season they ought to be dry. Our opinion may not have much weight, when opposed to that of such an experienced Officer as General D'Aguilar, but time will prove whether it is correct or not.[8]

The newspaper also considered the orientation and tight clustering of the three blocks of buildings to be a grave mistake.

> The arrangement of the buildings also, we think, bad. They are in three ranges immediately behind each other facing the N.E. and S.W. During the N.E. monsoon, the front row will have the full benefit of a bracing wind, the second row will be partly deprived of it by the hills, the third will have little or none. In the S.W. monsoon, any slight breeze that may find its way through the gorge of the hills will only benefit the back row; the other two being in a dead calm in a low damp valley.[9]

When malaria eventually struck in 1848, it caught the new regime by surprise. Staveley ordered an inquiry. In the meantime, the Board of Ordnance in London initiated corresponding investigations. This correspondence was collected into a short folio and placed within the War Office and entitled 'Hong Kong Murray Barracks—unhealthiness of—alterations. Sketches *From Ordnance Correspondence Barracks (Foreign) Eastern 1849*'.[10] A letter from Lieutenant Colonel John Walter, dated Hong Kong, 30 June 1848, seemed to have been the first notice the colony recorded of a growing crisis.[11] Staveley had now placed Walter in charge of the barracks and men of the 95th. Walter's superiors would later praise him for the 'unremitting manner he has watched over the discipline, interior economy, comfort and well-being of the Regiment since the command of it has devolved upon him'.[12] On 5 July, a board of medical officials met at the barracks and examined several suspected rooms and those adjoining. Staveley then wrote to the master-general and Board of Ordnance on 21 July with their preliminary findings.[13]

On 11 October, the Board of Ordnance met in London to discuss the 'sickness which has prevailed in the Murray Barracks at Victoria, Hong Kong whilst occupied by the 95th Regt. and on the state of the Ablution Rooms; as well as the Huts adjacent to that Barracks'.[14] The Board had received no information from the new commanding Royal Engineer in Hong Kong, Lieutenant-Colonel George Phillpotts. So, the inspector-general of fortifications (or IGF), now Major-General Sir John Fox Burgoyne, sought the advice of the man who might know the situation best, the barrack designer himself, Major Edward Aldrich. Aldrich had returned to England in 1847 and was now the commanding Royal Engineer of the 'London District'. This outbreak must have been of great embarrassment to Aldrich, and he was obliged to set out a prompt and detailed reply. Dated 21 October, his careful set of observations would form the basis of further discussion with Hong Kong's military leading to a series of measures, some of which would be priced and acted upon the following year. Notably, there had been growing confidence in the general health of the colony since 1845. The barrack sickness was in danger of dissolving this

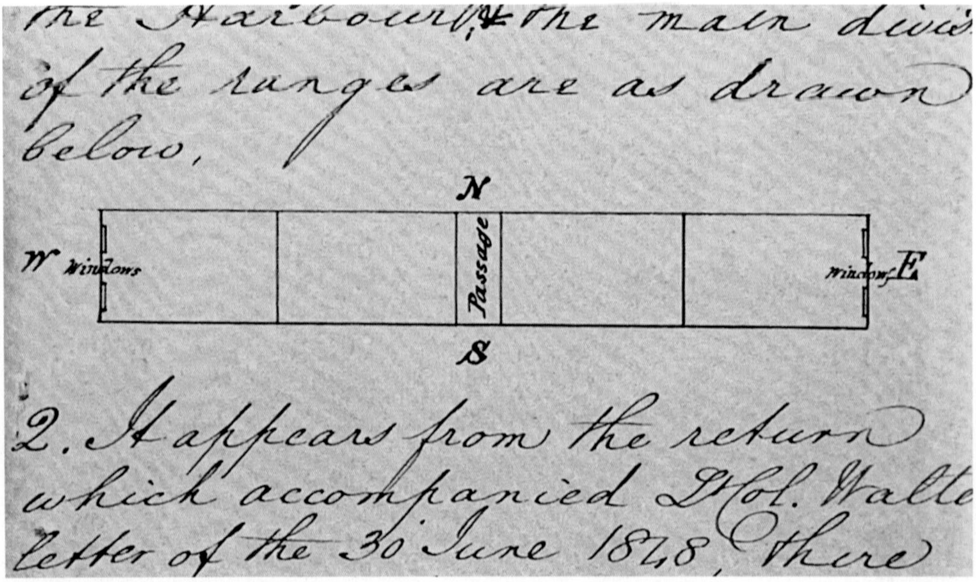

Fig. 6.3. Maj. E. Aldrich, Plan Diagram of the B or C Ranges, 1848. Ink on paper. © The National Archives, Kew (WO 44/594).

recent optimism and fear of its fragile containment was becoming an acute political and economic threat. Nevertheless, the localised measures believed by both Aldrich and subsequently his replacement as architect–engineer, Lieutenant-Colonel Phillpotts, to rectify and make safe the situation reveals new-found confidence in the application of specific procedures and technologies to the problem of malaria.

This letter, the first of three that Aldrich would formally address to the IGF on the issue, was in response to the quarter master general's letter of 9 October.[15] In his analysis, Aldrich noted two critical locations where the malarial fever was present within the blocks. To help illustrate this, he first sketched the anatomy of the identical B and C ranges of barracks—a plan indicating the source of the outbreak (**fig. 6.3**).

Using statistical data gleaned from the medical records, Aldrich noticed that sickness within the B and C ranges of barracks had been confined to two precise areas. The first and most afflicted area was on the lowest level through, as he argued, the 'improper occupation of the rooms in the Basement [ground] Floor', which had been used as quarters for the staff sergeants. This use was not part of Aldrich's design intent. He had designed the ground floor to be free of human occupancy at night.[16] Second in extent of seriousness seemed to be the first-floor dormitories at the gable ends of the buildings that had been placed above the 'Washing or Ablution Rooms'. These spaces saw significantly more sickness than those rooms in the middle of each block (**fig. 6.4**). In his sketch, Aldrich noted that these ends contained an additional pair of windows and which would, therefore, 'receive a much greater body of miasma than the occupation of the latter rooms'.[17] The problem, as he saw it, was that soldiers threw open the windows and the protective jalousies 'to obtain every breath of air' at night, placing their lives in jeopardy. Understandably, he refused to agree with Phillpotts and Staveley that the cause may have been dampness within the washrooms below from rooms 'contiguous to the Ablution Rooms' (**fig. 6.5**). Such an acknowledgement would have implied negligence.[18] Inconveniently, each range's floor plans lodged in London's War Office explicitly showed a pair of communicating stairs directly linking the washrooms to the troublesome gable ends of the dormitory rooms above.

Aldrich recommended two solutions, something he would add to later, 'derived from residence in the West Indies'.[19] The first seemed straightforward: to keep the gable windows and the lower division of windows on the south side (the mountain-facing side) of the C Range firmly closed from sunset to sunrise. The second suggestion was somewhat more peculiar. Aldrich believed that the nearby firing of an artillery gun twice a day with blank rounds would positively affect the nature of the air around the barracks rendering it less harmful.

> I have spoken of the stagnation of air of the Climate at Hong Kong during the S.W. Monsoon, & I beg to remark that any circumstance even theoretically that may induce the impure air of miasma to mix with the pure air, without incurring expense, must be considered advantageous to be adopted, and therefore I am of opinion looking to a practice followed in the East Indies, that of the morning & evening Gun during the S.W. Monsoon at Hong Kong were fired at a convenient position to the rear of the Barracks, & against the side of the Hill rising immediately behind the Barrack, it might conduce by the concussion of air thus obtained in that locality, to produce the beneficial result required.[20]

This remarkable recommendation would be treated with utmost seriousness by both the Treasury and the War Office and was described by them as one of 'several simple and inexpensive solutions'.[21]

Phillpotts eventually wrote to London, enclosing his own belief as to remedial approaches. He responded to Aldrich's thoughts, though in the main, he followed those of a new investigative panel of experts in Hong Kong who assembled on three separate occasions in March 1849. This panel had gathered at the request of the War Office, concerned that 'it is not shewn that any steps have been taken to trace the mortality consequent upon the occupation of these Barracks, whether attributable to their position or construction, or to circumstances of a local nature, capable of being remedied'.[22] Calling themselves the 'Board of Officers', they met on 7, 8, and 10 March. The board comprised of four doctors: Dr. Huntly George Gordon (assistant surgeon, 95th Regiment); Dr. John Newton (surgeon, Ceylon Rifles); Dr. W. Home (staff surgeon, 2nd class); and Dr. Andrew Fergusson (deputy inspector-general of hospitals). The board also included Lieutenant-Colonel John Walter (95th Regiment) and Lieutenant-Colonel Henry Simmonds (Ceylon Rifles), and was presided over by Phillpotts himself.[23]

The board revisited all the rooms previously inspected by the medical officers back in July. A 'cement skirting' had already been applied by Phillpotts to the damp washroom walls adjacent to the internal ground floor rooms and, together with improved drainage, this was thought sufficient to meet this problem.[24] The board's findings, based upon monthly statistics of the invalided during the summer of 1848, pieced together a detailed spatial survey, across both floor level and position, of sickness spreading through the B and C ranges (**fig. 6.6**). Statistics revealed that the number of men admitted to the military hospital was smaller in the B Barracks (the block constructed northwards and therefore nearer to the sea) than that of the C Barracks (southwards and closer to the rear hill). Twenty-seven men were admitted from B compared to thirty-seven from C in June, 114 compared to 181 in July, while in August, no comparative data was available as Staveley had, by then, instructed to evacuate most of the C Barracks.[25] Statistical 'returns' revealed more victims on the east side than on the west within the B Barracks, but about the same on both wings within the C Barracks. By these directional peculiarities, the board felt it could discount recent earthworks dug to form the parade ground to the west as the cause of the outbreak.[26] Upturned soil had long been thought to be a chief source of malaria in Hong Kong. This dismissal revealed a dramatic shift and open attentiveness to other causes by 1849. Likewise, more patients were observed to have been admitted to hospital who had slept on the first floor (that is, the middle floor) of the C Barracks than on its upper floor, whereas there was almost no difference in floors within the B Barracks.[27]

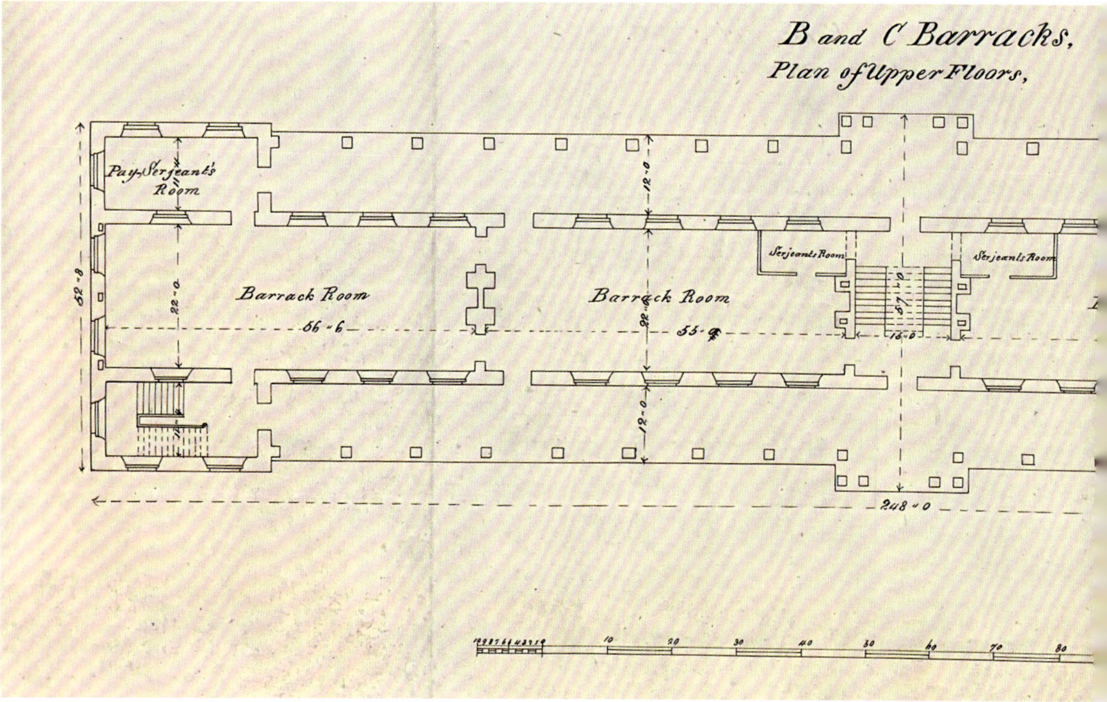
B and C Barracks,
Plan of Upper Floors,
Pay Serjeant's Room
Barrack Room
Barrack Room
Serjeants Room
Serjeants Room
52-8
22-0
12-0
56-6
248-0
16-0
10
20
30
40
50
60
70
80

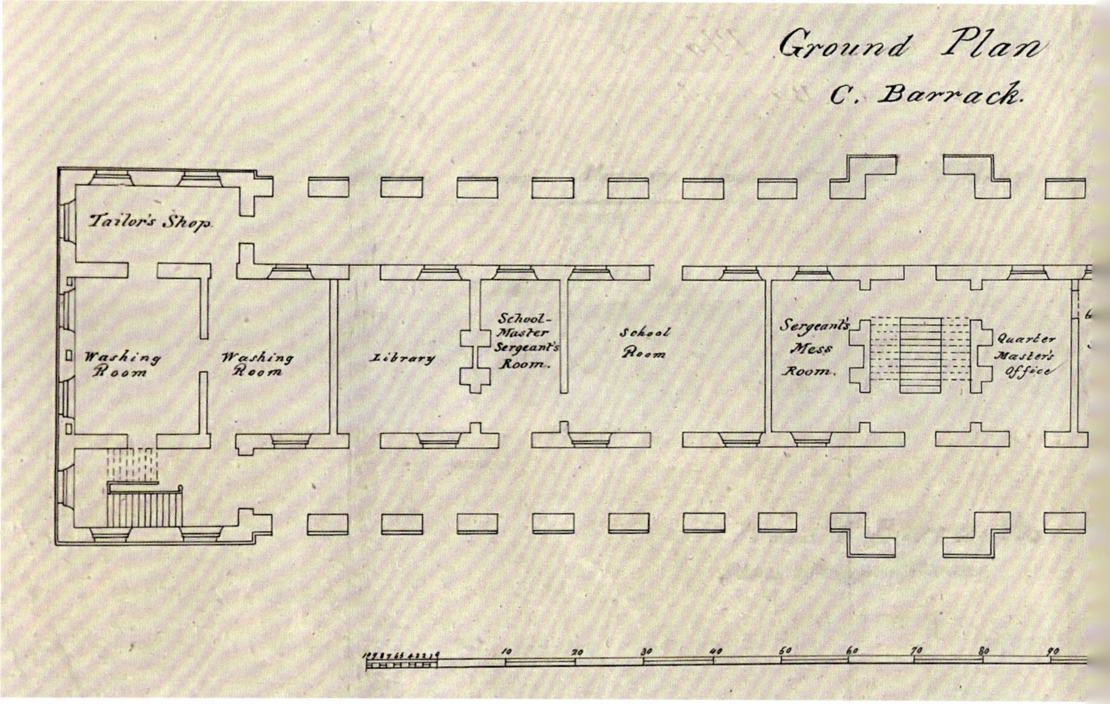
Ground Plan
C. Barrack.
Tailor's Shop
Washing Room
Washing Room
Library
School-Master Sergeant's Room.
School Room
Sergeant's Mess Room.
Quarter Master's Office
10
20
30
40
50
60
70
80
90

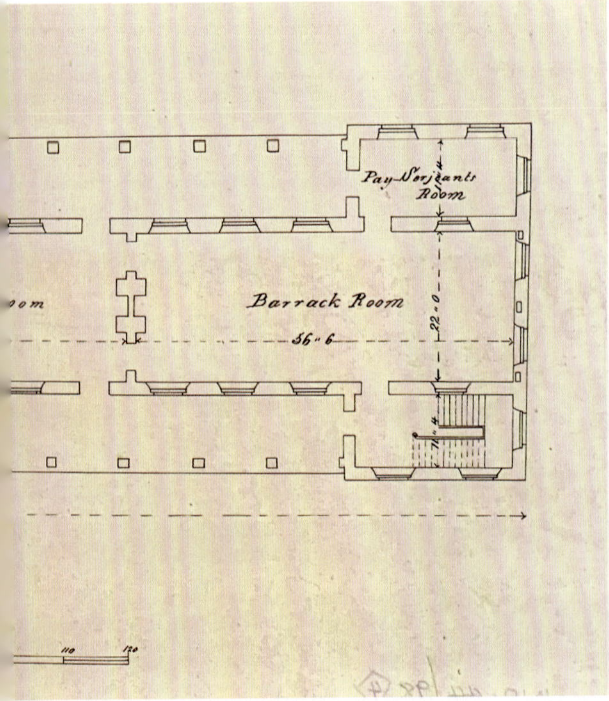

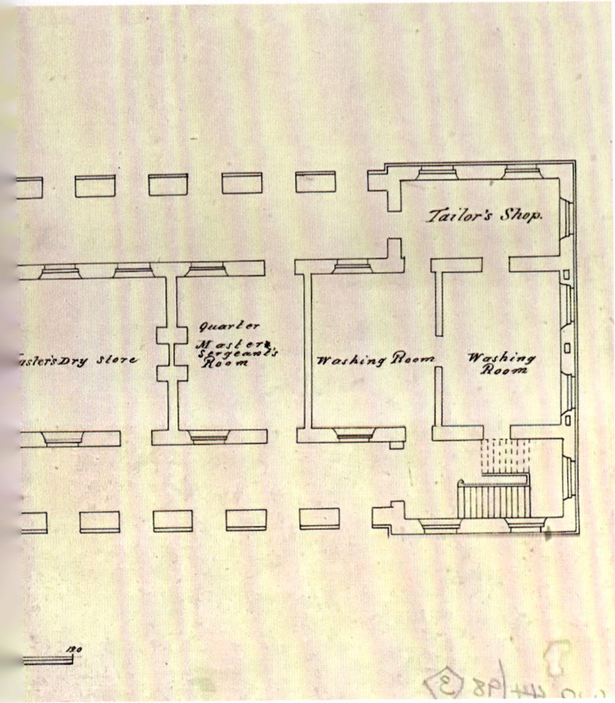

▲**Fig. 6.4.** Maj. E. Aldrich, 'B and C Barracks. Plan of Upper Floors', 1846. Ink on paper. © The National Archives, Kew (MFQ 1/37).

◄**Fig. 6.5.** Maj. E. Aldrich, 'Ground Plan. C Barracks', 1846. Ink on Paper. © The National Archives, Kew (MFQ 1/37).

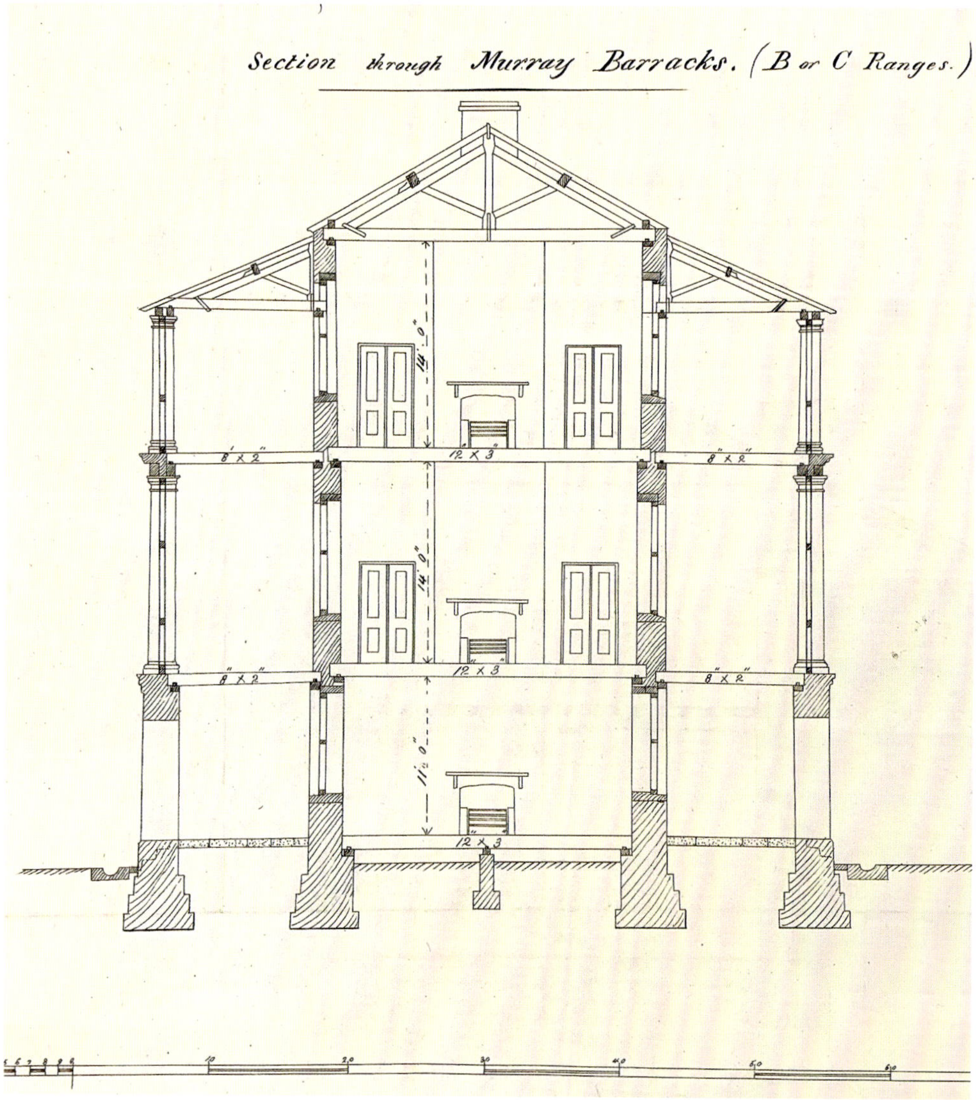

Fig. 6.6. Maj. E. Aldrich, 'Section Through Murray Barracks. B or C Ranges', 1846. Ink on paper. © The National Archives, Kew (MFQ 1/37).

The board also noted that the centres of both barrack ranges were healthier than at the ends. From this, they 'inferred the necessity of verandahs at the ends of the barracks and wire gauze to the end windows, as well as the South windows of the C Range'.[28] Major-General Fanshawe, assistant IGF, also thought wire gauze an appropriate measure.

'I am not aware of any better preventative,' he wrote to the secretary to the Ordnance in October 1848, 'than the use of wire gauze windows which prevents drafts and mitigates malaria without absolutely excluding a current of air.'[29] This fascinating approach to miasma protection, more so as there was absolutely no sense yet as to a relationship between malaria and mosquitoes, was now a standard remedial response for buildings in the tropics. The concept developed from medical theories about a preference for continuous perforation compared with ventilation derived from standard window openings, but it often came at a cost to the fabric of a building. The barrack master in Hong Kong, Colonel H. H. Farquharson, lamented the damage inflicted by this remedial practice. 'The General has at length decided in giving up Gillespie's Temporary Barracks,' he had written in consternation to Aldrich in March 1846. 'If so, something must be done to the upper room floors, which all those damned doctors of the 98th [Regiment] recommended to be perforated & bored through—all along the room over the passage!!! & which was executed by your department.—This in repairing will cost some dollars I guess.'[30]

One of the first to experiment with retrofitting wire-gauze to windows on barracks were captains Smyth and Brandreth, two Royal Engineers working in the West Indies in the 1830s. The use of wire gauze seems to have been first recommended to Brandreth by an army medical officer, Dr. Arthur, 'to mitigate the effect of marsh miasma'.[31] Smyth concurred,

> At the suggestion of Captain Brandreth, Royal Engineers, iron wire blinds were ordered to be tried in the new hospital at Demarara, and were demanded from England, but they were not supplied during the period I was in the colony. When referred to by Captain Brandreth on this subject, I fully concurred in the opinions he expressed, having for many years in my own quarters in Canada (at Isle aux Noix) and in Demarara, used frames of wood, with leno or mosquito net stretched on them in the opening both for windows and doors, not only with a view to exclude insects, but also to exclude the miasmata. In several hospitals in Italy fine wire gauze has been placed in the windows instead of glass, and it has proved efficacious in arresting the miasmatic current.[32]

Brandreth recounted the case in 1827 of a ship, the *Magnificient*, lying in the English harbour of Antigua, its occupants struck with 'marsh fever'. Medical officers found that one side of the vessel, 'the windward ports', admitted too much breeze, so much so that they covered patients in bunting, which relieved the situation. Brandreth surmised from this that 'it may be that the wire gauze simply sifts, or as it were dilutes the body of

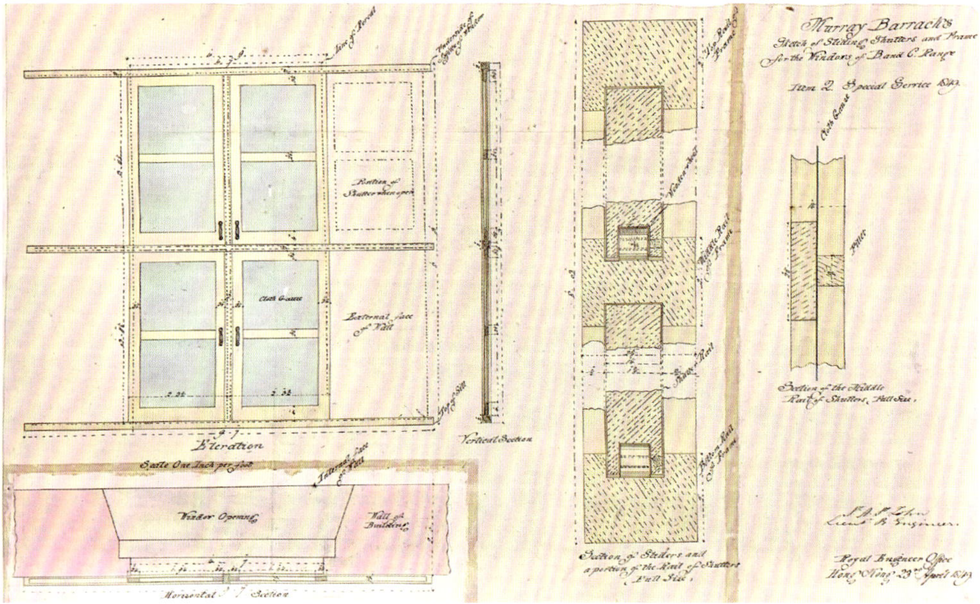

Fig. 6.7. Lt. S. A. St. John, 'Sketch of Sliding Shutters and Frame for the Windows of B and C Range', 1849. Pen and wash on paper. © The National Archives, Kew (MFQ 1/962).

malaria, and renders its operation on the human frame less obnoxious, when introduced in particles through the net-work, than in a compact stream through the open window'.[33] And so, through experimentation, he found that a mesh size of 1/24th of an inch proved the most effective and selected copper wire as this was the most resistant to saline action from the sea air.[34] Repurposing these findings for other regions, the British military later observed this gauge to match readily-available mosquito netting.

Such was the case in Hong Kong. Phillpotts and Staveley both considered retrofitting the barrack windows with mesh as one of two remedial items so essential to the ensured health of the troops that they did not wait for sanction from the Board of Ordnance in London (**fig. 6.7**).[35] In his 'Report and Estimate' for the 'Special Service No. 1', Phillpotts detailed how these panels of mesh fitted. 'The shutter to be filled in with Stout gauze or Musquito netting and secured by a fillet of wood nailed to the rebate of the shutter.'[36] As mosquito netting was used to 'sift' the gaseous miasma entering the window as if a tea strainer, the mesh material selected would be an inexpensive cloth rather than copper.

The board of officers at the Murray Barracks were able to condense their observations on this topography of sickness into one fascinatingly precise paragraph.

> It appears, however, that more men were admitted from the south side of C Barrack than from the north side, more from the north side of C Range than from the south side of B Range, and the smallest number from the north side of B Range; the number being 309, 165, 133 and 129—from which there is every reason to believe that the cause of the disease, whatever it may have been, originated to the southward of the Barracks—which is in some measure confirmed by the fact that in the Officers' Barracks, which are situated about 80 yards distant to the northward of B Range, only one case of fever occurred.[37]

Fig. 6.8 illustrates the relative distances and elevations across the Murray Barracks. An 'enclosing wall' to the westward end of the B and C ranges alongside the barrack yard (and not present by the Officers' Quarters) was believed to restrict the free circulation of air and so was recommended to be replaced by iron railings 'open to the surface of the ground'.[38] More strenuously recommended was the resurfacing of the ground immediately south of the C Range with a material called *chunam*. This material—the name derived from the Tamil word *cunnam* meaning lime or ground mortar—could be found on indigenous architecture in and around Madras. It had subsequently been appropriated for use across British India to simulate stone. It was made of burnt seashells and applied as stucco to 'shoddy brick and woodwork . . . to make it look like stone'.[39] For flooring, mixed with a stone aggregate, it could appear as terrazzo. The *chunam* or lime plaster, when polished, gave off an impressive sheen as if smooth marble. And it was this property that led to its use as a hygienic surfacing material, considered sheer and easy to clean. 'Chunaming' would become a commonly understood verb used by the military in the tropics to describe a method of dealing with unhealthy exposed surface conditions beside a building. The board recommended that the ground be covered extensively with this 'chunam or cement' (**fig. 6.9**), and it would form the second item Phillpotts and Staveley would act upon without awaiting sanction from London,

> . . . because the present state of the surface of this ground is of a loose porous nature, in consequence of which the rain penetrates to some depth, and the whole becomes saturated with moisture, upon which the action of the Sun's rays, or the atmospheric heat, causes a great evaporation in the hot months, and converts the atmosphere of this part of the Barrack Square into a kind of Vapour Bath.[40]

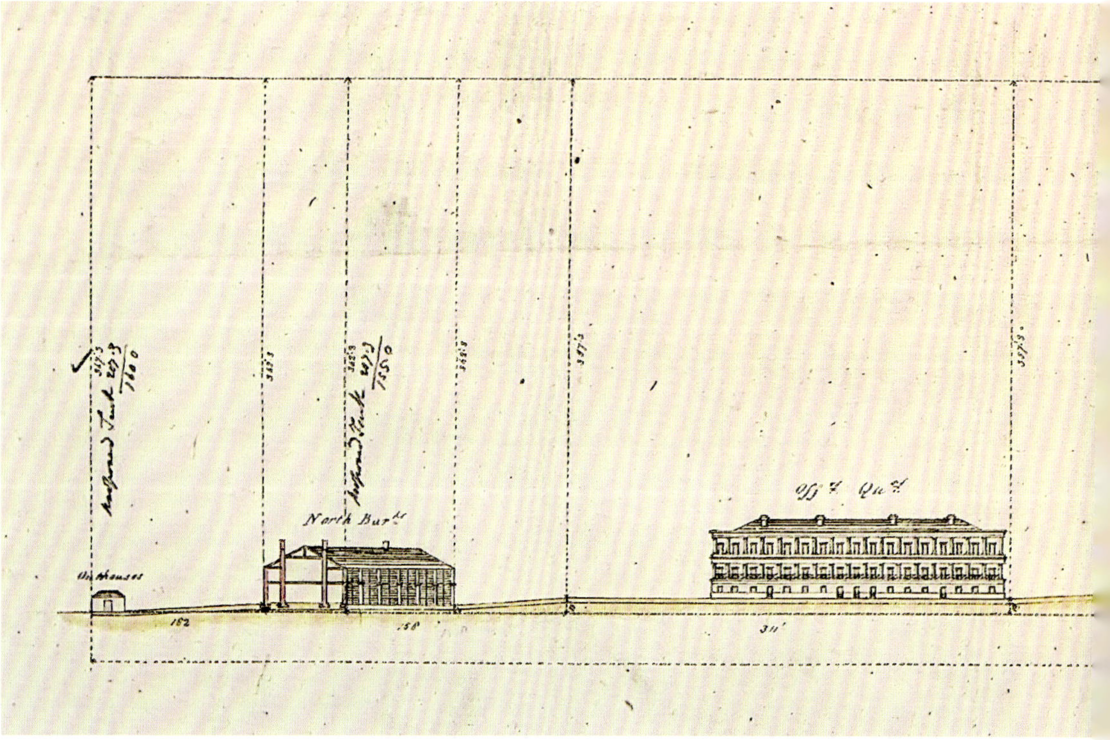

Both measures, the gauze to the windows and the 'chunaming' of the ground, were estimated to cost a hefty £502. 11s. 6d.[41] A third and concluding set of measures suggested by the board included converting the open nullah running by the Murray Barracks into a 'sewer of masonry' since this nullah ran down from the Albany Barracks and its 180 occupants were passing their effluence to the unfortunate soldiers below.

It is noteworthy how close in pattern these recommendations were to a request made by an anonymous medical expert writing to the *Friend of China* almost five years earlier, in June 1844. These measures suggest that approaches to protect against malaria within building interiors were increasingly consistent among empirically observant medics.

> . . . I therefore earnestly recommend sleeping on a second floor, or if this is not practicable, on a floor well raised on timbers over the ground previously well chinamed.

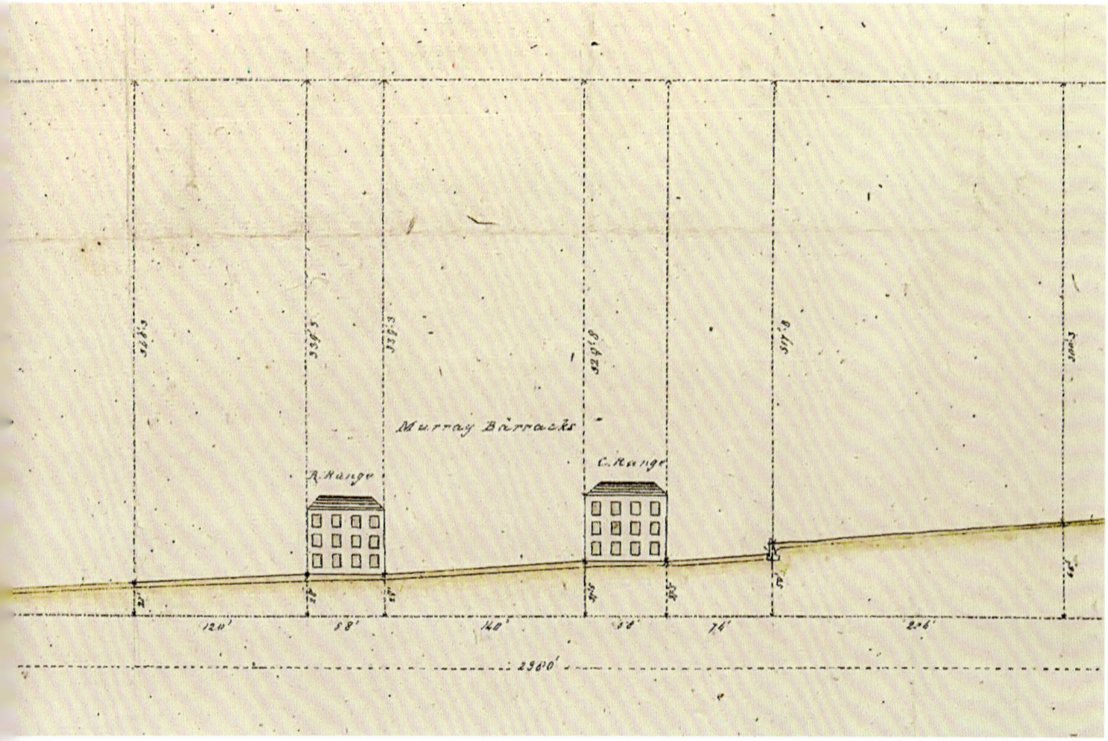

Fig. 6.8. Lt. J. J. Wilson, Site Section Across the Murray Barracks (detail), 1849. Pen and wash on paper. © The National Archives, Kew (MFQ 1/962).

> Sleeping in the open air, or even verandahs, is dangerous: several have met their death in this way. And the vicinity of damp places, and uncultivated spots, as ravines and valleys, are unquestionably fruitful sources of malaria, and should not be approached late in the evening.
>
> . . . Besides the above, there are other precautionary measures which must not be neglected, such as an immediate change of our clothes and shoes,—frequent ablution by cold sponging or the shower bath without rubbing, . . .'
>
> Yours respectfully
> MEDICUS
> Victoria, June 10th, 1844.[42]

Another measure recommended by the board was to plant trees to act as wind breaks for the road behind and south of the C Barracks in order to block cold mountain drafts seen as a

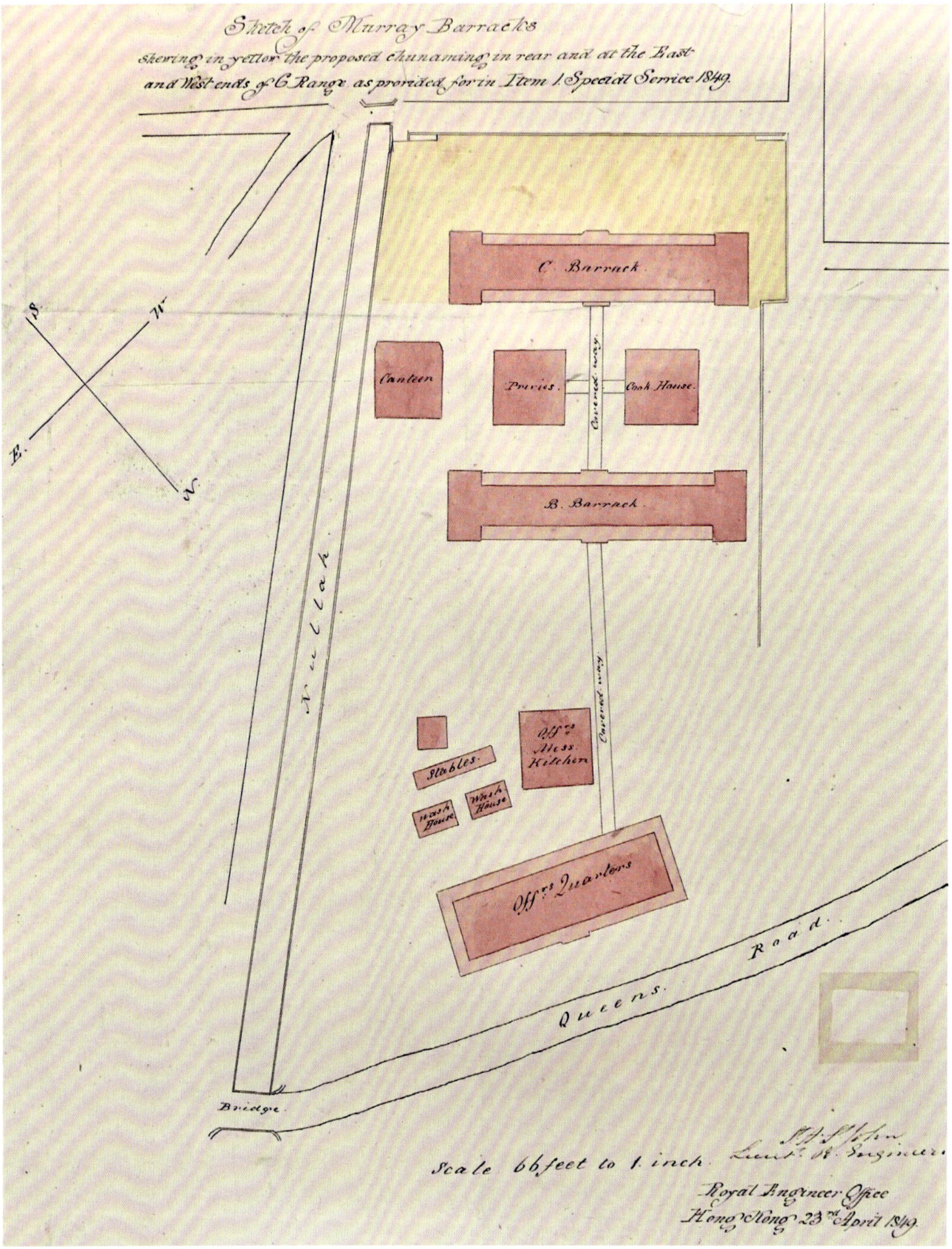

Fig. 6.9. Lt. S. A. St. John, 'Shewing in Yellow the Proposed Chunaming' to the Rear and Sides of the C Range, 1849. Pen and wash on paper. © The National Archives, Kew (MFQ 1/962).

potential source of miasma. Finally, the board requested that London sanction the hiring of two vessels during the hot season to be moored in the harbour. The floating overspill would allow the army to decant half of a garrison if necessary, enabling the doubling of space (and the volume of air) per person within each dormitory. Each ship could also act as a refuge in the event of another fever attack.[43] Unsurprisingly, officials rejected this rather expensive request.

Aldrich responded furiously to these findings. He was upset to discover that the board limited their recommendations to remedying deficiencies in and around his buildings, thereby all but holding him accountable. His lengthy memorandum criticised the results as illogical since, he complained, they did not consider an outbreak within the nearby house of Alexander Johnston, now a billeted residence for troops. He cited Dr. Fergusson's earlier letter to London, in which the doctor stated that he was convinced that both the B and C ranges *and* Johnston's house were 'the fully proved source of the disease'.[44] Fergusson continued:

> . . . had the Board in the first instance fully taken into consideration the direction of the Wind in Hong Kong during June, July & August the S.W. Monsoon, the altitude, situation, enclosure of Mr. Johnston's House by the Murray Barracks and of the Albany Barracks, the reasons and conclusions mentioned in their report would have been found inapplicable to all these positions.[45]

In his defence, Aldrich cited the contoured survey of part of the island by Lieutenant Thomas Bernard Collinson. He used it as evidence to show that height, orientation, and relative openness or enclosure were not to blame. Aldrich was referring not to the 1845 *Ordnance Map* but the slightly earlier, extraordinarily detailed survey produced by the young Royal Engineer and presently deposited at the London office of the IGF (**fig. 6.10**). Collinson's exquisitely made and colour-coded, extensively contoured survey of the area surrounding Cantonment Hill and Government Hill was the first of several he produced for the military in 1844 for their various installations. Collectively they may be seen to serve as a precursor to his published *Ordnance Map* of the island the following year.[46] It must be regarded among the finest detailed surveys made of the island in the nineteenth century. On it can be seen the positions of verandas, external walls, paths, steps, and watercourses. Contours are light blue, red represents government houses and property, purple is private houses, yellow is for the proposed works, while 'black' (or grey) is for 'mat or wooden houses'. It is the most meticulous layout of an extensive area of Hong Kong to have survived from the 1840s.

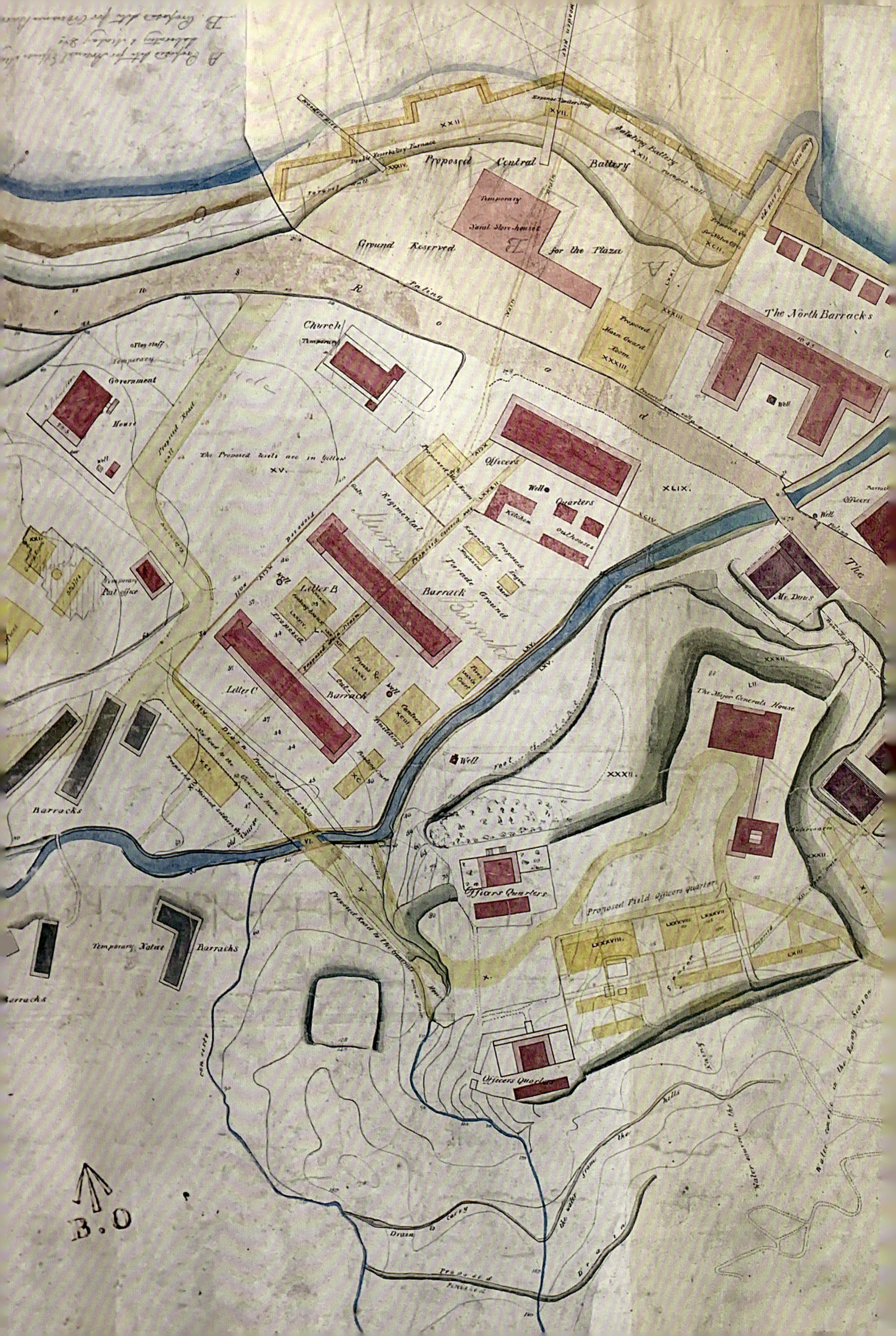

Proposed Central Battery
Temporary
Naval Store-house
Ground Reserved for the Plaza
Paling
R o a d
Church
Temporary
Flag staff
Government
House
Well
The North Barracks
Proposed
Main Guard
Room
XXXIII
The Proposed Roads are in Yellow
XV.
Proposed Road
Officers
Quarters
Well
Kitchen
Outhouses
XLIX.
Regimental
Parade Ground
Barrack
Letter B
Letter C
Canteen
Barracks
Temporary Post office
Well
XXXII
The Major Generals House
Officers Quarters
Proposed Field Officers quarters
LXXXVIII
Temporary Native Barracks
Barracks
Officers Quarters
the water from the hills
B. O

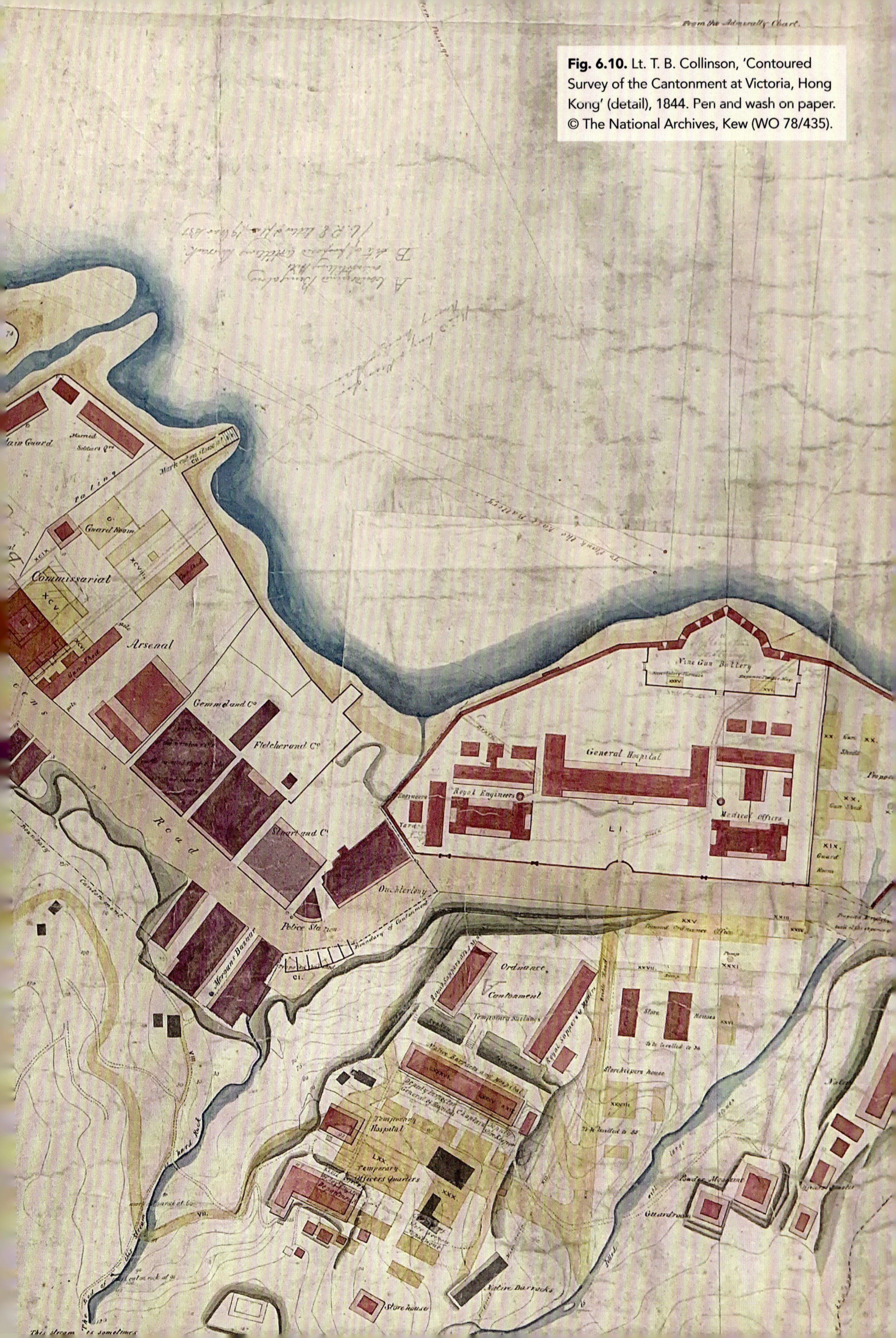

Fig. 6.10. Lt. T. B. Collinson, 'Contoured Survey of the Cantonment at Victoria, Hong Kong' (detail), 1844. Pen and wash on paper. © The National Archives, Kew (WO 78/435).

Aldrich argued that the survey threw into doubt the conclusions reached by the Board of Officers. According to Collinson's map, the situation, orientation, and enclosure of Johnston's house (upper left on the survey) were markedly different from that of the B and C ranges of barracks. Johnston's property had an enclosed gallery on its north and west sides, had no enclosing wall and was 'fully open to every gust of wind'.[47] Notwithstanding the differences in these two properties, Fergusson had identified them as a source of the disease. Aldrich then pointed out that it made it hard to explain the case of the Albany Barracks, positioned some way above. If anything, its situation seemed even more perilous than that of the C Range below. Yet it had escaped an outbreak.

> The Albany Barracks . . . is about 330 feet above mean water, and is 2000 feet nearer to the top of the mountain than C Range of Barracks, and also South of it.—The Building has only a gallery on the North side, has no wire gauze blinds, and has no area in the East, South and West sides levelled for the freer admission of air.—The surface of the ground round it is not covered with Chunam, and Granite Chips, and is of similar description to the surface of the ground round B & C Ranges. Yet there was no fever in this Barrack.[48]

Aldrich, of course, dismissed criticism that the gable ends of his B and C ranges needed verandas, insisting that the mountain's orientation and proximity to the rear protected these sides from the 'influence' of the rising and setting sun.[49] In considering the healthfulness of residents in the Albany Barracks, Aldrich regarded both wire gauze to the windows and 'chunaming' to the ground outside as costly and unnecessary. Instead, he suggested a cheaper application of 'Asphalte or Metallic Lava'.[50] Another dilemma was that the army had constructed solid walls to Barrack Square along its western flank in order to block liquor smugglers from passing 'samshoo' to European soldiers. In addition, the solid wall has been conceived to 'screen the privies' from nervous parishioners visiting the nearby colonial church to protect their sensibilities. Nevertheless, such a wall was seen now as a dangerous impediment to healthy air flow.[51] At the heart of Aldrich's veiled defence of his barracks design was a deeply held belief that both the earlier fevers of 1841 to 1844 and now the 1848 attack were importations into Hong Kong from outside of the island. Neither period, he maintained, had accumulated sufficient evidence to demonstrate any localised 'source' of disease upon the island, nor now upon any inherent failing in the architectural design of the barracks themselves.

> The sickness in 1848 in Hong Kong was partial in its effects—it occurred during the S.W. Monsoon.—The troops occupying Murray's Barracks in 1846 & in 47 were healthy, and it therefore appears to me that the Fever that existed in Hong Kong among the Troops previous to Murray Barracks having been built, and also from all the papers &c., I have seen relative to the Fever of 1848, that the Troops suffered from an Epidemic not attributable to any local miasma, and in its effects more attributable to the state of health or predisposition to attack of the Soldier, before the Epidemic set in, than to any other cause.[52]

Aldrich's opinion on the subject would hold sway with the IGF, doubtless assisted by the cost-effectiveness of his solutions to address the outbreak. Three days later, the IGF himself would scribble in the margin of an earlier letter from Phillpotts that

> This is one of those embarrassing cases arising from the usual attempt to attribute Fevers among the Troops that will occur in all tropical climates, & seemingly to fix on peculiar situations, to matters of arrangement and construction of Barracks. . . . I have no faith in the sweeping and expensive attentions that are usually recommended rather for a change of good effect, than one of any sound principles.[53]

His 'sound principles', however, reflected one of a multitude of opinions that through the noise of disagreement and debate had dragged Hong Kong through its nadir years and into a post-fever city of relative optimism and physical magnificence.

Conclusion

Just before malaria made its sudden and unwelcome return to the colony, Colonel Phillpotts and his wife joined a large picnic tour to Kowloon on 20 March 1848. It was, of course, an uninvited excursion, being in Chinese territory. Organised by the chief magistrate, Major William Caine, such trips allowed the army to scout stretches of enemy land informally. The party was carried across the harbour in three large lorchas. Once they landed, they formed a long column of travellers. This trip was especially bold, the route taking them several miles northwest into the hinterlands and up into the Kowloon mountains. The officers' wives were carried on bamboo sedan chairs while the party was armed, gun-carrying lascars positioned at the head and rear. The justification was the chance of some sport with a recently sighted tiger, but Kowloon as a conceptually vast landscape was considered wild, untamed, and dangerous (**figs. 6.11a** and **6.11b**).[54] Only three days earlier, the departing governor, Sir John Davis, and his military entourage had gone on a picnic to the southern side of Hong Kong Island, to Chek Chue, 'to examine a site for a new fort'. Phillpotts, the new commanding engineer, also made sure to attend that event. This kind of 'picnic reconnaissance' had become a flagrant habit of the British as they began to ache and stretch within the cramped compass of Hong Kong Island. The Kowloon party, after a champagne supper on board a Chinese boat moored by the Lei Yue Mun Pass, arrived back on the island at nine that evening, surprised to greet the arrival of their new governor, George Bonham.[55]

As we know, the ambitions of the officers to explore beyond the confines of the island were met now by a return of that cankerous malignancy set within the confines of their architecture. Yet, the barrack fever that soon followed in 1848 must be seen for what it was against the broader historical context of Hong Kong's first end-of-the-decade, its *fin de la décennie*: a mere blip. It may have temporarily tamped down and distracted from the expansive ambitions of the colony's settlers. But, throughout the debates over remedial measures—site-specific versus broader environmental—no one now questioned the certainty of colonial Hong Kong's further densification and expansion, let alone its survival. Bonham was the first governor to consider property as the quintessential free-market tool to subsidise much government spending through a more robust and vigorous mechanism of leasehold legislation and land rates taxation. Consequently, this rapid urban stimulation led to an overwhelming sense by city inhabitants that the northern stretch of the island would not be enough space to live upon. Yet, there it was, 'empty' Kowloon, teasingly sunlit in front of them. The armed picnic and sporting parties to Kowloon continued, of course, foreshadowing the colony's desired expansion across the harbour in the 1860s after another horrendous war with China. Malaria had become a recurrent, ephemeral, yet accepted component of life in the region, even if its causes were not collectively understood or universally agreed upon. Importantly, though, it was no longer thought to jeopardise the settlement's survival and growth.

As shown throughout this book, identifying and remedying the perceived pathologies of the colony was subjective, contested, ideological, and developmental. These approaches shifted and transformed across the early years of Hong Kong's history, catalysing reactions and bold assertions that interacted with the small island's land and climate to produce particular ways of fabricating an environment. The instability of these contestations gave

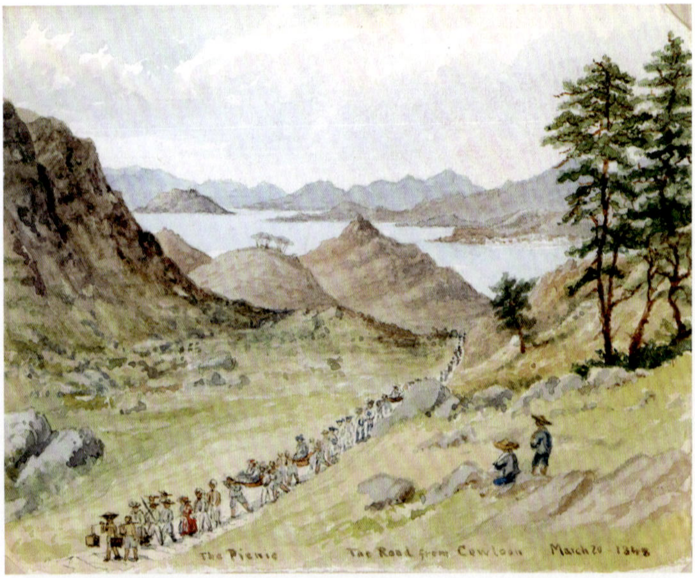

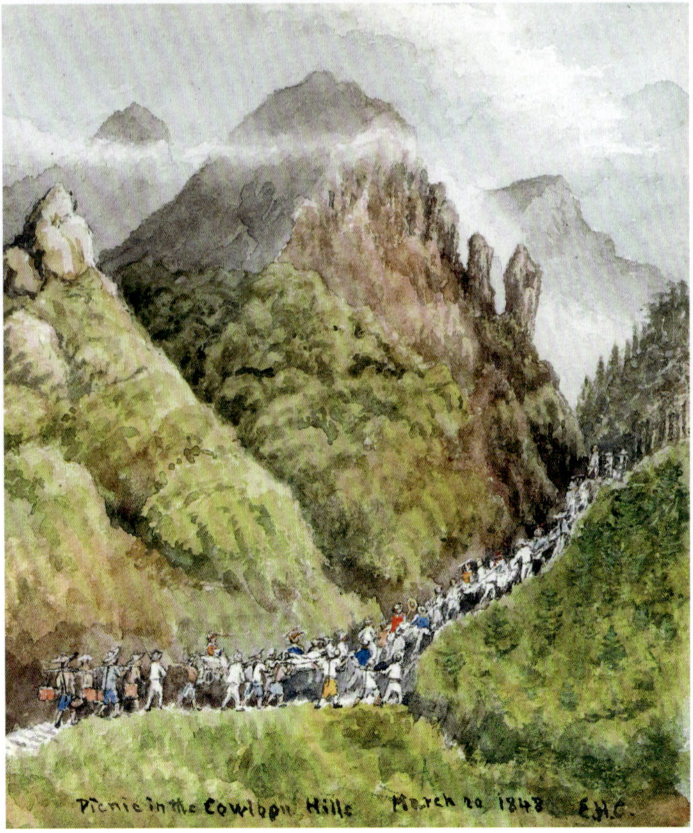

▲**Fig. 6.11a.** Dr. E. Cree, 'The Picnic. The Road from Cowloon', 20 March 1848. Watercolour on paper. © National Maritime Museum, Greenwich, London (CRJ/11).

◀**Fig. 6.11b.** Dr. E. Cree, 'Picnic in the Cowloon Hills', 20 March 1848. Watercolour on paper. © National Maritime Museum, Greenwich, London (CRJ/11).

dynamic propulsion to the planning and construction of Victoria and to constructing its critical social discourse. This discourse demanded a more committed government and the growth of municipal voices within an interdependent community.

We have seen, for example, how the perception and remedial measures taken in addressing health concerns, particularly those thought to be linked to malaria as miasma, were integrated into a broader set of socio-political issues. From 1841 to 1844, due to political uncertainty and related individual concerns about personal and emotional long-term investment upon the island, a mantle of doubt and fear seemed to extend itself upon the very terrain of the land itself. This undifferentiated geography of fear changed following the outbreak of 1843—the Hongkong Fever—replaced by a precise set of rules about where and how to build. Nevertheless, arguments continued, and through the subsequent years from 1844 to 1846, as a visually cohesive city emerged, thoughts shifted within the community towards commerce, leisure, and society. Miasmas remained a threat, but these were now considered containable. 1846 and 1847 were a particularly healthy pair of years, especially for the unfortunate military, who had always seemed to be the canaries in the mine for Hong Kong—barometers of an approaching hot season's ailments. Substantial barracks had, at last, been built for almost all the troops stationed on the island. Meanwhile, a programme of comfortable billeting was now in place to compensate those that remained without shelter. Yet, the outbreak of 1848 shocked and surprised some who had, by now, considered Hong Kong's urban miasmas to have been kept in check.

The barracks outbreak revived old fears about latent threats posed by Hong Kong's terrain, the orientation of its buildings, and their disposition. And it raised further questions about the means and methods of construction. However, the very localised nature of the outbreak and the miniaturisation of focus meant that containment and subsequent remedial measures could easily be handled. Another attack of malaria would occur in 1850, but, as with 1848, Hong Kong's natural terrain would no longer be considered an irredeemable feature. The community finally laid Martin's haunting condemnation of Hong Kong as a permanent source of sickness to rest. The colonisers now possessed the confidence to improve the island through extensive irrigation projects and infrastructure, afforest the hillsides, control diseases through a plethora of policies, and eventually remove the perceived threats posed by this natural terrain. In so doing, they were preparing the ground, so to speak, for emerging modern political approaches within the second half of the nineteenth century, approaches that considered nature as little more than a passive resource for mass social advancement. Victoria could be said to finally reach some state of critical mass by the late 1840s, more seriously accepted as an important trading port and now visually looking the part to elicit such confidence. This pull resulted, between the years 1848 to 1853, in Hong Kong seeing the first significant boom in its population, increasing across this period by over eighty per cent, due principally to an influx of Chinese—their numbers swelling from 20,228 to over 38,000, with European numbers climbing more modestly from 642 to 776.[56] This rapid influx was directly due in part to the California Gold Rush (1848–1855), beginning Hong Kong's enduring reputation as a significant transit point for the global migration of Chinese.[57]

The perceived link between modest changes in altitude and surviving the Hongkong Fever fed into newer statistical methods employed by the home government in the later epidemics of cholera that swept along Western Europe in 1848–1849 and 1853–1854. Organisations such as the Registrar-General's Office in London began to correlate disease with topographical elevations, finding 'that the mortality of the cholera epidemic is highest on the land at the low mouths of rivers, and generally on the low ground of towns'.[58] In turn, these approaches—linking land, elevation, and proximity to stagnant water—would shape the sanitary procedures of Europeans in Shanghai beginning in the 1850s. It would also influence British-controlled Tientsin (Tianjin) in the 1860s and their compulsive drive to eliminate marshes and block up trenches, such as with that Chinese city's perimeter moat.[59] However, Hong Kong did not just provide itself as a test case for nearby colonial settlements to learn from. It quickly became an essential part of Britain's widening imperial network beyond the compass of the five China Treaty Ports. It stitched itself into a 'global thalassocracy', one of the more significant beads on the string of a growing maritime empire.[60] For instance, militarily, a natural link in the sharing of knowledge between Hong Kong and Mauritius would develop due simply to a coeval early stage in their respective colonial development (the building of a British military citadel at Port Louis in 1835, for example), as can be read in the often interlaced War Office files in the National Archives at Kew.

As the bias of this research has leaned in favour of charting the *physical* development of Hong Kong during these first formative years, more research is needed to explore the city's social development. Under Governor Pottinger and especially Governor Davis, a disjointed set of ordinances slowly coalesced into a coherent legal and regulatory structure, providing an embryonic policy framework for the colony. Davis was primarily known and, to a large extent, despised as a governor who revelled in issuing ordinances and imposing new taxes. Both his Registration Ordnance (no. 17 of 1844) and Police Assessment Bill (no. 2 of 1845), the latter an ordinance to raise revenue based upon property assessment, had an enormous impact upon the European and Chinese communities and added fuel to calls for greater involvement from the former community in the affairs of municipal governance.

A deeper examination of the Chinese and other communities of Hong Kong at this time is also needed. Regarding race and creed, the colony's earliest years were surprisingly cosmopolitan, arguably more so than in present-day Hong Kong. For instance, Parsees, Hindus, Sikhs, and Malays occupied positions in both the mercantile community and the armed forces. It would also be a mistake to consider the Chinese community on the island as a socially and geographically homogenous entity. Punti, Hakka, and Hokkien natives to the south and east of the island were joined by Tanka and Cantonese in the city itself, along the Lower Bazaar and Tai Ping Shan to the west. Subsequently, wealthier Chiu Chow (Chaozhou) merchants settled to the east, where they initially set up alongside East Point. What also needs examining is how, even within the European community itself, there was a swelling in the ranks of the middle and working classes during these first years that would spark concerns about issues of social welfare and increasingly ascribe the affliction of malaria as a 'poor man's disease'.

Nevertheless, the decisions shown to have corresponded in part to governmental reactions to malaria, particularly the forcible relocation of Chinese residents from Upper Bazaar to the western Tai Ping Shan district in 1844, would fossilise into a clear bifurcation of the city along racial lines. Future regulatory instruments that followed would reinforce this imposed geographical divide. One such example was Governor John Bowring's radical Brothel Licensing Ordinance (no. 12 of 1857), an ordinance which anticipated the home government's first Contagious Diseases Act by seven years. The ordinance imposed the registration of prostitutes and brothels, the product of which was to both formalise and legitimise racial segregation across an east-west divide. Purely Chinese-serving brothels were permitted along the west end of the town, and those serving European clients were reserved along the east.[61] What the authorities *neglected* was equally discriminatory, for example, the discrepant long-term lack of piped fresh water to the western section of the town.[62] This disregard, coupled with unsanitary conditions, would culminate in the wholesale government-ordered destruction of Tai Ping Shan itself in 1894 following a most virulent and deadly outbreak of the bubonic plague. In turn, policy reactions to this event would profoundly influence future building regulations and even the shape of speculative development in Chinese housing.[63] Therefore, we can now trace a clear historical thread between a 'solution' to malaria in 1844 and the 'solution' to the plague precisely fifty years later.

Regarding the physical construction of Hong Kong, historians can undoubtedly make more headway in investigating both the private and public worlds constructed. A separate investigation, for instance, deserves to be made into the connective tissue of programmes concerning the public works—specifically, an almost Foucauldian interrelationship between barracks, hospitals, and prisons—developing seemingly contradictory architectural impulses of surveillance yet separation. These programmes actively learned from each other, from the natural island terrain upon which they sprang, and from local and international imperial experiences. Growing sophistication in dealing with approaches to hygiene in Britain and the attaching to this of a social and moral set of imperatives (what might be described as the crafting of a 'Victorian consciousness') plays a large part in this story. So does the experimentation with tropicalised methods of construction and form that acted as rudimentary environmental science projects for a global empire.

But, of course, the emerging acceptance of 'germ theory' would upend everything. A shift towards the microscopic study of the bacterium paralleled the erosion of older rule-of-thumb approaches to health management. The eventual dismissal of miasma theory (though it would take a surprisingly long time to be entirely relinquished by most medics) would also, in effect, lead to the weakening of the physical built form of a city as a singularly essential component of survival. Certainly, particular building components would continue to be regarded as inducible to well-being. The veranda, for instance, would exert a relentless pull on the minds of the tropical inhabitant as a necessary appendage of comfort and a much-needed tempered zone in a period still without access to the electric fan. The veranda of a building, extending to the ground and linked into a civic relationship with its neighbour, would form the 'arcade'. Increasingly, the health of the body would become that of the town, and the means of constructing a building to preserve human life would give way to the planning and making of the total urban system itself—that is, the birth of modern town planning.

Colonial Hong Kong may have been a mistake of history, an unloved consequence of a trade war between two civilisations that shared little respect or understanding for each other. But once determined to become a modern settlement, a significant problem had to be solved: how to make a solitary rock, initially important due only to its harbour, habitable? Malaria may not have been the only baneful emergent property of ill-contrived occupation and the relentless, heedless development of the island, but it was significantly important. For it has been shown through an intense chain of events that an urban community and an island colony were manifestly given shape by meeting a hidden threat. Through examining the relationships between sickness and shaping, this account has charted the fall and rise of a new city. Yet, out of repeated crises, a renewed, reinvigorated 'form' would follow 'fever', definitively stamping a spatial and social imprint upon its volatile society long into the next century.

Notes

1 Alan Harfield, *British and Indian Armies on the China Coast* (Farnham, Surrey: A. and J. Partnership, 1990), 57.

2 Ibid.

3 Ibid.

4 Ibid., 60.

5 Ibid., 61. Casualty figures are taken from the returns published in the *China Mail* during this period (undated).

6 'Annex B', ibid., 77. This observation is based on the 'returns' given by the *China Mail* (undated).

7 Ibid., 61.

8 *Friend of China* 'Extra', 20 Dec. 1845.

9 Ibid.

10 The National Archives, Kew [hereafter NA]; War Office [hereafter WO] 44/594.

11 WO 44/594, as recorded by Maj. Edward Aldrich in his letter dated 21 Oct. 1848.

12 Harfield, *British and Indian Armies*, 64. Originally in Col. H. C. Wylly, *History of the 1st and 2nd Battalions: The Sherwood Foresters* (London, 1929), 408–409.

13 WO 44/594, Horse Guards to Butler (Ordnance), 9 Oct. 1848.

14 WO 44/594, Fanshawe (Assist. IGF) to Byham (Secretary to the Ordnance), '. . . relative to the unhealthiness of the Murray Barracks at Victoria, Hong Kong', 24 Oct. 1848.

15 WO 44/594. The other two are subsequently dated 18 June and 24 Aug. 1849.

16 WO 44/594, Aldrich to the IGF, 21 Oct. 1848.

17 Ibid.

18 Ibid.

19 Ibid.

20 Ibid.

21 WO 44/594, Trevelyan (Treasury) to The Secretary at War, 23 Aug. 1849; re-quoted by WO 44/594, War Office to The Secretary of the Board of Ordnance, 29 Aug. 1849. The East Indies' practice of blank

rounds of heavy artillery fired at dawn and dusk most likely fumigated the air of mosquitoes by cannon smoke.

22 WO 44/594, Maule (War Office) to Staveley, 4 Dec. 1848.

23 WO 44/594, 'Proceedings of a Board of Officers assembled by order of the Honourable Major General Staveley . . . to report on matters connected with the Murray Barracks', 7 Mar. 1849.

24 Ibid., 3.

25 Ibid., 9–10.

26 Ibid., 10–11.

27 Ibid., 11–12.

28 Ibid., 11.

29 WO 44/594, Fanshawe (Assist. IGF) to Byham (Secretary to the Ordnance), 24 Oct. 1848.

30 WO 44/98, Col. H. H. Farquharson, Barrack Master, to Major E. Aldrich, Commanding Royal Engineer, 14 Mar. 1846.

31 Capt. H. R. Brandreth R.E., 'XIX.—Memorandum relative to a System of Barracks for the West Indies, recommended by Colonel Sir C. F. Smith C.B., R.E., and approved by the Master-General and Board of Ordnance', *Papers on Subjects Connected with the Duties of the Corps of Royal Engineers* [hereafter *Professional Papers*], vol. 2 (London, 1838): 245.

32 Captain John Smyth R.E., 'XVIII.—On the Construction of Barracks for Tropical Climates', *Professional Papers*, vol. 2 (London: 1838): 235–236.

33 Brandreth, 'Memorandum', 245.

34 Ibid., 246.

35 WO 44/594, as acknowledged by Grey (Colonial Secretary) to Staveley, 16 Aug. 1849.

36 WO 44/594, 'Report and Estimate', Phillpotts to the IGF, 24 May 1849.

37 WO 44/594, 'Proceedings', 12–13.

38 Ibid., 7, 13.

39 Jan Morris with Simon Winchester, *Stones of Empire: The Buildings of the Raj* (Oxford: Oxford University Press, 1983), 18.

40 WO 44/594, 'Proceedings', 6–7.

41 WO 44/594, Phillpotts to the IGF, 24 May 1849.

42 *Friend of China*, 22 June 1844.

43 Ibid., 15–17.

44 WO 44/594, as quoted by Aldrich to the IGF, 13 June 1849.

45 Ibid., 2.

46 WO 78/435, T. B. Collinson, 'Contoured Survey of the Cantonment at Victoria, Hong Kong', 1844, and countersigned by Major Aldrich on 31 Aug. 1845. The four other military surveys by Collinson are WO 78/472, 'Plan of Green Island, Hong Kong', 1844; 'Contoured Survey of the Cantonment at Chuck Chu (Stanley), Hong Kong', 1844; 'Plan of Kellets Island, Hong Kong', 1844; and 'Contoured Survey of the Cantonment of Sywan and the Lyeemoon', 1845, all countersigned by Aldrich on 18 July 1846.

47 WO 44/594, Aldrich, 13 June 1849, 2–3.

48 Ibid., 4.

49 Ibid., 2.

50 Ibid., 6, 8.

51 Ibid., 7.

52 Ibid., 10.

53 WO 44/594, Marginalia of the IGF, 16 June 1849 (on letter from Phillpotts to the IGF dated 3 Mar. 1849).

54 National Maritime Museum, Greenwich, London [hereafter NMM]; CRJ/11, Private Journal of E. H. Cree, 20 Mar. 1848. Evidence of firearm-carrying lascars is shown in the two adjacent watercolours.

55 Ibid.

56 Ka-Che Yip, *Disease, Colonialism, and the State: Malaria in Modern East Asian History* (Hong Kong: Hong Kong University Press, 2009), 14.

57 John M. Carroll, *Edge of Empires: Chinese Elites and British Colonials in Hong Kong* (Cambridge, MA: Harvard University Press, 2005), 14. As Elizabeth Sinn muses provocatively, 'What might have happened if the discovery of gold in California had occurred in 1838, rather than 1848'? Elizabeth Sinn, *Pacific Crossing: California Gold, Chinese Migration, and the Making of Hong Kong* (Hong Kong: Hong Kong University Press, 2012), 10.

58 William Farr, *Seventeenth Annual Report of the Registrar-General of Births, Deaths, and Marriages in England* (London: Longman, Brown, Green an Longmans, 1856), 88; see also Kerrie L. MacPherson, *A Wilderness of Marshes: The Origins of Public Health in Shanghai, 1843–1893* (Hong Kong: Oxford University Press, 1987), 41.

59 MacPherson, *A Wilderness of Marshes*, 68–82; Ruth Rogaski, *Hygenic Modernity: Meanings of Health and Disease in Treaty-Port China* (Berkeley and Los Angeles: University of California Press, 2004), 83–87.

60 As Daniel Headrick writes: 'But only once has there been a truly global thalassocracy, a nation whose fleet and merchant marine were dominant on almost all the seas of the world. This was Great Britain in the nineteenth century.' Daniel R. Headrick, *The Tools of Empire: Technology and European Imperialism in the Nineteenth Century* (New York: Oxford University Press, 1981), 174–175; see also Robert Home, *Of Planting and Planning: The Making of British Colonial Cities* (London: E & FN Spon, 1997), 71.

61 Philippa Levine, 'Modernity, Medicine, and Colonialism: The Contagious Diseases Ordinances in Hong Kong and the Straits Settlements', *Positions*, vol. 6, no. 3 (Winter 1998): 676; and Philip Howell, 'Prostitution and Racialised Sexuality: The Regulation of Prostitution in Britain and the British Empire before the Contagious Diseases Acts', *Environment and Planning D: Society and Space*, vol. 18 (2000): 329.

62 It was a clerk in the Royal Engineers, S. B. Rawlings, who first proposed a reservoir at Pok Fu Lam, completed in 1864, to be fed to the western half of the city where the Europeans lived, bypassing the Chinese population. See Daniel R. Headrick, *The Tentacles of Progress: Technology Transfer in the Age of Imperialism, 1850–1940* (New York: Oxford University Press, 1988), 149–150.

63 Cecilia L. Chu, 'Combatting Nuisance: Sanitation, Regulation, and the Politics of Property in Colonial Hong Kong', in Robert Peckham and David Pomfret, eds., *Imperial Contagions: Medicine and Cultures of Planning in Asia* (Hong Kong: Hong Kong University Press, 2013), 17–36; and, more recently, Cecilia L. Chu, *Building Colonial Hong Kong: Speculative Development and Segregation in the City* (London: Routledge, 2022).

Map of Victoria, Hong Kong, 1843

Two Years into Colonisation

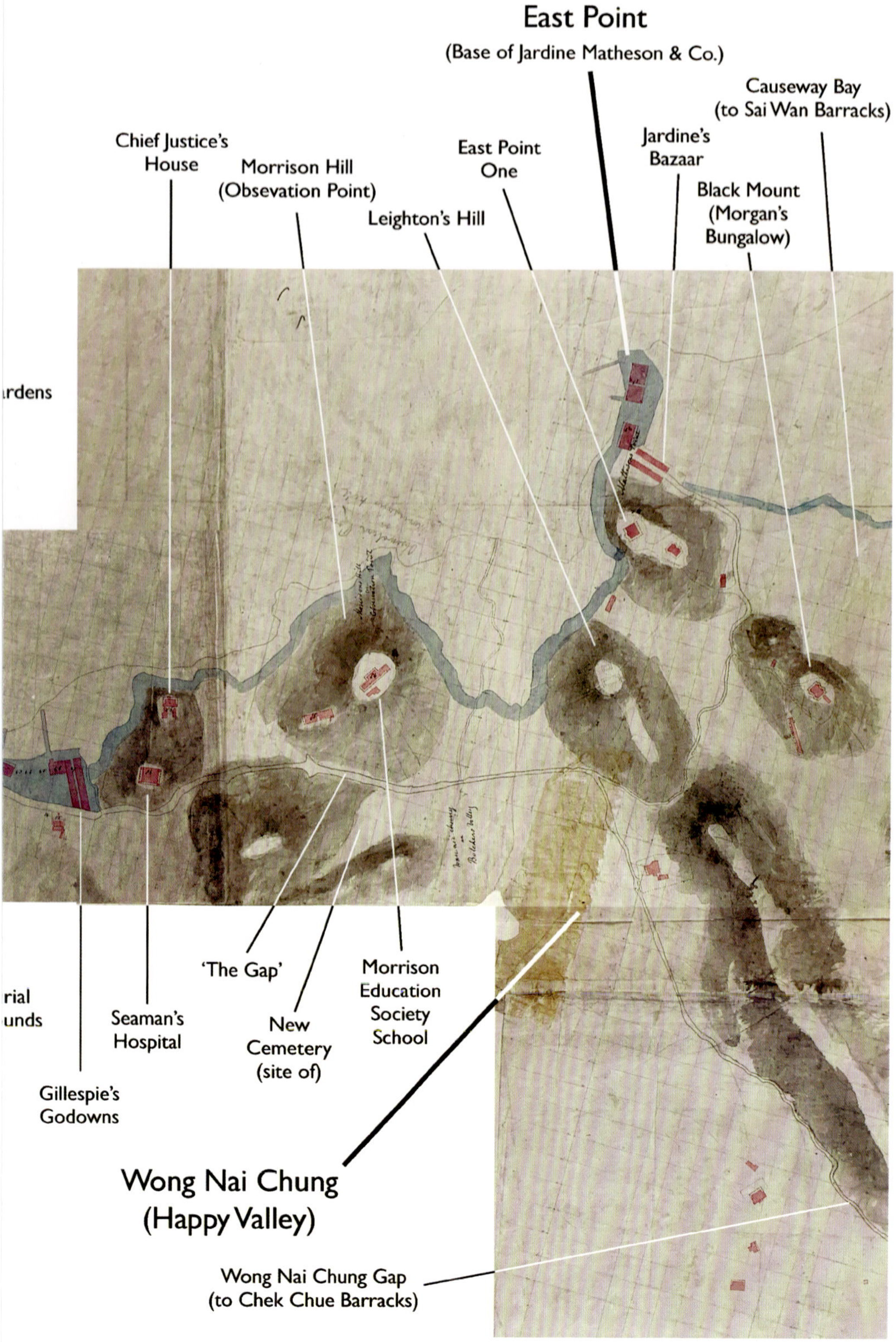

Bibliography

Primary Sources

A. Manuscripts

The National Archives, Kew, London (NA)

Colonial Office (CO)

129 Series *Hong Kong, Original Correspondence*

CO 129/1 (1842)
CO 129/2 (1843)
CO 129/3 (1843)
CO 129/4 (1843)
CO 129/5 (1844)
CO 129/6 (1 Jan.–31 July 1844)
CO 129/7 (1 Aug.–31 Dec. 1844)
CO 129/9 (1844)
CO 129/10 (1841–1844)
CO 129/11 (1 Jan. 1845–30 Apr. 1845)
CO 129/12 (1 May 1845–31 July 1845)
CO 129/13 (1 Aug. 1845–31 Dec. 1845)
CO 129/16 (1 Jan. 1846–30 June 1846)
CO 129/17 (1 July 1846–31 Dec. 1846)
CO 129/18 (1846)
CO 129/20 (1 May–31 Aug. 1847)

131 Series	*Hong Kong, Sessional Papers*	
	CO 131/1 (1844–1847)	
133 Series	*Hong Kong Miscellanea, Blue Books of Statistics, etc.*	
	CO 133/2 (1845)	
	CO 133/6 (1849)	
	CO 133/7 (1850)	

War Office (WO)

7 Series	*Various Departmental Out-Letters, 1715–1862*	
	WO 7/118	Clerks of Sub-Divisions, N–Z, 1813–1817
44 Series	*Ordnance Office and War Office Correspondence, 1682–1873*	
	WO 44/67	Correspondence, East Indies, 1841–1846
	WO 44/68	Correspondence, East Indies, 1847–1855
	WO 44/97	Hong Kong (1), 1844–1847
	WO 44/98	Hong Kong (2), 1844–1847
	WO 44/593	Barracks, Eastern, 1837–1848
	WO 44/594	Barracks, Eastern, 1849–1855
78 Series	*Maps and Plans, 1627–1953*	
	WO 78/115	Ten Outline Sketches of the Island of Hong Kong, 1846
	WO 78/118	Ordnance Map of Hong Kong, 1845
	WO 78/435	'Contoured' survey, Cantonment at Victoria, Hong Kong, 1844
	WO 78/472	'Contoured' surveys (Green Island, Stanley, Kellet's Island, Sai Wan), Hong Kong, 1845
	WO 78/479	Plan of Victoria, Hong Kong, 1845

Admiralty (ADM)

1 Series	*Admiralty, Ministry of Defence, Navy Department: Correspondence and Papers, 1660–1976*	
	ADM 352/412	Chart of Part of the Coast of China and Adjacent Islands, 1771
	ADM 1/5530	Mediterranean, China and East Indies, 1843

Foreign Office (FO)

233 Series *Consulates and Legation, China: Miscellaneous Papers and Reports, 1727–1951*

FO 233/185 Entry Book of Local Proclamations, and Official Notes, to and from Chinese Authorities, 1844–1849

925 Series *Maps and Plans, 1700–1944*

FO 925/2427 Plan of Hong Kong. MS. In Sir H. Pottinger's 'Superintendent', 1842

Maps and Plans (MFQ, MPG, MPH, MR 1)

MFQ Series *Maps and Plans, Flat Storage, Extracted from Various, 1565–1962*

MFQ 1/37 Plans/Sections of Murray Barracks & North Barracks, 1845–1846 (WO 44/98)

MFQ 1/962 Remedial work to Murray Barracks, 1849 (WO 44/594)

MPG Series *Maps and Plans, Flat Storage, Extracted from CO, 1612–1949*

MPG 1/156 Part Plan of the City of Hong Kong and Surrounding Country, 1843 (CO 129/2)

MPG 1/158 Four Plans and Elevations of 'Green Bank', 1850 (CO 129/35)

MPH Series *Maps and Plans, Flat Storage, Extracted from WO, 1661–1945*

MPH 1/867 Mauritius, Ceylon, Hong Kong, Cornwall, 1831–1855 (WO 44/68)

MPH 1/899 Military sites and Cantonments, Hong Kong, 1844–1846 (WO 44/97)

MR 1 Series *Maps and Plans, Rolled Storage, Extracted from Various, 1500–1966*

MR 1/381 Architectural Plans, Drawings, Plans, and Chart of Buildings and Harbours in Hong Kong, 1843 (ADM 1/5530)

Department of Manuscripts and University Archives, Cambridge University Library, Cambridge (CUL)

Jardine Matheson Archives (JMA)

C5 Series 'Private "Out" Correspondence of James Matheson'

C5/6 Nov. 1840–May 1841

C5/7 May–Dec. 1841

C6 Series 'Private "Out" Correspondence of Alexander Matheson'

C6/1 Aug.–Nov. 1841, Feb. 1842

	C6/2	Jan.–June 1842
	C6/3	July 1842–Jan. 1845
C15 Series	General Insurance Letter Books	
	C15/2	May 1845–Dec. 1846
	C15/3	Jan. 1847–Oct. 1848
	C15/5	Oct. 1850–Dec. 1851

Caird Library and Archive, National Maritime Museum, Greenwich, London (NMM)

Private Illustrated Journal of Dr. E. H. Cree (CRJ)

CRJ/5	Volume 5 (1841)
CRJ/7	Volume 7 (1843)
CRJ/8	Volume 8 (1844)
CRJ/10	Volume 10 (1846–1847)
CRJ/11	Volume 11 (1848)
CRJ/12	Volume 12 (1849)

Hong Kong Public Records Office, Hong Kong (HKPRO)

T. B. Collinson (Lt.). 'Transcripts of Correspondence of Lieut. Thomas Bernard Collinson RE, Dec. 1838–29 Mar. 1846.' HKMS 140-1-1.

National Library of Australia, Canberra (NLA)

Papers of Edward Ashworth, Notebook (Mfm M602)

File 3	8 May 1844(–25 Feb. 1845)

United Kingdom Hydrographic Office Archive, Taunton (UKHO)

SVY Series	Hydrographic Survey and Incoming Data, ca. 1620–2016	
	SVY/A/y13Bb4	Book A: Survey, 1810–1813

B. Newspapers and Journals

Newspapers

Canton Press, 23 Jan. 1841–16 Mar. 1844.

Canton Register, 12 Jan. 1841–23 May 1843 (renamed) *Hongkong Register*, 18 July 1843–22 Dec. 1846.

China Mail, 6 Mar. 1845–5 Feb. 1846.

Friend of China, 24 Mar. 1842 (amalgamating as) *Friend of China and Hongkong Gazette*, 23 Mar. 1843–5 Jan. 1856.

Journal Articles

The Builder, vol. 3, no. 130 (2 Aug. 1845); vol. 5, no. 230 (3 July 1847).

'Art. VIII. Some account of Her Majesty's Twenty-Sixth, or Cameronian Regiment, from its formation to the present time.' *The Chinese Repository*, vol. 12, no. 3 (Mar. 1843): 145–166.

'Art. III. Religious and charitable institutions in Hong Kong: churches, chapels, schools, colleges, hospitals, &c.' *Chinese Repository*, vol. 12, no. 8 (Aug. 1843): 441–442.

'Art. IV. Record of criminals, European and Chinese, lodged in jails at Hongkong, from 9th of August, 1841, to the 18th of September 1843.' *Chinese Repository*, vol. 12, no. 10 (Oct. 1843): 534–535.

'Art. V. Sickness and deaths in Hongkong; remarked upon by a member of the Church of England, in a letter to the Editor of the Chinese Repository.' *The Chinese Repository*, vol. 12, no. 11 (Nov. 1843): 145–166.

'Art. V: Notices of Hongkong: situation, shape and extent of the island . . .' *Chinese Repository*, vol. 14, no. 6 (June 1845): 291–298.

'1843 Principal Events.' *Historical and Statistical Abstract of the Colony of Hong Kong 1841–1930*, 3rd ed. Hong Kong: Noronha & Co., 1932.

C. Published Sources

Abel, Clarke. *Narrative of a Journey in the Interior of China, and of a Voyage to and from that Country, in the Years 1816 and 1817.* London: Longman, Hurst, Rees, Orme, and Brown, 1818.

Aldrich, Edward (Maj.). 'VI.—Description of the Mat Covering Sheds used at Hong-Kong in the erection of the Ordnance Buildings, and of the mode adopted by the Chinese in transporting and raising heavy Weights for these Buildings', 153–155. *Papers on Subjects Connected with the Duties of the Corps of Royal Engineers*, vol. 10. London: John Weale, 1849.

Ashworth, Edward. 'Memoranda Concerning the Erection, by Native Artizans [sic], of an English House in China, Designed and Superintended by the English Architect', under 'Chinese Architecture', 1–69. *Architectural Publication Society: Detached Essays and Illustrations Issued During the Years 1850–51.* London: Thomas Richards, 1853.

Brandreth, H. R. (Capt.). 'XIX.—Memorandum relative to a System of Barracks for the West Indies, recommended by Colonel Sir C. F. Smith C.B., R.E., and approved by the Master-General and Board of Ordnance', 239–246. *Papers on Subjects Connected with the Duties of the Corps of Royal Engineers*, vol. 2. London: J. Barker, 1838.

Cates, Arthur. 'The Dictionary of Architecture, A Retrospect, 1848–1892.' *Dictionary of Architecture*. London: Architectural Publication Society, 1892.

Cree, Edward H. *Naval Surgeon: The Voyages of Dr. Edward H. Cree, Royal Navy as Related in His Private Journals, 1837–1856*, edited by Michael Levien. New York: E. P. Dutton, 1981.

Cunynghame, Arthur (Capt.). *An Aide-de-Camp's Recollections of Service in China*. London: Saunders and Otley, 1844.

Farr, William. *Seventeenth Annual Report of the Registrar-General of Births, Deaths, and Marriages in England*. London: Longman, Brown, Green an Longmans, 1856.

Fortune, Robert. *A Journey to the Tea Districts of China*. London: John Murray, 1852.

Hunter, William C. *The 'Fan Kwae' at Canton before Treaty Days 1825–1844*. Shanghai: Oriental Affairs, 1882.

Johnston, A. R. 'Note on the Island of Hong-Kong.' *Journal of the Royal Geographical Society of London*, vol. 14 (1844): 112–117.

Legge, James. 'The Colony of Hong Kong—From a lecture by the Rev. James Legge, D.D., L.L.D., on Reminiscences of a Long Residence in the East, Delivered in the City Hall, November 5, 1872.' *The China Review*, vol. 3 (1874): 163–176.

McPherson, D., M.D. *Two Years in China: Narrative of the Chinese Expedition from its Formation in April, 1840, till April, 1842*. London: Saunders and Otley, 1842.

Ouchterlony, John (Lt.). *The Chinese War: An Account of All the Operations of the British Forces from the Commencement to the Treaty of Nanking*. London: Saunders and Otley, 1844.

Smyth, John (Capt.). 'XVIII.—On the Construction of Barracks for Tropical Climates', 233–238. *Papers on Subjects Connected with the Duties of the Corps of Royal Engineers*, vol. 2. London: J. Barker, 1838.

Tarrant, William (attrib.). 'Brief Description of the Town of Victoria, with Remarks on the various Trades, Institutions &c. prepared as an accompaniment to the Hongkong Almanack and Directory for 1848.' *The Hongkong Almanack and Directory for the Year 1848*. Hong Kong, 1848.

Tarrant, William. *Hongkong Part 1: 1839 to 1844*. Canton: Friend of China, 1861.

Thompson, John. *Hong Kong Illustrations of China and its people*, vol. 1. London: Sampson Low, Marston, Low, and Searle, 1873.

Wilson, John, M.D. *Medical Notes on China*. London: John Churchill, 1846.

Secondary Sources

A. Published Sources

Arnold, David. 'Introduction: Tropical Medicine Before Mansion.' In *Warm Climates and Western Medicine: The Emergence of Tropical Medicine, 1500–1900*, edited by David Arnold, 1–19. Amsterdam: Editions Rodopi, 1996.

Bremner, G. A., Johan Lagae & Mercedes Volait. 'Intersecting Interests: Developments in Networks and Flows of Information and Expertise in Architectural History.' *Fabrications*, vol. 26, no. 2 (2016): 227–245.

———. 'Tides that Bind: Waterborne Trade and the Infrastructure Networks of Jardine Matheson & Co.' *Perspecta*, vol. 52 (2019): 31–47.

Carroll, John M. *Edge of Empires: Chinese Elites and British Colonials in Hong Kong*. Cambridge, MA: Harvard University Press, 2005.

Chan, Wai Kwan. *The Making of Hong Kong Society: Three Studies of Class Formation in Early Hong Kong*. Oxford: Clarendon Press, 1991.

Chang, Jiat-Hwee. *A Genealogy of Tropical Architecture: Colonial Networks, Nature and Technoscience*. Abingdon, Oxon.: Routledge, 2016.

Cheng, Kris. 'HKU Urges Heritage Status for Oldest Boundary Stone Ever Discovered in Hong Kong.' *Hong Kong Free Press*, 17 Dec. 2015.

Chu, Cecilia L. 'Combatting Nuisance: Sanitation, Regulation, and the Politics of Property in Colonial Hong Kong.' In *Imperial Contagions: Medicine and Cultures of Planning in Asia*, edited by Robert Peckham and David Pomfret, 17–36. Hong Kong: Hong Kong University Press, 2013.

———. 'Contagious City: The Bubonic Plague and the First Urban Renewal Scheme in Hong Kong.' *HKIA Journal*, vol. 76 (2020): 25–29.

———. *Building Colonial Hong Kong: Speculative Development and Segregation in the City*. London: Routledge, 2022.

Clavell, James. *Tai-Pan*. New York: Dell Publishing, 1966.

Cowell, Christopher. 'The Hong Kong Fever of 1843: Collective Trauma and the Reconfiguring of Colonial Space.' *Modern Asian Studies*, vol. 47, no. 2 (March 2013): 329–364.

———. *Edward Ashworth, Artist & Architect: Fourteen Watercolour Studies of Hong Kong & Macau, 1844–46*. Sydney: Hordern House, 2014.

———. 'Borrowed Verses: Code and Representation Within the First Travelogue of the City of Hong Kong, 1841–42.' In *Late Victorian Orientalism: Representations of the East in Nineteenth-Century Literature, Art and Culture from the Pre-Raphaelites to John La Farge*, edited by Eleonora Sasso, 133–162. London: Anthem Press, 2020.

———. 'Hong Kong, Fever and Form: How Disease Shaped the First Layout of the Colonial City.' In 'Hygiene · Control', *HKIA Journal*, vol. 76 (2020): 20–24.

Crisswell, Colin N. *The Taipans: Hong Kong's Merchant Princes*. Hong Kong: Oxford University Press, 1981.

Decaudin, Maxime. 'Founding the Barren Rock: Landscape Transformations and Discourses in Nineteenth-Century Colonial Hong Kong.' *Journal of the LUCAS Graduate Conference* (2019): 38–75.

Denison, Edward, and Guang Yu Ren. *Modernism in China: Architectural Visions and Revolutions*. Chichester, West Sussex: John Wiley & Sons, 2008.

Diamond, A. I. 'Major-General T. B. Collinson, Royal Engineers' (File Note), *Hong Kong History Workshop*. Hong Kong: Department of History, The University of Hong Kong, Dec. 1984.

Eitel, E. J. *Europe in China: The History of Hong Kong from the Beginning to the Year 1882*. Hong Kong: Kelly and Walsh / London: Luzac & Co., 1895.

Empson, Hal. *Mapping Hong Kong: A Historical Atlas*. Hong Kong: Government Information Services, 1992.

Endacott, G. B. *A History of Hong Kong*. London: Oxford University Press, 1958.

———. *A Biographical Sketch-Book of Early Hong Kong*. Singapore: Eastern Universities Press, 1962.

———. *An Eastern Entrepôt*. London: Her Majesty's Stationery Office, 1964.

Evans, Dafydd M. E. 'Jardine, Matheson & Company's First Site in Hong Kong.' *Journal of the Hong Kong Branch of the Royal Asiatic Society*, vol. 8 (1968): 149–153.

———. 'Hong Kong's First Government House.' *Journal of the Hong Kong Branch of the Royal Asiatic Society*, vol. 8 (1968): 156–160.

———. 'Chinatown in Hong Kong: The Beginnings of Taipingshan.' *Journal of the Hong Kong Branch of the Royal Asiatic Society*, vol. 10 (1970): 69–78.

———. 'The Foundation of Hong Kong: a Chapter of Accidents.' In *Hong Kong: The Interaction of Traditions and Life in the Towns*, edited by Marjorie Topley, 11–41. Hong Kong: Hong Kong Branch of the Royal Asiatic Society, 1975.

Farris, Jonathan Andrew. *Enclave to Urbanity: Canton, Foreigners, and Architecture from the Late Eighteenth to the Early Twentieth Centuries*. Hong Kong: Hong Kong University Press, 2016.

Foucault, Michel. 'The Eye of Power.' In *Power/Knowledge, Selected Interviews & Other Writings, 1972–1977*, edited by Colin Gordon, 146–165. New York: Pantheon, 1980.

Gharipour, Mohammad, and Caitlin DeClercq, eds. *Epidemic Urbanism: Contagious Diseases in Global Cities*. Chicago: University of Chicago Press, 2021.

Ghosh, Amitav. *Flood of Fire*. London: John Murray, 2015.

Hamilton, Shelia E. *Watching over Hong Kong: Private Policing 1841–1941*. Hong Kong: Hong Kong University Press, 2008.

Harfield, Alan. *British and Indian Armies on the China Coast*. Farnham, Surrey: A. and J. Partnership, 1990.

Harrison, Mark. 'Tropical Medicine in Nineteenth-Century India.' *The British Journal for the History of Science*, vol. 25, no. 3 (Sep. 1992): 299–318.

———. *Disease and the Modern World: 1500 to the Present Day*. Cambridge: Polity Press, 2004.

———. 'Disease and Medicine in the Armies of British India, 1750–1830: The Treatment of Fevers and the Emergence of Tropical Therapeutics.' In *British Military and Naval Medicine, 1600–1830*, edited by Geoffrey L. Hudson, 87–118. Clio Medica, vol. 81. Amsterdam; New York: Rodopi, 2007.

Hawkins, R. S. (Lt. Col.). 'Far Eastern Outpost.' *The Royal Engineers Journal*, vol. 82 (Mar. 1968): 37–47.

Headrick, Daniel R. *The Tools of Empire: Technology and European Imperialism in the Nineteenth Century*. New York: Oxford University Press, 1981.

———. *The Tentacles of Progress: Technology Transfer in the Age of Imperialism, 1850–1940*. New York: Oxford University Press, 1988.

Ho, Pui-Yin. *Challenges for an Evolving City: 160 Years of Port and Land Development in Hong Kong*. Hong Kong: The Commercial Press, 2004.

Home, Robert. *Of Planting and Planning: The Making of British Colonial Cities*. London: E & FN Spon, 1997.

Howell, Philip. 'Prostitution and Racialised Sexuality: The Regulation of Prostitution in Britain and the British Empire before the Contagious Diseases Acts.' *Environment and Planning D: Society and Space*, vol. 18 (2000): 321–339.

Iu, Kow-Choy. 'The Cultivation of the "Incense Tree" (Aquilaria Sinensis).' *Journal of the Hong Kong Branch of the Royal Asiatic Society*, vol. 23 (1983): 247–249.

Jensen Carr, Sara. *The Topography of Wellness: How Health and Disease Shaped the American Landscape*. Charlottesville, VA: University of Virginia Press, 2021.

Keswick, Maggie, ed. *The Thistle and the Jade: A Celebration of 150 Years of Jardine, Matheson & Co.* London: Octopus Books, 1982.

King, Frank H. H. 'Martin, Robert Montgomery.' *Oxford Dictionary of National Biography*, vol. 36, 974–975. Oxford: Oxford University Press, 2004.

King, Frank H. H., and Prescott Clarke, eds. *A Research Guide to China-Coast Newspapers, 1822–1911*. Cambridge, MA: Harvard University Press, 1965.

Ko, Tim-Keung. 'A Review of development of Cemeteries in Hong Kong: 1841–1950.' *Journal of the Hong Kong Branch of the Royal Asiatic Society*, vol. 41 (2001): 241–280.

Lau, Alfred Y. K. 'An Outline of the Urban Development of Sai Ying Pun in the Nineteenth Century.' *Journal of the Hong Kong Branch of the Royal Asiatic Society*, vol. 35 (1995): 59–73.

Levine, Philippa. 'Modernity, Medicine, and Colonialism: The Contagious Diseases Ordinances in Hong Kong and the Straits Settlements.' *Positions*, vol. 6, no. 3 (Winter 1998): 675–705.

Lo, Hsiang-Lin. *1842 nian yi qian zhi Xianggang ji qi dui wai jiao tong* (Hong Kong and Its External Communication before 1842). Hong Kong: Institute of Chinese Culture, 1959.

Luk, Gary Chi-Hung. 'Occupied Space, Occupied Time: Food Hawking and the Central Market in Hong Kong's Victoria City during the Opium War.' *Frontiers of History in China*, vol. 11, no. 3 (2016): 400–430.

Macpherson, Kerrie L. *A Wilderness of Marshes: The Origins of Public Health in Shanghai, 1843–1893*. Hong Kong: Oxford University Press, 1987.

Marshall, P. J. 'The White Town of Calcutta under the Rule of the East India Company.' *Modern Asian Studies*, vol. 34, no. 2 (May 2000): 307–331.

Mo, Timothy. *An Insular Possession*. London: Chatto & Windus, 1986.

Morris, Jan, with Simon Winchester. *Stones of Empire: The Buildings of the Raj*. Oxford: Oxford University Press, 1983.

Morse, H. B. *The International Relations of the Chinese Empire, Vol. I: The Period of Conflict, 1834–1860*. London: Longmans, Green, and Co., 1910.

Munn, Christopher. 'The Chusan Episode: Britain's Occupation of a Chinese Island, 1840–46.' *The Journal of Imperial and Commonwealth History*, vol. 25, no. 1 (Jan. 1997): 82–112.

———. *Anglo-China: Chinese People and British Rule in Hong Kong, 1841–1880*. Richmond, Surrey: Curzon, 2001.

Oxley, D. H. (Lt. Col.). *Victoria Barracks 1842–1979*. Hong Kong: British Forces Hong Kong, 1979.

Packard, Randall M. *The Making of a Tropical Disease: A Short History of Malaria*. Baltimore: Johns Hopkins University Press, 2007.

Peckham, Robert. 'Hygienic Nature: Afforestation and the Greening of Colonial Hong Kong.' *Modern Asian Studies*, vol. 49, no. 4 (July 2015): 1177–1209.

Platts, Una. 'Ashworth, Edward, 1814–1896.' In *Nineteenth Century New Zealand Artists*. Christchurch: Avon Fine Prints, 1980.

Porter, Roy. *The Greatest Benefit to Mankind: A Medical History of Humanity from Antiquity to the Present*. London: Harper Collins, 1997.

Ride, Lindsay, and May Ride. *An East India Company Cemetery: Protestant Burials in Macao*. Hong Kong: Hong Kong University Press, 1996.

Roskam, Cole. *Hong Kong: Uncertain City*. Hong Kong: University of Hong Kong Press, (anticipated) 2024.

Sayer, G. R. *Hong Kong 1841–1862: Birth, Adolescence and Coming of Age*. London: Oxford University Press, 1937.

———. *Hong Kong 1862–1919: Years of Discretion*. Hong Kong: Hong Kong University Press, 1975.

Sinha, Ria. 'Fatal Island: Malaria in Hong Kong.' *Journal of the Royal Asiatic Society Hong Kong Branch*, vol. 58 (2018): 55–80.

Sinn, Elizabeth. *Power and Charity: The Early History of the Tung Wah Hospital*. Hong Kong: Oxford University Press, 1989.

———. 'Beyond "Tianxia": The "Zhongwai Xinwen Qiribao" (Hong Kong 1871–1872) and the Construction of a Transnational Chinese Community.' *China Review*, vol. 4, no. 1 (Spring 2004): 93–95.

———. *Pacific Crossing: California Gold, Chinese Migration, and the Making of Hong Kong*. Hong Kong: Hong Kong University Press, 2012.

Smith, Carl T. *Chinese Christians, Elites, Middlemen, and the Church in Hong Kong*. Hong Kong: Oxford University Press, 1985.

———. *A Sense of History: Studies in the Social and Urban History of Hong Kong*. Hong Kong: The Hong Kong Educational Publishing Co., 1995.

Starling, Arthur E., et al., eds. *Plague, SARS, and the Story of Medicine in Hong Kong*. Hong Kong: Hong Kong University Press, 2006.

Sullivan, Louis. 'The Tall Office Building Artistically Considered.' *Lippincott's Magazine* (March 1896): 403–409.

Taylor, W. A. *Crown Lands: A History of Survey Systems*. Victoria, British Columbia: Registries and Titles Department, 1975.

Tsai, Jung-Fang. *Hong Kong in Chinese History*. New York: Columbia University Press, 1993.

Weiler, John. 'Colonial Connections: Royal Engineers and Building Technology Transfer in the Nineteenth Century.' *Construction History*, vol. 12 (1996): 3–18.

Welsh, Frank. *A History of Hong Kong*. London: Harper Collins, 1993, rev. ed. 1997.

Worboys, Michael. *Spreading Germs: Disease Theories and Medical Practice in Britain, 1865–1900*. Cambridge: Cambridge University Press, 2000.

Wylly, H. C. (Col.). *History of the 1st and 2nd Battalions: The Sherwood Foresters*. London, 1929.

Yeoh, Brenda S. A. *Contesting Space in Colonial Singapore: Power Relations and the Urban Built Environment*. Kuala Lumpur: Oxford University Press, 1996.

Yip, Ka-Che, ed. *Disease, Colonialism, and the State: Malaria in Modern East Asian History*. Hong Kong: Hong Kong University Press, 2009.

Zhuo, Nansheng. *Zhongguo jindai baoye fazhan shi, 1815–1874* (The Development of Chinese Newspapers in the Modern Period, 1815–1874). Taipei: Zhengzhong shuju, 1998.

B. Doctoral Dissertations

Decaudin, Maxime. '"A Barren Rock": An Environmental History of the Landscapes of the British Colonization of Hong Kong, 1794–1898.' PhD diss., Centre André Chastel, Université Paris-Sorbonne, 2021.

Rehman, Nida. 'Epidemiological Landscapes: The Spaces and Politics of Mosquito Control in Lahore.' PhD diss., University of Cambridge, 2020. https://doi.org/10.17863/CAM.62263

Weiler, John Michael. 'Army Architects: The Royal Engineers and the Development of Building Technology in the Nineteenth Century.' PhD diss., University of York, 1987. https://etheses.whiterose.ac.uk/4272

C. Exhibition

Kwok, Ying (curator). *Contagious Cities: Far Away Too Close*. Tai Kwun Contemporary. Supported by The Wellcome Trust. 26 Jan.–21 Apr. 2019.

Index

References to images are in *italics*.